IMMUNOLOGICAL TOLERANCE

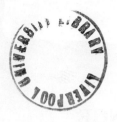

ACADEMIC PRESS RAPID MANUSCRIPT REPRODUCTION

Proceedings of an International Conference Held at
Brook Lodge, Augusta, Michigan
April 27 - May 1, 1974

IMMUNOLOGICAL TOLERANCE

MECHANISMS AND POTENTIAL THERAPEUTIC APPLICATIONS

Edited by

DAVID H. KATZ, M.D.

BARUJ BENACERRAF, M.D.

Department of Pathology
Harvard Medical School
Boston, Massachusetts

ACADEMIC PRESS   New York San Francisco London
A Subsidiary of Harcourt Brace Jovanovich, Publishers

ACADEMIC PRESS, INC.
111 Fifth Avenue, New York, New York 10003

United Kingdom Edition published by
ACADEMIC PRESS, INC. (LONDON) LTD.
24/28 Oval Road, London NW1

Library of Congress Cataloging in Publication Data
Main entry under title:

Immunological tolerance.

Proceedings of an international conference held at
Brook Lodge, Augusta, Mich., Apr. 27-May 1, 1974.
Bibliography: p.
1. Immunological tolerance–Congresses.   2.   Immuno-
therapy–Congresses.   3.   Immunosuppressive agents–
Congresses.   I.   Katz, David H., ed.   II.   Benacerraf,
Baruj, Date   ed.   [DNLM: 1.   Immune tolerance–
Congresses.   QW504 I361 1974]
RM276.I45   615'.36   74-16469
ISBN 0–12–401650–2

CONTENTS

111507

General Discussion—Session II

Session III: Mechanisms of B Cell Tolerance—*Hugh McDevitt, Chairman*

General Discussion—Session III

Session IV: Mechanisms of T Cell Tolerance—*William Weigle, Chairman*

PARTICIPANTS

Dr. Gordon Ada
John Curtin School of Medical
   Research
Australian National University
Canberra, A.C.T., 2600
Australia

Dr. Anthony C. Allison
Clinical Research Centre
Watford Road, Harrow
Middlesex HA1, 3UJ
England

Dr. Richard Asofsky
Laboratory of Microbial Immunity
National Institute of Allergy and
   Infectious Diseases
National Institutes of Health
Bethesda, Maryland 20014

Dr. Michael K. Bach
Hypersensitivity Diseases Research
The Upjohn Company
Kalamazoo, Michigan 49001

Dr. Phillip Baker
Laboratory of Microbial Immunity
National Institute of Allergy and
   Infectious Diseases
National Institutes of Health
Bethesda, Maryland 20014

Dr. Antony Basten
Department of Bacteriology
Immunology Unit
The University of Sydney
Sydney, N.S.W. 2006
Australia

Professor Baruj Benacerraf
Department of Pathology
Harvard Medical School
25 Shattuck Street
Boston, Mass. 02115

Dr. Yves Borel
Department of Medicine
Tufts University School of
   Medicine
Boston, Mass. 02111

Dr. Sven Britton
Division of Immunobiology
Karolinska Institute
Wallenberg Laboratory
104 05 Stockholm 50
Sweden

Sir Macfarlane Burnet
Department of Microbiology
University of Melbourne
Parkville 3052
Victoria, Australia

Dr. Jacques Chiller
Scripps Clinic and Research
   Foundation
476 Prospect Street
La Jolla, California 92037

Dr. Bernhard Cinader
Department of Medical Cell
  Biology
University of Toronto
Toronto 181, Ontario
Canada

Dr. Henry Claman
Department of Medicine
University of Colorado Medical
  Center
4200 East Ninth Avenue
Denver, Colorado 80220

Dr. Sheldon G. Cohen, Chief
Allergy and Immunology Branch
Extramural Programs
National Institute of Allergy and
  Infectious Diseases
National Institutes of Health
Bethesda, Maryland 20014

Dr. Erwin Diener
MRC Transplantation Unit
University of Alberta
Edmonton, Alberta
Canada

Dr. David Dresser
National Institute for Medical
  Research
The Ridgeway, Mill Hill
London NW7 1AA
England

Dr. Marc Feldmann
Department of Zoology
University College London
Gower Street
London WCIE 6 BT
England

Dr. Richard K. Gershon
Department of Pathology
Yale Medical School
New Haven, Connecticut 06510

Dr. Karl-Erik Hellström
Department of Pathology
University of Washington
Seattle, Washington 98195

Dr. Leonore A. Herzenberg
Department of Genetics
Stanford University School of
  Medicine
Stanford, California 94305

Dr. James G. Howard
The Wellcome Research
  Laboratories
Langley Court
Beckenham
Kent BR3 3BS, England

Dr. John H. Humphrey
National Institute for Medical
  Research
The Ridgeway, Mill Hill
London, NW7 1AA, England

Dr. David H. Katz
Department of Pathology
Harvard Medical School
25 Shattuck Street
Boston, Mass. 02115

Dr. Sidney Leskowitz
Department of Pathology
Tufts University School of
  Medicine
Boston, Mass. 02111

Dr. Rose Mage
Laboratory of Immunology
National Institutes of Allergy and
  Infectious Diseases
National Institutes of Health
Bethesda, Maryland 20014

Professor Hugh O. McDevitt
Department of Medicine
Stanford University School of
  Medicine
Palo Alto, California 94304

Dr. Graham Mitchell
The Walter and Eliza Hall
  Institute of Medical Research
Royal Melbourne Hospital
Victoria 3050, Australia

Dr. Erna Möller
Division of Immunobiology
Karolinska Institute
Wallenberg Laboratory
104 05 Stockholm 50
Sweden

Dr. Göran Möller
Division of Immunobiology
Karolinska Institute
Wallenberg Laboratory
104 05 Stockholm 50
Sweden

Professor G. J. V. Nossal
The Walter and Eliza Hall
  Institute of Medical Research
Royal Melbourne Hospital
Victoria 3050, Australia

Dr. William E. Paul
Laboratory of Immunology
National Institutes of Allergy and
  Infectious Diseases
National Institutes of Health
Bethesda, Maryland 20014

Dr. David W. Scott
Department of Microbiology and
  Immunology
Duke University Medical Center
Durham, North Carolina 27710

Dr. Gregory W. Siskind
Department of Medicine
Cornell University Medical School
New York, New York 10021

Dr. Richard T. Smith
Department of Pathology
University of Florida Medical
  School
Gainesville, Florida 32601

Dr. Tomio Tada
Department of Pathology
School of Medicine
Chiba University
Chiba, Japan

Dr. R. B. Taylor
Department of Pathology
University Medical School
University Walk
Bristol, BS8 1TD
England

Dr. William Terry
National Cancer Institute
National Institutes of Health
Bethesda, Maryland 20014

Dr. Emil R. Unanue
Department of Pathology
Harvard Medical School
25 Shattuck Street
Boston, Mass. 02115

Dr. Byron Waksman
Department of Microbiology
Yale Medical School
New Haven, Connecticut 06510

Dr. William O. Weigle
Scripps Clinic and Research
  Foundation
476 Prospect Street
La Jolla, California 92037

PREFACE

Immunological tolerance has stimulated the curiosity of immunologists for decades in a highly teleological sense, because, on the one hand, it is well understood that it is nature's provision to allow the complex mammalian organism to coexist within itself, and, on the other hand, although the phenomena have been reasonably well defined, the cellular and molecular mechanisms underlying them remain largely enigmatic.

The contents of this book represent the proceedings of a conference held at Brook Lodge, Michigan, April 27–May 1, 1974, at which time we were privileged to bring together many of the investigators who have actively contributed to furthering our knowledge and understanding of immunological tolerance. It will be immediately clear to the reader that the conference was structured in a way to consider phenomena of tolerance and immune suppression as interrelated entities with a certain degree of emphasis on the possible common cellular mechanisms involved. The results of the conference do not make the cellular and molecular mechanisms underlying tolerance and suppression any less enigmatic, but, rather, do place a realistic and sharp perspective on where we must focus our subsequent investigative energies in order to answer the unresolved questions. Perhaps more important is the fact that, as will be apparent to the reader, we have now reached the stage at which our laboratory models have become sufficiently well understood to permit us to consider seriously the clinical applicability of our rapidly advancing technology in this area.

The recognition of the role of the thymus-derived or T lymphocyte as a regulatory cell for immune responses endowed with the capacity to both facilitate and suppress the functions of other T lymphocytes and bone marrow-derived B lymphocytes in reactions of cell-mediated and humoral immunity has clearly deepened our understanding of the control mechanisms involved in these responses. However, we are now faced with the increasing complexity that this understanding places on the concept of specific immunological tolerance. It is, indeed, a more realistic concept that we are forced to recognize and deal with and certainly in keeping with evolutionary trends to diverge from the simple to the more highly integrated system as the ladder extends further up the tree. We can no longer justify the simpler connotation of immunological tolerance as the deletion of specific clones of immunocompetent lymphocytes due to mechanisms unknown, for while such clonal deletion probably does, in fact, occur under certain circumstances, the existence of other pathways to the same functional end—namely, specific unresponsiveness—can be demonstrated experimentally and probably also plays an important physiologic role in the induction and/or maintenance of tolerance. The role of suppressor T cells is particularly important, as it is pointed out in these proceedings, as an alternate pathway to specific unresponsiveness in populations of both T and B lymphocytes, and we are left with the general impression that the origin and maintenance of self-tolerance, perhaps the most enigmatic of all questions, reflects the operation of both clonal deletion and suppressor T cell mechanisms. The precise nature of these mechanisms will hopefully be delineated to a greater extent by the time of the next tolerance conference.

In closing, we wish to acknowledge the outstanding efforts of Ms. Candace H. Maher in the organization and planning of this conference. Mrs. Annette Benacerraf for her secretarial assistance during the conference and Ms. Deborah Maher for her tireless work in the preparation of this book. This conference was made possible by the support of the National Institute of Allergy and Infectious Diseases, the National Institutes of Health, and the Upjohn Company, which also made available to us the luxurious and serene setting of Brook Lodge.

David H. Katz
Baruj Benacerraf

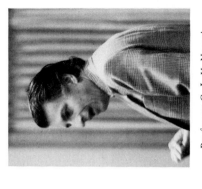

Professor G. J. V. Nossal

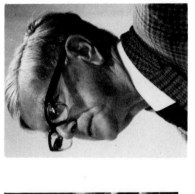

Sir MacFarlane Burnet

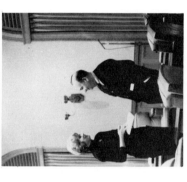

Erna Möller   Baruj Benacerraf

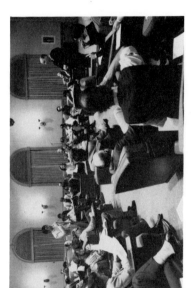

Conference In Session

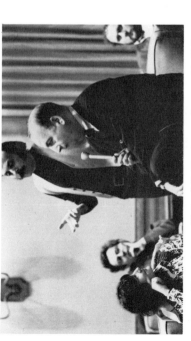

Leonore A. Herzenberg   Richard K. Gershon   Jacques M. Chiller

Michael K. Bach   Baruj Benacerraf

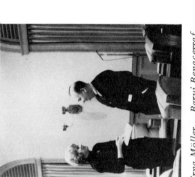

Dr. Graham F. Mitchell

T CELL TOLERANCE

RICHARD T. SMITH, CHAIRMAN

FACTORS INFLUENCING THE RATE OF INDUCTION
OF TOLERANCE BY BOVINE GAMMA GLOBULIN

D.W. Dresser

National Institute for Medical Research
Mill Hill, London NW7 1AA

INTRODUCTION

Antibody production and immunological tolerance are good systems for studying cellular differentiation despite their overt complexity. The advantages of the systems lie in the specific handle afforded by antigen and in the temporal reference point of exposure to antigen or adjuvant. Nossal has pointed out that immunological tolerance can be discussed in terms of a decision between two alternative pathways for an individual lymphocyte (1) (see Fig. 1). Such concepts of stimulation of a differentiating cell, down one or two or more alternative pathways, are commonplace in embryology and epigenetics. Known inducers range from diffusable substances acting at long range to substances dependent on cell-cell contacts (2).

Differences in the rate of entry into a state of immunological unresponsiveness after the administration of tolerogen (tolerance-inducing form of antigen) exist (3-6). Sometimes these differences can be accounted for by different methods of measuring responsiveness (precipitation, antigen elimination, plaques), sometimes to different protocols (intact animals, cell transfers, in vitro) and sometimes to the antigen (immunogenic/non-immunogenic, protein/carbohydrate). However, in a series of classical experiments, Chiller and his colleagues in cell transfer experiments have shown that real differences exist in dose sensitivity and rate of entry into a state of unresponsiveness, between tolerance induction in T and in B lymphocytes (4, 5, 7) and in further experiments differences between spleen and bone marrow B cells have been demonstrated (6).

Since all mechanisms demonstrated in disrupted systems must eventually be related to physiological reality in intact animals, it was decided that a study of factors affecting the rate of induction in intact mice would be made. Experiments have been started in an attempt to measure the induction of tolerance in different lines of B cells; some preliminary results are included here. If observed differences can be ascribed to differences at the cellular level, then it may be possible to gain insight into the variety of tolerance induction mechanisms which may operate in normal development.

MATERIALS AND METHODS

Male mice of the CBA/H strain which were free of Tyzzer's disease were used in these experiments (8). Thymectomy of 3-5 week old mice and reconstitution with syngeneic fetal liver was carried out as described previously (9). A whole body dose of 800-850 röntgens was delivered from a ^{60}Co source at a rate of about 40 röntgens per minute. In some experiments a population of helper T cells sensitive to DNP was raised by painting the shaved belly of the mice with DNFB (10).

Bovine gamma globulin (Ethanol fraction II, Armour, BGG) was refractionated on DEAE cellulose (DE 32; 0.02M phosphate buffer, pH 7.4). This material (B G) was used for tolerance induction after centrifugation at 30,000 Xg for 30-40 minutes or for immunization after either: a) alum precipitation (BA), or b) heat aggregation by a midification of a published method (11) (65^{0} for 2 hours followed by 0^{0} for 2-24 hours and finally, one or two washed in 0.9% NaCl). Purified antibody from bovine or porcine anti-mouse-lymphocyte serum (ALSAb) was prepared from ALS by first preparing a DEAE globulin fraction and then eluting antibody from glutaraldehyde-fixed thymocytes (anti-T) or spleen cells from thymectomized-reconstituted mice (anti-B) (12, 13).

T cells were primed (educated) against B G (EdT) (14) by injecting 70 x 10^{6} CBA thymus cells plus 250 g HaB intravenously into lethally irradiated syngeneic recipients. A week later the spleens of these mice were harvested, and the cells used as a source of EdT (yield 3-4 x 10^{6} cells/spleen).

The LHG assay was carried out using the slide method (15). Class specific developing sera was prepared, absorbed and tested as described earlier (9) but received an additional absorption with B G-Sepharose. For use as target cells sheep erythrocytes (SRBC) were coated with B G by the methodology of Hosono and Maramatsu (11) with the modifications that the $CrCl_3$ is dissolved in 0.9% NaCl (immediately before use), 2.5 mg B G per ml of solution are used and all solutions are kept at 0^{0} until homogenous mixing of all components is obtained. After 1 hour at 37^{0} with very gentle stirring, the coated SRBC are washed three times in Hank's

4

solution containing 0.5% Difco gelatin (HG). HG was used for suspending cells (PFC and target cells) used in these experiments.

The coprecipitation assay for anti-5563-idiotype antibodies was described by Iverson (10). The antigen-binding capacity (ABC or Farr) assay was a modification of the methodology used by Mitchison and his colleagues for serum albumins (16). For bovine and porcine gamma globulins it is necessary to use ethanol-fractionated material refractionated on DEAE-cellulose. The ammonium sulfate is diluted to 32% saturation (at 4°) with 0.15 M borate buffer at pH 8.4. This ABC assay could be considered as a direct precipitation in high salt concentration: it is about ten fold more sensitive than coprecipitation with a very strong antiserum to mouse gamma globulins, and more than ten fold as sensitive as direct precipitation in 0.15 M borate buffer. $B\gamma G$ was labelled with ^{125}I by the standard method (17). Isoelectric focusing (IEF) was carried out by the method of Phillips and Dresser (19, 20) using $B\gamma G$ coated SRBC and an anti-γG_1 developing serum in the indicator layer.

RESULTS

Rates of tolerance induction.
Different rates of tolerance induction have been reported by workers using the same or similar antigens in the same species of experimental animal. These differences may reflect different experimental protocols, for instance, in experiments in intact animals total responsiveness often declines slowly (3), whereas experiments involving the transfer of cells to irradiated recipients, usually result in a much more rapid rate of tolerance induction (4, 5). In intact animals it is difficult to determine whether it is the T or the B arm of the response which is the primary target of the tolerogen. In the cell transfer protocols which allow in vitro manipulations and various admixing of cells, analysis of tolerance at the cellular level is practicable. It was this latter protocol which allowed Chiller and colleagues to demonstrate differences between T and B and between spleen B and bone marrow B cells.

In Fig. 2 it can be seen that in intact mice the rate of tolerance induction to $B\gamma G$ is slow when responsiveness is measured by the elimination technique and faster when responsiveness is measured by the ABC assay. In experiments in intact animals such as these, it is impossible to know

5

whether it is T cells or B cells or both which are the effective limiting factor causing a decline in responsiveness. If T cell help is a necessity for a response to manifest itself, it should be possible to raise a population of helper cells to a determinant not normally on the tolerogenic molecule and then couple this determinant to the immunogenic challenging form of the antigen. In this protocol it can be argued that an observed unresponsiveness must be due to tolerance induction in B cells (21). As a consequence of this, T cell help to DNP was raised in mice prior to the induction of tolerance to $B\gamma G$ by painting them with DNFB. Subsequently, the mice were challenged with alum-precipitated $DNP_6B\gamma G$ and the response to $B\gamma G$ measured. The observed rate of tolerance induction (in B cells) is the same as that seen in mice challenged with $B\gamma G$ (BA) in the normal way.

The rate of tolerance induction by 5563 idiotype, also measured in DNFB painted mice, was substantially the same as for $B\gamma G$. The observed difference between elimination and ABC protocols could possibly be due to the two assays measuring different kinds of antibody, each kind (class) manifesting its own rate of tolerance induction. At the level of the B cells, the differences can be in whole or in part due to primary B cell class differences or to a secondary effect reflecting differences in T cell dependence.

Although age has a profound effect on the rate of loss of a state of tolerance (22, 23, 24, 3), it can be seen in Fig. 3 that age has at best a marginal effect on the rate of induction of tolerance. It is possible that very old mice enter a state of tolerance more slowly than younger mice. Mice thymectomized 2 1/2 months previously as young adults but not reconstituted enter a state of tolerance at a similar rate to that seen in intact mice of the same age (Fig. 4). These mice are deficient in T_1 cells (25) but retain enough T cells (T_2) for controls not injected with tolerogen to mount as good a response to a challenge with immunogenic $B\gamma G$, as do normal (intact) mice. It is clear from this result that an earlier suggestion that a functional thymus might be necessary for tolerance induction (3), is wrong. Thymectomized-reconstituted control mice fail to respond to immunogenic $B\gamma G$ (see next section).

T-dependence.
If an antigen is generally only capable of stimulating a class of antibody which is T dependent, then it is important to know if there are any situations where such T

6

dependence can be by-passed. With antigens such as sheep RBC and ØX 174, this can be done by using very high doses of antigen in conjunction with a powerful adjuvant (9, 26). In the response to sheep RBC, the γM response seems to be partially T independent. The dependence of the γG_{2a} and γG_1 responses are almost complete in the absence of adjuvant. Coprecipitation tests of anti-BγG-immunized mice show that the response to BγG is more than 90% γG_1. ALSAb (both bovine and porcine) is a highly immunogenic form of soluble gamma globulin. In Figs. 5 and 6 it can be seen that despite the use of very high doses of ALSAb, thymectomized/reconstituted (T^-) mice failed to respond to a degree detectable by the ABC assay.

Class differences in tolerance induction.

Experiments (unpublished) have partly confirmed the suggestion of Hosono and Muramatsu (11) that after immunization with heat-aggregated gamma globulin (HaB), an early peak of developable (indirect) γM plaques can be detected. Somewhat later, at about 12 days after priming, a more conventional γG response was seen by these workers who used a polyspecific-developing serum in their experiments. In Mill Hill CBA mice it has been shown, using highly specific developing sera (anti-μ; anti-γ_1; anti-γ_{2a}; anti-γ_{2b}; anti-Fab), that a peak of indirect γM plaques occurs at day 3, followed by an early γG_1 peak at day 5 with another γG_1 peak at day 10 (plus some γG_2). Figure 7 shows that the plaques have different morphologies. Splenic indirect γM plaques are induced best by an intraperitoneal injection of 100 μg alum-precipitated BγG (BA) and the γG plaques by 1mg HaB injected intravenously. These challenge procedures have been used in the tolerance experiments illustrated in Figs. 8, 9 and 10, where it can be seen that the tempo of tolerance induction (and perhaps in some cases concomitant immunization) differ between indirect γM, early γG_1 and late γG_1 (and γG_2). After a tolerance induction time of 14 days (t.14), the simple direct relationship between the degree of indirect γM tolerance and the dose of tolerogen contrasts with the more complex relationship seen especially clearly in the induction of tolerance in the early γG_1 response.

Using a cell transfer protocol, spleen cells have been exposed to particle-free BγG in vivo, at two dose levels, for different lengths of time before being transferred with antigen (250 μg HaB) and BγG-educated T cells, intravenously into lethally irradiated syngeneic mice. In this situation it seems likely that any observed tolerance effect will be the result of B cell tolerance. Figure 11 shows that with high doses of tolerogen (3 mg), the γG_1 response in the spleen (only a trace of γG_2 classes seen in controls) declines rapidly between days 3 and 6, whereas with a lower dose of tolerogen (60 μg), there is evidence of a slight immunization effect. This experiment confirms for BγG a cadence of tolerance induction in B cells previously demonstrated for human γG in other strains of mice.

It would be interesting to know if the early γG_1 and the late γG_1 responses are made by the same line of cells or are made by two physiologically distinct lines of B cell. The isoelectric spectrum of a population of antibody molecules may be a "finger print" which could in certain circumstances be a marker for the product of a particular clone of B cells (27). If a similar pattern occurs frequently in different individual animals, such a "finger print" cannot of course be a clonal marker, although it may be an effective method of detecting a particular sub-class of gamma globulin. Although CBA mice immunized with 32 μg to 3.2 mg of HaB show extremely heterogenous γG_1 and γG_{2a} responses, a dose of 3.2 μg stimulates γG_1 responses with a reasonably restricted heterogeneity.

Using mice immunized with this low dose of HaB, Dr. J.M. Phillips and I have run day 6 and day 12 sera from individuals side by side of an IEF plate. Figure 12 shows that the same γG_1 spectrum seems to predominate in the two bleeds; differences between the spectra of different individuals can be seen as well. If the response to the low dose of antigen used in this experiment is eventually shown to stimulate early and late γG_1 in a similar way to higher doses of HaB, then we would conclude that this result is compatible with both early and late γG_1 being made by the same line of cells. If this were so, it might imply that the late γG_1 is dependent on more than one antigen hit and perhaps could be considered as a secondary type of response.

DISCUSSION

The experiments described briefly in this paper confirm the supposition that observed differences in the rate of induction of immunological tolerance (paralysis) have two main sources. These are: 1) differences of technique and experimental protocol; and 2) differences in the target cells.

In the $B\gamma G$-CBA system used here, there are gross differences between results derived from elimination, ABC (Farr) and plaque assays. The elimination assay may measure overall responsiveness including all classes of humoral response together with cell-adherent antibodies, whereas the ABC assay may only measure serum-γG antibodies. In contrast, the plaque assay measures the number of cells secreting a soluble antibody irrespective of whether or not that antibody is physiologically stable or functional in vivo. Furthermore the plaque method only reflects the response in the organ assayed, although the dissection of that response into its component classes is easier and more accurate to carry out than it is for secreted serum antibody.

A further technical contribution to different rates of tolerance induction lie in the experimental protocols employed. In intact animals feedback loops and cell interactions may exist which could be altered or absent in vitro or in irradiated recipients of populations of washed cells whose normal microanatomical relationships have been disrupted.

The cellular targets of a tolerogen differ. Chiller and Weigle and their colleagues have shown very clearly that tolerance to human γG in T cells and B cells require different doses of tolerogen and that the rates of tolerance induction are different (4, 5 and 7). They have also shown in further cell transfer experiments that a population of B cells in spleen enter a state of unresponsiveness more quickly than a population of B cells in bone marrow (6). This last difference may reflect the state of maturity of B cells in the two organs. Consideration of the maturity of the target cell may be of importance in any consideration of how a tolerogen "turns off" or kills a line of potentially responsive cells, and also in considerations of the ontogeny of the immune response in relation to aberrations such as autoimmunity. A cell transfer experiment reported in this paper shows that spleen B cells of CBA mice become unresponsive to $B\gamma G$ in a manner similar to that demonstrated for human γG.

The results of experiments in which particle-free (deaggregated) $B\gamma G$ was shown to induce a specific state of immunological tolerance, while animals injected with the

9

same antigen together with a powerful adjuvant induced a state of active immunity, compelled the author to propose a "two stimulus" model of immunocyte maturation (28, 29). Figure 13a outlines the essentials of such an hypothesis. The adjuvant (non-specific) stimulus is proposed as a necessary addition to the specific antigenic stimulus for triggering the differentiation of antibody-forming cells. The adjuvant stimulus can originate from a substance such as endotoxin or pertussis organisms injected independently but in temporal terms concomitantly with the antigen; or it can originate from the intrinsic adjuvanticity of the antigenic molecule itself. Subsequently, a model was proposed which suggested that the adjuvant stimulus was mitogenic (18, 30, 31); compelling evidence that this mechanism operates the tolerance-immunity switch does not yet exist, although there is recent evidence which is compatible with the hypothesis (32). The general schema outlined above has been elaborated and integrated into a more general immunological theory by Bretscher and Cohn (33, 34).

Howard and Mitchison in their recent thought provoking review (35) have dismissed the two stimulus (two signal) hypothesis and have suggested an alternative which they believe offers a more satisfactory explanation of the experiments of Diener and Feldmann (36, 37) and of Howard and colleagues (38, 39). Howard and Mitchison's hypothesis is outlined in simple form in Fig. 13b. They propose that a tolerance stimulus kills off cells which have bound antigen. The difference between simple stimulation of an inbuilt "go" trigger and killing the cell by some sort of antigenic stangulation is the presence of a cross-linking antibody in the Feldmann/Diener experiments and a sufficient concentration of highly polymerized-polysaccharide antigen in the Howard experiments. A somewhat similar "alloallergic" killing model of immunological tolerance at the cellular level was proposed many years ago by Chase (40).

It is not impossible that "tolerance" will turn out to be a generic term covering several mechanisms or alternative pathways, each of which can result in antigen specific immunological unresponsiveness. These alternatives may include: 1) cell modulation in the absence of an adjuvant (mitogenic) stimulus; 2) direct cell killing or opsonation by antigen or by antigen cross linked by certain kinds of antibody; 3) antigen-specific suppressor T cells similar to the mechanism proposed for allotype suppression; and 4) antibody feedback (42, 43). Different mechanisms or combination of mechanisms may operate simultaneously in different kinds of lymphocyte.

The immune mechanism like other systems of cellular differentiation is a Gordian knot which may be resolved at one level by experiments with an Alexandrian protocol, but which will have to be patiently unravelled piece by piece if the matrix of feedback, direct cellular interaction and cellular change are to be understood. A degree of acceptance of the dogma of clonal selection is implicit in both alternatives outlined in Fig. 13; for example, this may be convenient but dangerous. Howard and Mitchison consider that the question of whether tolerance induction means cell "killing" or cell "turn off" is an irrelevance from the point of view of the acquisition of a state of antigen specific unresponsiveness. In terms of practical immunology this may be so but to those workers interested in tolerance induction as a complex model of cellular differentiation, albeit one with a convenient handle for its manipulation, the question is indeed relevant. The alternative to killing off unwanted pre-differentiated cells is that cells are switched into another epigenetic pathway before differentiation is irreversible. The alternative pathway may perhaps be one for which the experimenter has at present no convenient means for detection.

ACKNOWLEDGMENT

I thank Miss A.M. Popham for excellent technical assistance.

REFERENCES

1. Nossal, G.J.V., _Prog. Immunol._ _1_:665, 1971.

2. Tiedmann, H., _Current Topics Dev. Biol._ _1_:85, 1966.
   Nieuwkoop, P.D., _Adv. Morph._ 10:1, 1973.
   Deuchar, E.M., _Adv. Morph._ 10:175, 1973.

3. Dresser, D.W., _Int. Arch. Allergy._ _35_:253, 1969.

4. Chiller, J.M., Habicht, G.S. and Weigle, W.O., _Proc. Nat. Acad. Sci._ (Wash.). _65_:551, 1970.

5. Chiller, J.M., Habicht, G.S. and Weigle, W.O., _Science._ _171_:813, 1971.

6. Chiller, J.M. and Weigle, W.O., _J. Immunol_. 110:1051, 1973.

7. Chiller, J.M. and Weigle, W.O., _Contemp. Topics, Immunobiology_. 1:119, 1971.

8. Anderson, H.R., Dresser, D.W. and Wortis, H.H., _Clin. Exp. Immunol_. 16:393, 1974.

9. Dresser, D.W., _Europ. J. Immunol_. 2:50, 1972.

10. Iverson, G.M., _Nature_ (London). 227:272, 1970.

11. Hosono, M. and Muramatsu, S., _J. Immunol_. 109:857, 1972.

12. Anderson, H.R. and Dresser, D.W., _Europ. J. Immunol_. 1:31, 1971.

13. Dresser, D.W., _Nature_ (London). 229:630, 1971.

14. Mitchell, G.F. and Miller, J.F.A.P., _J. Exp. Med_. 128:821, 1968.

15. Dresser, D.W. and Greaves, M.F., Ch. 27 in "Handbook of Experimental Immunology", Ed. D.M. Weir (2nd Ed.), Blackwell, 1973.

16. Mitchison, N.A., _Proc. Roy. Soc. B._ (London). 161:275, 1964.

17. Hunter, W.M. and Greenwood, F.C., _Nature_ (London). 194:495, 1962.

18. Dresser, D.W., _Immunology_. 9:261, 1965.

19. Phillips, J.M. and Dresser, D.W., _Europ. J. Immunol_. 3:524, 1973.

20. Phillips, J.M. and Dresser, D.W., _Europ. J. Immunol_. 3:738, 1973.

21. Iverson, G.M. and Dresser, D.W., _Nature_ (London). 227:274, 1970.

22. Mitchison, N.A., "Colloque International sur les Problemes Biologiques des Greffes", Univ. de Liege, p. 239, 1959.

23. Claman, H.N.O., Talmage, D.W., Science. 141:1193, 1963.

24. Taylor, R.B., Immunology. 7:595, 1964.

25. Cantor, H., Simpson, E., Sato, V.L., Fathman, C.G. and Herzenberg, L.A., submitted to Cellular Immunology, 1974.

26. Tao, T.W., personal communication.

27. Askonas, B.A., Williamson, A.R. and Wright, B.E.G., Proc. Nat. Acad. Sci. (Wash.) 67:1398, 1970.

28. Dresser, D.W., Immunology. 5:378, 1962.

29. Dresser, D.W. and Mitchison, N.A., Adv. Immunol. 8:129, 1968.

30. Dresser, D.W., Proc. IV Int. Congr. Pharm. 4:176, 1969.

31. Taub, R.N., Krantz, A.R. and Dresser, D.W., Immunology. 18:171, 1970.

32. Coutinho, A., Gronowicz, E., Bullock, W.W., Möller, G., J. Exp. Med. 139:74, 1974.

33. Bretscher, P. and Cohn, M., Science. 169:1042, 1970.

34. Bretscher, P., Transplant. Rev. 11:217, 1972.

35. Howard, J.G. and Mitchison, N.A., Progr. Allergy. In press.

36. Diener, E. and Feldmann, M., J. Exp. Med. 132:31, 1970.

37. Feldmann, M. and Nossal, G.J.V., Transpl. Rev. 13:3, 1972.

38. Howard, J.G., Christie, G.H. and Courtenay, B.M., Proc. Roy. Soc. B. 180:347, 1972.

39. Howard, J.G., Transpl. Rev. 8:50, 1972.

40. Chase, M.W., <u>Ann. Rev. Microbiol</u>. <u>13</u>:349, 1959.

41. Herzenberg, L.A., Chan, E.L., Ravitch, M.M., Riblet, R.J. and Herzenberg, L.A., <u>J. Exp. Med</u>. <u>137</u>:1311, 1973.

42. Rowley, D.A., Fitch, F.W., Stuart, F.P., Köhler, H. and Cosenza, H., <u>Science</u>. <u>181</u>:1133, 1973.

43. Hellström, I. and Hellström, K.E., <u>Int. J. Cancer</u>. <u>4</u>: 587, 1969.

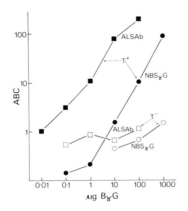

Fig. 5. The inability of soluble BγG or ALSAb (plus
4×10^9 pertussis - all i.p.) to immunize T⁻ (thymectomized
reconstituted) mice, T⁺ indicates sham-reconstituted controls. In a similar experiment using alum-precipitated porcine γG and alum-precipitated porcine ALSAb, both plus pertussis, there was no detectable antibody in T⁻ mice even
with a dose of ALSAb of 1 mg.

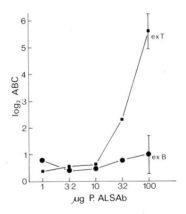

Fig. 6. Porcine ALS was divided into two aliquots; one
was absorbed with CBA thymocytes and the other with spleen
cells from T⁻ mice. ALSAb was prepared reciprocally from
similar cells after glutaraldehyde fixation. The ALSAb was
injected i.p. as a solution (without pertussis, which makes
only a slight difference). It can be seen that the anti-T
material is more immunogenic than the anti-B. This result
is compatible with the view that T-cell help is only marginally concerned with antigen concentration at the surface
of the B cell.

17

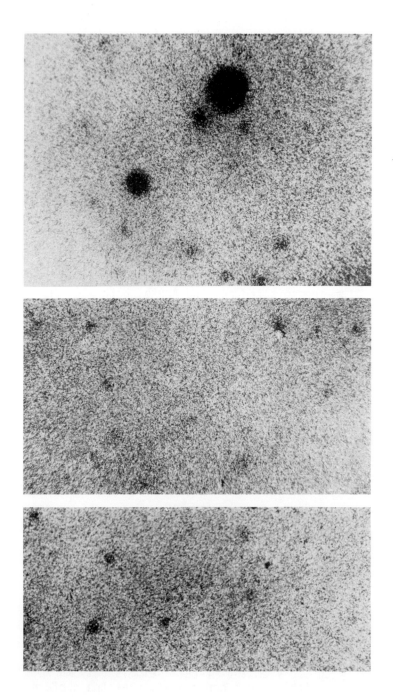

Fig. 7. Anti-BγG plaque morphology, with left to right, indirect γM; early γG₁ and late γG₁ plaques.

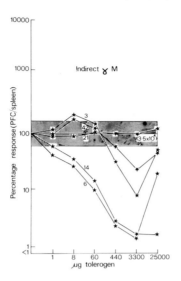

Fig. 8. Induction of tolerance to different doses of BγG after different tolerance induction times, which are indicated (days) on each curve. The geometric mean number of plaques per spleen in 5 groups of 4 animals is indicated on the 100% line; the shaded area represents the standard deviation of the control value expressed as a percentage of the mean. Indirect γM after challenge with 100 μg alum-precipitated BγG i.p.

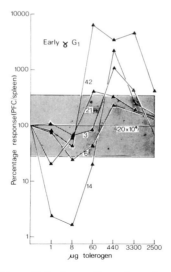

Fig. 9. As Fig. 8 but early γG₁ after 1 mg HaB intravenously.

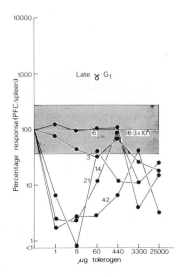

<u>Fig. 10</u>. As Fig. 9 but late γG_1.

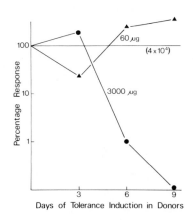

<u>Fig. 11</u>. The γG_1 plaque response in lethally irradiated recipient mice, 11 days after the transfer of spleen cells (70×10^6) from normal or tolerogen-treated donors. The different dose levels of tolerogen and the different times of exposure to tolerogen are indicated on the graph. Each mouse received in addition to spleen cells 250 μg HaB and 3.7×10^6 BγG-educated T cells, i.v.

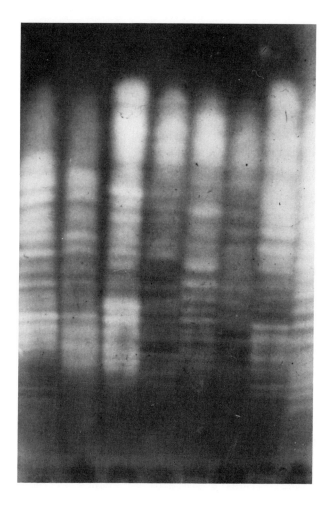

Fig. 12. The IEF spectra of γG_1 anti-BγG antibodies from 4 individual mice primed with 3.2 µg of HaB, i.v. Each pair of spectra represent respectively on the left a day 6 bleed and on the right a day 12 bleed from each individual.

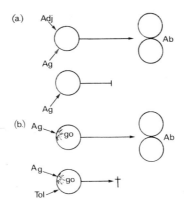

Fig. 13. This figure illustrates in a simplified form alternative mechanisms of immune induction and tolerance. In the two stimulus (signal) hypothesis (a), the triggering of immune differentiation depends on a specific (antigenic) stimulus accompanied by a non-specific (adjuvant-mitogenic?) stimulus. A cell capable of detecting and receiving an antigenic stimulus (tolerogenic) but which does not receive an adjuvant stimulus is "turned off" or killed.

In contrast, (b), Howard and Mitchison have suggested that adjuvant is largely irrelevant as a decision-making stimulus and that the antigen-receptor is an intrinsic "go" signal. In their model a state of tolerance is induced by the elimination of clones of responding cells through the cytotoxicity or opsonizing effect of antigen or antigen-antibody complexes.

DISCUSSION FOLLOWING DAVID DRESSER

G. MÖLLER: In your ALS experiments with anti-T and anti-B sera where only anti-T was immunogenic, did you study whether anti-B induced tolerance?

DRESSER: No.

G. MÖLLER: This is most important because anti-T and anti-B most likely have the same antigenic determinants. Therefore, what appears important is the cell with which the substance binds to rather than differences in structure between immunogens and tolerogens.

DRESSER: I agree that it will be very important to follow this up by doing the appropriate experiment.

TAYLOR: In your experiments do you think tolerance occurred at the T or B cell level or both?

DRESSER: In the experiments using elimination and antigen-binding capacity to measure the response, where fairly large (1/2 - 1 mg) doses of tolerogen were used, the evidence is, I think, that both T and B cells are made tolerant. However, the experiments carried out more recently using the plaque assay and doses of tolerogen as low as 1 μg have not yet been extended far enough to answer your question.

LESKOWITZ: If I interpreted your data correctly, you demonstrated significant tolerance induction with doses of BGG as low as 1 μg. Yet, tolerance with these doses is not demonstrable by other techniques such as immune clearance. How do you account for these discrepancies?

DRESSER: Mainly because the observed tolerance was in the γ G response. At a tolerogen dose of 1 μg there is absolutely no effect on the indirect γM response. The The elimination assay presumably measures all kinds of antibody irrespective of class.

FELDMANN: I was interested in the difference between the high immunogenicity of ALS eluted from T cells compared with that eluted from B cells, as these experiments remind me of those of Reber and Riethmüller who have reported similar results using anti-Ig antibody. They found that anti-Ig eluted from T cells is highly immunogenic, while that from B cells is not. They interpreted their results as indicating that a "helper" factor was eluted from T cells, but not from B cells. Have you looked to see if anything elutes with the ALS from T cells; as this could be a helper factor as suggested by Reber and Riethmüller.

DRESSER: No, I have not. However, I must remind you that the immunoabsorbent cells were fixed with 0.25% glutaraldehyde, so if such a factor does exist, it is resistant to this treatment. We certainly ought to investigate this point.

DIENER: Did you test the tolerant cells for the presence of suppressor T cells by treating them with anti-θ serum and complement before transfer?

DRESSER: No. In the transfer experiment shown, T cells were increased by the addition of educated T cells since the question being asked concerned tolerance induction in the B cell line. Anti-θ experiments will certainly have to be done.

MITCHELL: Can you elaborate on the T cell-dependence/independence of indirect IgM PFC and whether you find such cells in the primary response to SRBC rather than BGG?

DRESSER: The concentration of anti-μ serum used in these experiments to develop indirect (anti-BγG)γM plaques completely (>97%) inhibits both background and actively acquired direct plaques to sheep RBC. The experiment to determine the T-dependence of the indirect γM response has not been done yet.

INTERACTIONS OF T AND B LYMPHOCYTES
IN SELF-TOLERANCE AND AUTOIMMUNITY

A.C. Allison

Clinical Research Centre
Harrow, Middlesex, England

Ehrlich (22) with his usual perceptiveness drew attention to the remarkable fact that, although vertebrates can
readily be immunized with cells or body fluids from other
animals, they do not as a rule make antibodies against their
own tissue constituents. He termed the phenomenon "horrow
autotoxus" but was unable to advance any satisfactory explanation for it. While developing the clonal selection theory
of immunity, Burnet (9) postulated that autoantigens ("self"
antigens) are either secluded from the immune system or that
potential antibody-forming cells exposed to autoantigens
early in the course of ontogenetic development are eliminated
or inactivated. Autoimmunity was thought to follow the proliferation of "forbidden clones" of lymphocytes with specificity for autoantigens.

Burnet's postulates attracted widespread interest but
have run into serious difficulties. With the development of
sensitive methods for quantitation, notably radioimmunoassay
antigens thought to be secluded have been demonstrated in
circulating blood. Thus, thyroglobulin is found in serum
from normal human newborns and adults in concentrations of
about 10-100 ng. per ml (59). Thyroglobulin will be taken
as a model autoantigen in this paper because of the ease with
which autoantibodies against this protein can be elicited,
for example, by immunization with autologous thyroglobulin
in the presence of Freund's complete adjuvant or by immunization with heterologous thyroglobulins in the absence of
adjuvant. Formation of autoantibodies against thyroglobulin
in experimental animals is often accompanied by thyroiditis.
Indeed, in subprimates the main antigen involved in the
development of autoimmune thyroiditis is thyroglobulin,
although in primates including man, microsomal antigens appear also to be involved.

Such autoimmune reactions are not confined to thyroglobulin; for example, immunization with isologous testicu-
lar or brain extracts leads to autoimmune orchitis or enceph-
alomyelitis. It is difficult to understand how such procedures could rapidly induce the proliferation of "forbidden

clones" of lymphocytes able to react with the appropriate autoantigens.

Tolerance in T and B lymphocytes.

Several findings of the past few years have allowed reconsideration of the problem. The first and most important is the distinction between thymus-dependent (T) and other (B) lymphocytes; the latter cells and their progeny responsible for antibody synthesis and release while the former partici- pate in cell-mediated immunity and exert helper effects in the formation of antibodies against most antigens (34, 47). The second relevant finding is that, in the absence of adju- vants, administration of native heterologous serum proteins in certain dosage schedules induces specific unresponsiveness so that treated animals are unable to form antibodies when the same proteins are inoculated in a highly immunogenic form together with adjuvants (21). Such specific unrespon- siveness can be induced by administration of a high dose or repeated administration of low doses of proteins such as heterologous serum albumin or immunoglobulin. It is shown by Taylor (55) for mice inoculated with bovine serum albumin and by Chiller et al (15) for mice inoculated with human immunoglobulin that low-dose unresponsiveness affects mainly T cells whereas high-dose unresponsiveness affects both T and B cells. This was demonstrated by testing immune res- ponses in irradiated syngeneic mice reconstituted with thymus and lymph node or bone marrow cells from normal and unres- ponsive donors. Thus, lymph node or bone marrow cells from low-dose unresponsive donors transferred to irradiated recip- ients together with normal thymus cells allowed the develop- ment of good immune responses in the recipients. After a high dose of antigen bone marrow cells also become unrespon- sive; moreover, unresponsiveness is rapidly induced and is persistent in T lymphocytes and is more slowly induced and transient in B lymphocytes.

These findings led to the postulate, made independently by Allison (3) and by Weigle (67), that with circulating soluble autoantigens, two types of tolerance are present. When antigens circulate in low concentrations such as thyro- globulin, there will be the equivalent of low-dose tolerance; specific T cells become unresponsive but specific B cells are present in normal numbers and are able to respond to autoantigens suitably presented to them. The B cells cannot respond to low doses of autologous thyroglobulin in the cir- culation in the absence of T cell help, but they can be stimulated by immunization with cross-reacting antigens, in

26

which case autoantibodies are made only against those auto-antigenic determinants shared with the cross-reacting anti-gens (Fig. 1). Alternatively, alloantibodies would be formed by immunization with autoantigens in the presence of suitable adjuvants which provide non-antigen-specific T cell stimula-tion (see 4). Other situations allowing stimulation of auto-antigen-reactive B cells are discussed below. In contrast, it can be postulated that by analogy with high-dose tolerance in the case of soluble autoantigens circulating in high dose such as serum albumin, both B and T cells become unrespon-sive. In that case no manipulation would give rise to auto-antibody formation.

The first type of tolerance is precarious, since it can easily be broken, for example, by infections. It is, there-fore, necessary that a second line of defence against auto-immunity be present, and Allison et al (5) suggested that this might be the development of populations of T lymphocytes able to suppress autoantibody formation. For these postu-lates to be tenable, it is necessary to provide evidence in support of the following points:-

1) The formation of antibodies against heterologous thyroglobulins and induction of autoimmune thyroiditis should be thymus-dependent;

2) B cells binding autologous thyroglobulin should be present in normal humans and experimental animals. Selective inactivation of these cells following binding of highly radioactive thyroglobulin should abrogate the capacity to form autoantibodies against thyroglobulin;

3) T lymphocytes should not react with native autolo-gous thyroglobulin, and autoimmune thyroiditis should be an antibody-mediated and not a T cell-mediated immunopatholog-ical reaction; and

4) Deprivation of T lymphocytes which exert suppressor effects should accelerate and accentuate thyroiditis.

The thymus dependence of antibody formation against thyroglobulin and development of thyroiditis.
Observations summarized in Table I show that in mice formation of antibodies against heterologous thyroglobulins, of cross-reacting autoantibodies to mouse thyroglobulins and the development of autoimmune thyroiditis are thymus depen-dent. Similarly, the formation of autoantibodies and

development of thyroiditis in mice immunized with mouse thyroid extracts in the presence of Freund's complete adjuvant are thymus-dependent (Table II). Valdutiu and Rose (62) and Claggett and Weigle (17) have recently also published reports that lethally irradiated mice reconstituted with syngeneic bone marrow cells (with or without treatment with anti-Θ serum and complement) fail to make antibody to mouse thyroglobulin and to develop thyroiditis. Autoimmune thyroiditis following immunization with thyroglobulin of the same species is also prevented by neonatal thymectomy in the chicken (26) and the rat (11).

TABLE I

THYMUS-DEPENDENCE OF FORMATION OF ANTIBODY AGAINST HETEROLOGOUS THYROGLOBULINS (HTg) AND MOUSE THYROGLOBULIN (MTg) AND THYROIDITIS

Mice	Antibody Responses		Thyroiditis**
	Anti-HTg*	Anti M-Tg*	
Intact	14.2 ± 3.7	12.5 ± 1.6	3.7 ± 0.8
TXBM	2.1 ± 0.9	1.2 ± 0.7	0.5 ± 0.3
TXBM + thymus	12.3 ± 2.4	10.2 ± 1.4	2.9 ± 0.8

Adult ♀ CBA mice. Experimental conditions of Rose et al (J. Immunol. 106:691, 1971).

TXBM - 6 week thymectomy, 750 R and reconstitution with anti-Θ-treated bone marrow cells ± thymus graft beneath the renal capsule.

* Passive hemagglutination of erythrocytes coated with mouse thyroglobulin by the chromic chloride method (log_2 ± standard error). Serum samples taken 28 days after first injection.

**Index based on the proportion of thyroid tissue replaced by mononuclear infiltrate. Total replacement = 5.0.

TABLE II

THYMUS-DEPENDENCE OF AUTOIMMUNE MURINE THYROIDITIS $\frac{0}{+}$ CBA
8 WEEKS

Mice	Anti-Tg	Thyroiditis
Intact	12.2 + 1.2	3.1 + 0.5
TXBM	1.7 + 1.0	0.4 + 0.3
TXBM + Thymus	10.3 + 1.4	2.6 + 0.6

Experimental conditions of Rose et al., J. Immunol. 106:691, 1971.

The presence of lymphocytes binding autoantigens.
If the hypothesis of self-tolerance presented above is correct, it should be possible to identify B cells capable of reacting with autoantigens circulating in low concentration, such as thyroglobulin or growth hormone, whereas neither B nor T cells able to react with autoantigens circulating in high concentration, e.g. serum albumin should be demonstrable. Experiments were, therefore, undertaken to determine by sensitive autoradiographic techniques the binding of homologous thyroglobulin and serum albumin by human lymphocytes (7). Peripheral blood lymphocytes from normal human subjects were allowed to bind high specific activity ^{125}I-human thyroglobulin and human serum albumin. The B lymphocytes were identified by their large amount of surface immunoglobulin as shown by binding of radioactive anti-immunoglobulin. Selective removal of B cells from the population of lymphocytes was achieved by passing them through columns of beads coated with antibody against human immunoglobulin. The B lymphocytes are retained on such columns, presumably because their large amount of surface immunoglobulin reacts with the antibody on the beads. Studies of the cells that have passed through the columns show marked depletion or absence of B lymphocytes.

Nine out of eleven normal subjects had peripheral blood

lymphocytes which bound ^{125}I-thyroglobulin (Table III). In contrast, no lymphocytes which bound human serum albumin were found in normal human subjects. Lymphocytes binding thyroglobulin were absent after passage through the column retaining B cells in three experiments and were markedly depleted in a fourth experiment. Thus, the antigen-binding cells are identified as B lymphocytes.

TABLE III

LYMPHOCYTES BINDING HOMOLOGOUS ^{125}I ANTIGENS IN NORMAL SUBJECTS (Ref. 7).

Type of labelled antigen ≠	No. of labelled cells*	
	Individual Subjects	Average**
Human thyroglobulin	175, 455, 150, 0, 100, 80, 380, 0, 500, 298, 240	216
Human serum albumin	0, 0, 0	0

*Number of labelled lymphocytes per 10^6 lymphocytes.

≠5 x 10^6 lymphocytes were reacted for 30 minutes with 270-500 ng. labelled antigen in a 0.5 ml volume. Autoradiographs were exposed for 8 to 24 days.

**Average calculated from the nine positive subjects.

Two general criticisms of the work carried out on antigen-binding cells are that the cells have been incubated with less than saturating amounts of labelled antigen or that they may represent cells producing low-affinity antibodies, which would not be eliminated during the development of self-tolerance. However, the concentrations of thyroglobulin used in our experiments are close to those in the circulation, and the binding is followed by radiation-induced elimination of cells producing autoantibodies against thyroglobulin as described in the next section. Thus, the conditions used for our experiments appear to identify the cells on which attention should be focused, namely, antigen-binding immunocompetent cells which are the precursors of cells producing reasonably high-affinity antibodies.

The finding of thyroglobulin-binding cells in human peripheral blood has been confirmed by Roberts et al. (45). These authors also reported the presence of thyroglobulin-binding cells in the thymus. The antigen-binding cells in thymus were thought to be B cells because of staining with fluorescein-labelled anti-globulin sera. However, there is some uncertainty about the results with thymus cells because the amount of antigen bound was rather small despite the use of much higher concentrations than in our experiments and because of lack of specificity of the anti-globulin preparations used.

Preliminary reports have also been published of the presence of lymphocytes binding thyroglobulins of the same species in rats (1) and mice (17). Since inbred animals were used, these observations show that the binding is due to autologous rather than isologous (allotypic) determinants as confirmed by the suicide experiments mentioned below.

The lack of binding of autologous serum albumin might well be due to receptor blockade following exposure to a high dose of antigen. However, when receptors were removed by protease digestion and the cells washed and cultured over night in medium containing fetal calf serum, surface immuno-globulins and binding of autologous thyroglobulin and hetero-logous albumin could be demonstrated, but no binding of auto-logous albumin appeared. Unanue (61) has reported the finding in mice of lymphocytes binding mouse growth hormone but not mouse serum albumin. Thus, the accumulated observations on antigen-binding cells are consistent with the view that these cells are present in the case of autoantigens that circulate in low dose, such as thyroglobulin and polypeptide hormones, but not in the case of proteins such as serum albumin which circulate in high dose.

These results are analogous to those reported for induction of unresponsiveness in experimental animals. Thus, following injection of tolerogenic doses of bovine serum albumin and of human gammaglobulin into mice decreases of antigen-binding cells in lymphoid tissues have been found (31, 38).

Suicide of thyroglobulin-binding cells.

Antigen-binding lymphocytes have been characterized in the mouse using radioiodinated antigens by Ada and by Sulitzeanu and their colleagues (see 1). Antigen-binding lymphocytes are primarily B lymphocytes; their number is not reduced by treating spleen cells with anti-theta serum and complement, and there are normal numbers of antigen-binding lymphocytes in the congenitally athymic (nu/nu) mouse. The antigen-binding cells are also the antigen-sensitive lymphocytes: radiation-induced death of lymphocytes which bind a highly radioactive antigen specifically abrogates the immune response to that antigen while leaving other immune responses intact.

Our demonstration that normal humans have B lymphocytes binding autologous thyroglobulin did not provide conclusive proof that these cells are able to respond to antigenic determinants in the circulating protein. Conceivably, the binding cells might have recognized determinants which were allotypic or exposed during the purification of the protein, or the cells might have had a rather low affinity for the protein and so be less easily rendered unresponsive in the course of ontogeny. The specific inhibition of binding by unlabelled protein and finding of a small number of cells binding a relatively large amount of antigen even when the concentration of the latter was very low makes these alternative explanations unlikely. Nevertheless, experiments were initiated together with G.L. Ada to ascertain whether the B lymphocytes binding thyroglobulin are the same as those producing autoantibodies when suitably stimulated. Lymphocytes from mature mice were allowed to bind highly radioactive heterologous or mouse thyroglobulin, and after over night incubation with the antigen, they were inoculated into lethally irradiated syngeneic recipients. These were then tested for their capacity to form antibodies against heterologous and autologous thyroglobulin determinants and against an unrelated antigen (toxoid) and to develop thyroiditis.

The results of representative experiments are shown in Tables IV and V. It is clear that when splenic lymphocytes undergo suicide following binding of heterologous thyroglobulins, the subsequent antibody response against these antigens as well as cross-reactive autologous determinants, is markedly impaired. When the suicide follows binding of autologous thyroglobulin, autoantibody formation is depressed, but the antibody response against heterologous thyroglobulin determinants remains intact. The specificity of the suicide is confirmed by the insignificant reduction of the response to an unrelated antigen, diptheria toxoid. The development of autoimmune thyroiditis in the mice closely parallels their capacity to make autoantibodies against thyroglobulin. Similar observations following suicide of mouse bone marrow cells with high specific activity thyroglobulin have recently been presented by Clagett and Weigle (17).

TABLE IV

SUICIDE OF LYMPHOCYTES BINDING HIGH SPECIFIC-ACTIVITY ^{125}I-THYROGLOBULIN, ADULT ♀ CBA MICE 750 R

Reconstitution	Antibody Responses			
	Mouse Tg	Heterologous Tg	DT*	Thyroiditis
Normal spleen cells	9.3 ± 2.7	11.6 ± 2.3	13.8 ± 3.7	2.9 ± 0.5
Spleen cells ^{125}I-HTg	1.5 ± 1.1	1.8 ± 0.9	12.9 ± 3.1	0.3 ± 0.2
Spleen cells ^{125}I-MTg	0.9 ± 0.7	10.3 ± 2.6	13.3 ± 2.0	0.2 ± 0.1

*Diphtheria toxoid

TABLE V

EFFECT OF SUICIDE OF LYMPHOCYTES BINDING HIGH-SPECIFIC ACTIVITY ^{125}I-MOUSE THYROGLOBULIN (MTg) ON AUTOIMMUNE THYROIDITIS ADULT ♀ CBA MICE 750 R

Reconstitution	Antibody responses		Thyroiditis
	Anti-MTg	Anti-DT	
Normal spleen cells	12.0 ± 2.2	14.0 ± 2.9	3.4 ± 1.2
Spleen cells ^{125}I - MTg	1.5 ± 0.8	13.3 ± 2.7	0.4 ± 0.2

These results provide strong evidence that the antigen-
binding B cells in normal animals are the cells which when
stimulated, for example, by immunization with heterologous
thyroglobulins or autologous protein in the presence of
Freund's complete adjuvant are able to respond by autoantibody formation. Moreover, the formation of such autoantibodies can lead to the genesis of autoimmune thyroiditis.

Lymphocytes in autoallergic thyroiditis.
Autoallergic thyroiditis in humans and experimental
animals is accompanied by infiltration of the gland with
mononuclear cells. In acute experimental thyroiditis moderate numbers of polymorphonuclear leukocytes are also present
especially in the mouse and guinea pig, but the later infiltrate is largely mononuclear. Initially, the infiltrating
cells are confined to the perifollicular connective tissue,
but damage to epithelial cells and replacement of follicles
by infiltrating cells ensues in severe cases. Although some
mononuclear phagocytes are identifiable, especially in regions of tissue damage, the majority of infiltrating cells
have the appearance of lymphocytes. Many are identifiable
as belonging to the B lymphocyte lineage by their surface
immunoglobulin or differentiation into antibody-secreting
cells including mature plasma cells. A relatively high proportion of these cells are making antibody against autologous
thyroglobulin. In rabbits developing thyroiditis suspensions
of cells recovered from the thyroid form hemolytic plaques
with erythrocytes coated with rabbit thyroglobulin (16). In
human cases of Hashimoto's disease plasma cells binding
fluorescein-labelled human thyroglobulin are readily demonstrable.

Thus, there are in the thyroid many cells of B lymphocyte lineage making antibodies against thyroglobulin. Indeed
the predominant site of synthesis of these antibodies is the
gland itself. The question arises whether T lymphocytes can
also become responsive against antigenic determinants in the
native protein, or whether helper effects are achieved by
T cells reactive against determinants in heterologous thyroglobulins (in the experimental situation) or determinants
in altered autologous thyroglobulin (in experiments with
autologous protein in complete adjuvant and possibly naturally occurring thyroiditis). The role of exposure of hidden
determinants in autologous tissues has been widely discussed
in relation to autoimmunity in general. Its relevance to
the present discussion is shown by the observation of Stylos
and Rose (54) that rabbits immunized intravenously with

papain digests of rabbit thyroglobulin make antibodies against the protein.

In most experimental situations available, evidence suggests that T lymphocytes respond to heterologous but not autologous thyroglobulin determinants. Thus, as shown originally by Romagnani et al (48), lymphocytes from guinea pigs immunized with bovine thyroglobulin produce macrophage migration-inhibiting factor (MIF) when challenged with bovine thyroglobulin but not (with a single exception) when challenged with guinea pig thyroglobulin. In the guinea pig activation of lymphocytes for MIF production by specific antigen is a property of T cells (68). In rabbits immunized with heterologous thyroglobulins, spleen cells and cells recovered from the thyroid likewise produced MIF when challenged with heterologous thyroglobulins but not when challenged with rabbit thyroglobulin (16). Observations of MIF production by cells from patients with thyroiditis challenged with human thyroglobulin are ambiguous since it is now known that human B cells are able to elaborate MIF.

Interaction of antibodies and effector cells in the pathogenesis of autoimmine thyroiditis.

After many unsuccessful attempts to transfer autoimmune thyroiditis by serum, Nakamura and Weigle (37) were able to transfer the disease in rabbits using serum from thyroidectomized donors. Autoimmune thyroiditis has likewise been transferred with serum in mice (62). The technical problems concern the timing of the transfer and absorption of antibody by the thyroid gland. During the course of immunization a high proportion of B cells reacting against homologous thyroglobulin are removed from the blood stream into the thyroid itself where they differentiate into antibody-secreting cells (16); most antibody is absorbed before it can enter the circulation. Transfer of autoimmune thyroiditis by antibodies among guinea pigs can also be achieved; if large quantities of serum are given, acute inflammatory reactions with infiltration of the thyroid by polymorphonuclear as well as mononuclear cells are observed. If repeated small doses of autoantibody are administered, the infiltration into the gland is largely mononuclear.

Thus, the available evidence suggests that autoimmune thyroiditis is an antibody-mediated rather than a cell-mediated immunopathological process. Since there is no indication that complement is involved in the pathogenesis of the disease (36), the question arises whether antibody col-

laborates with antibody-dependent effector cells (K cells)
in damaging thyroid epithelial cells (Fig. 2). For this
hypothesis to be plausible, it must be shown first that K
cells can lyse target cells passively sensitized with thyroglobulin and antibody and, second, that K cells accumulate
in the gland during the course of the disease.

Ringertz et al. (40) induced thyroiditis by immunization
of guinea pigs with homologous thyroglobulin in complete
Freund's adjuvant. In the presence of sera from such animals, chicken erythrocytes coated with thyroglobulin were
lysed by lymphoid cells from normal guinea pigs. The presence in patients with Hashimoto's disease of lymphoid cells
cytotoxic for target cells coated with human thyroglobulin
was reported by Podleski (43) and the underlying mechanism
was analyzed by Calder et al. (12). Decomplemented sera from
28 out of 39 patients with Hashimoto's disease, but not normal sera, sensitized chicken erythrocytes coated with thyroglobulin for lysis by normal human peripheral blood cells.

Dr. R. Diamond and I have found considerable K cell
activity in populations of cells recovered by protease
treatment of surgically removed Hashimoto thyroid tissue.
These cells lysed chicken erythrocytes coated with rabbit
antibody.

Thus, in the course of autoallergic thyroiditis, there
is an accumulation in the thyroid of cells of the B lymphocyte lineage-making antibody against thyroglobulin and
against microsomal (possibly plasma membrane) antigens.
Hence, a relatively high local concentration of these antibodies is achieved as well as some antibody that spills over
into the circulation. Precipitates of immunoglobulin and
thyroglobulin are formed close to the bases of thyroid epithelial cells. There is no evidence that T lymphocytes reactive against autoantigenic determinants play any role in
the pathogenesis of autoallergic thyroiditis, and damage to
epithelial cells may result from attack by K cells on the
bases of epithelial cells sensitized by autoantibodies.
Possibly this occurs because of thyroglobulin or other antigenic determinants associated with their basal plasma membranes.

Helper effect in induction of autoantibodies against
erythrocytes.
It is reasonable to ask whether the model developed for
autoimmune thyroiditis is also applicable to other auto-

immune responses. Full discussion of this problem is beyond the scope of this paper, but some observations on autoimmune hemolytic anemia will suffice to illustrate the analogy. Playfair and Clarke (42) have found that repeated inoculations of mice with rat erythrocytes leads to the production of autoantibodies against erythrocytes. Helper T cells reacting against common antigenic determinants appear to be involved, since thymectomy abolished autoantibody formation. The strain which responded best was C57Bl in aging members of which a relatively high incidence of erythrocyte autoantibodies has been reported (30). These authors have shown that complexes of some erythrocyte antigens and antibodies accumulate in the kidneys from which it appears that small amounts of the antigens may normally circulate in soluble form, thereby inducing selective T cell unresponsiveness.

Suppression of autoimmune responses by T cells.

If tolerance to autoantigens is due to selective T cell unresponsiveness, it is inevitably precarious since it can easily be abrogated. It is, therefore, likely that an additional "fail-safe" mechanism for preventing autoimmunity should exist. A second hypothesis put forward by Allison et al. (5) is that T cells can exert specific feedback control on the synthesis of antibodies by B cells and that relaxation of this control--especially in aging humans and experimental animals--may be an important factor in the development of autoimmunity. A role of T cells in immunological surveillance against malignant cells is supported by observations of an increased incidence of tumors (especially those that are virus-induced) in experimental animals with depressed cell-mediated immunity (2) and the raised probability of developing lymphoreticular neoplasms in humans with immunodeficiency syndromes or immunosuppressed after kidney transplantation. Immunological reactions are known to be subject to feedback control, the most fully studied case being the specific inhibition of antibody formation by administration of antibody (60). We suggest that a similar inhibition can be exerted by T cells, and that this provides a surveillance mechanism against aberrant immune reactions (Fig. 3).

Evidence summarized by Allison and others (5) comes from experiments with NZB mice which develop a Coombs-positive hemolytic anaemia from about the age of 4 months. If spleen cells are transferred from old to young NZB mice, about one half of the recipients show positive Coombs tests which usually disappear in a few weeks (Fig. 4).

If the recipients are given antilymphocytic globulin (ALG), more develop positive Coombs tests and these remain positive usually until the death of the animals. The simplest explanation of these results is that T cells in the young animals exert an inhibitory influence on the B cells from the spleens of old animals that are producing antibody against homologous erythrocytes as shown by the arrow in Fig. 4 and that T cell control is abolished by ALG administration. In keeping with this interpretation, transfer of thymus cells from 2 week old NZB mice monthly to NZB's from the age of 1 month significantly delays the onset of positive direct Coombs test (Fig. 5). Further evidence for the positive nature of the controls comes from experiments in which spleen cells from NZB mice are transferred into irradiated BALB/c mice; the recipients develop positive Coombs tests only if treated with ALG (20). Adoptive transfer of renal disease within the NZB/NZW strain is likewise achieved only in ALG-treated recipients (19).

Thus, suppression of autoantibody formation in adoptive transfer experiments dominates over expression, but the suppression can be relieved by ALG. Additional evidence for a role of suppressor T cells in this situation comes from experiments in collaboration with Playfair in which spleen cells from NZB mice were transferred to irradiated NZB recipients. No positive Coombs tests were observed in the recipients unless the transferred cell population was treated with anti-theta serum and complement in which case recipients rapidly developed autoantibodies against erythrocytes.

In general, evidence has accumulated that NZB mice and some of their hybrid offspring are especially prone to develop autoimmunity for two reasons. Their T cells are usually resistant to tolerance induction as judged by reactions against foreign serum proteins and erythrocytes. Moreover, their T cell function declines rapidly with age as judged by capacity to mount graft-versus-host reactions and in other ways. Hence, there is a combination of both factors favoring autoimmunity.

Teague and Friou (57) have found that aging mice of strain A frequently develop antibody against deoxyribonucleoprotein (anti-nuclear factor-ANP). Transfers of thymus cells from young to old syngeneic animals that had developed ANF resulted in decreased levels or disappearance of ANF. These workers have also suggested that cells in the thymus and spleen of young mice may participate in homeostatic control of autoantibody formation and that this control may be less effective in aging animals. The age-dependence of autoantibody formation in humans is well documented.

Some of the most convincing evidence for a role of T cells in delaying or suppressing autoimmune reaction comes from studies of spontaneous autoimmune thyroiditis in chickens and mice. Leghorn chickens of the obese strain develop severe autoimmune thyroiditis. Wick et al (66) found that neonatal bursectomy reduces or prevents the the disease. Neonatal thymectomy, on the other hand, leads to earlier on-set and increased severity of thyroiditis (64, 66).

Spontaneous thyroiditis of autoimmune type also occurs in old Buffalo strain rats. Neonatal thymectomy considerably increases the number of animals with thyroiditis (49). Penhale et al (41) reported that Wistar rats neonatally thymectomized and given repeated sublethal doses of radiation to deplete residual T cells frequently develop autoimmune thyroiditis. Some strains of mice also show thyroiditis following neonatal thymectomy (34).

The dual role of T cells in autoimmunity is nicely il-lustrated by thyroiditis in which T cell helper effects favoring autoimmunity are delicately balanced against T cell suppressor effects controlling autoimmunity. Penhale (40) has recently found that Wistar rats severely depleted of T cells by thymectomy and repeated inoculations of anti-lympho-cytic serum (ALS) develop less thyroiditis than those thymec-tomized and irradiated. Thus, some residual T cell helper function may be required for the development of autoimmune thyroiditis.

In view of recent evidence that helper T cells are more radioresistant than suppressor T cells (Benacerraf, private communication), it is of interest that thymectomy followed by irradiation should result in a higher incidence of thy-roiditis than thymectomy followed by ALS. The former may affect primarily the suppressor cell population while the latter affects both suppressor and helper cells.

In all of these situations genetic factors exert a strong influence. In addition to thyroiditis, obese chickens show increased incidences of autoantibodies to liver and kidney (65). The autoimmune disorders of NZB mice are ob-viously under genetic control. The ability of mice to res-pond to injections of mouse thyroglobulin is largely deter-

mined by a gene linked to the major histocompatibility (H-2)
locus at or close to the Ir locus (56). Thymus cells from
a poorly responding strain reduced the response of lethally
irradiated mice reconstituted with live marrow cells from a
high-responder strain (63). Thus, genetic control may be
manifested through the suppressor function of the thymus
rather than its role in providing helper cells. This type of
genetic dissection may facilitate analysis of the two functions of T cells in autoimmunity.

Effects of haptens and drugs.

As mentioned above, another way in which the requirement
for specifically reactive T cells can be bypassed is to sen-
sitize an animal against a hapten (such as oxazolone or
dinitrophenol) and couple the hapten to host constituents
before re-injection into the same or a syngeneic animal.
Such procedures have been used to produce autoantibody against
thyroglobulin (67) and antibody against specific (idiotypic)
determinants of a monoclonal immunoglobulin in a syngeneic
system. This may be the way by which in human patients exposure to certain drugs is followed by autoantibody production. Two possible examples are the formation of autoantibodies against red cells (often directed against Rh blood
groups) in patients treated with α-methyldopa and the presence of antinuclear factors in patients treated with hydral-
lazine, isoniazid, procaineamide and other drugs (13). The
postulate is that patients will have T cell reactivity
against the drugs or their matabolites and that the drugs or
metabolites should be associated as haptens with erythrocyte
membranes or nucleoproteins, respectively. Both these postulates are testable, especially since the formation of anti-
nuclear factors can be reproduced in experimental animals exposed to appropriate drugs.

Allogeneic cell stimulation, adjuvants and autoantibody formation.

Injections of allogeneic immunocompetent cells under
conditions that produce mild graft-versus-host reactions abolish the need for cooperation of carrier T cells in a hapten-
carrier system (27, 28). Evidence has accumulated that in
such animals host T cells are stimulated in a non-antigen-
specific fashion. If the model of tolerance presented above
is correct, inoculations of allogeneic cells should stimulate
the formation of autoantibodies. Boyse et al. (8) reported
that mice injected with allogeneic cells produce autoantibodies against thymocytes. Cannat and Varet (14) and Fialkow
Gilchrish and Allison (24) have found that repeated injections

40

of Fl mice with parental cells rapidly induces the formation of antinuclear antibodies; allotype markers were used to establish that these were produced by host and not donor B cells. These results support the view that allogeneic cell stimulation can result in autoantibody formation, and the role of this pehnomenon in chronic graft-versus-host disease deserves further study.

The role of adjuvants in eliciting autoantibody formation in experimental animals is well known. Many adjuvants stimulate proliferation of T cells, and T cells are required for the increase by several adjuvants of antibody formation by B cells (see 4). Freund's complete adjuvant may in addition exert a carrier effect if mycobacterial antigens are able to form complexes with host antigens. The human counterpart is the finding of antinuclear and other autoantibodies in leprosy--in which patients carry a heavy mycobacterial load, which may have adjuvant activity--and also in malaria, syphilis and other infections (Refs. in 5).

Virus infections.
It follows from what has been said that, if it were possible to bypass the requirement for T cells responsive against autoantigens, autoantibody formation might be elicited. One way by which this might be achieved is by virus infection. Virus-specific antigens are often found on the membranes of infected host cells, and host antigens in the envelopes of lipid-containing viruses. Thus, virus antigens and autoantigens could form common immunogenic units which function in a manner analogous to the hapten-carrier system.

An analogous principle has been used by Lindenmann and Klein (24) to increase immunity against tumor-specific antigens by immunizing mice with influenza virus grown in the tumor cells. Harboe and Haukenes (25) have found that ckickens immunized with influenza virus containing an antigen from the chorioallantoic cells in which it was cultured produce autoantibody against the same antigen present in liver and bile. Tonietti et al. (58) have reported that infection of NZB, NZW and NZB/NZW hybrid mice with polyoma virus or lymphocytic choriomeningitis virus accelerates the onset of autoimmune manifestations and increases their incidence. As infectious mononucleosis infections wane, a variety of autoantibodies is often found, and human infections with several other viruses including influenza, measles, varicella, Coxsackie and herpes simplex viruses are sometime followed by autoallergic manifestations including antibody-

mediated thrombocytopenia and positive Coombs tests (see 5).
The development of cold autoagglutinins often directed
against the I blood group after Mycoplasma pneumoniae infections may have a similar explanation.

Multiplication and differentiation of lymphocytes.
In the course of normal ontogenetic development, many
different cell types--whether they are precursors of neurons,
muscle cells, erythrocytes, granulocytes or other specialized
cells--multiply and then differentiate. Often fully differentiated cells such as neurons or granulocytes lose the
capacity to synthesize DNA and multiply. The same appears
to be true of cells of the B lymphocyte lineage. The precursors certainly synthesize DNA and multiply when suitably
stimulated, but fully differentiated cells, antibody-secreting plasma cells, appear to have lost the capacity to synthesize DNA and multiply. Available evidence suggests that
the two processes, DNA synthesis and differentiation to
antibody secretion, are independent (33). Thus, in populations of mouse B lymphocytes (nude spleen cells) stimulated
by lipopolysaccharide, DNA synthesis as well as antibody
synthesis and secretion occur. Marked inhibition of DNA
synthesis by hydroxyurea does not interfere with increased
synthesis and secretion of immunoglobulin. Conversely,
antibodies with specificity for mouse immunoglobulin inhibit
the maturation of mouse B cells into antibody-secreting cells
but they enhance rather than depress DNA synthesis.

These observations allow reappraisal of the suggestion
by Sterzl (53) and others that "exhaustive differentiation"
of lymphocytes with specificities against certain antigenic
determinants may play a role in tolerance induction. The
concept can be discussed first with reference to thymus-
independent antigens, and later the implications for thymus-
dependent antigens will be considered. Thymus-independent
antigens stimulate specific clones of B lymphocytes (bearing
receptors for their antigenic determinants) to multiply and
differentiate into antibody-secreting cells. There is, in
addition, a non-specific mitogenic effect of several thymus-
independent antigens (18). It is reasonable to suppose that
thymus-independent antigens vary in the efficiency with
which they stimulate DNA synthesis and multiplication on the
one hand and differentiation into antibody-secreting cells
on the other. Some, such as levan, may strongly stimulate
differentiation, so that a very high proportion of the progeny of clones of cells with receptors for levan are stimu-

lated to differentiate (Fig. 6). The result would be a good primary response and then exhaustive differentiation resulting in no secondary response (Fig. 7).

Other thymus-independent antigens, such as pneumococcus polysaccharide and endotoxin of Gram-negative bacteria, would be less powerful stimuli to differentiation so that although no large population of memory cells accumulates, some B lymphocytes able to respond to secondary antigenic stimulation persist (Fig. 8). The result is a slight increase in antigen-binding cells following primary immunization and a secondary immune response of magnitude approximately equivalent to the primary.

With yet other thymus-independent antigens such as those of Brucella abortus, the stimulus to multiplication would be stronger than that to differentiation so that some build up of a memory population and increased secondary response is observed (Fig. 7).

These hypotheses are testable. For example, it should be possible with the electronic cell sorter to obtain populations of B lymphocytes with surface receptors for levan. Incubation of these cells with levan should provide a powerful stimulus to differentiation. In vitro exposure of such cells to levan would be expected to result in elimination of clones of cells able to respond to this antigen when transferred to syngeneic, irradiated recipients. In vitro assays of clone size, using methods analogous to those developed by Luzzatti et al. (32), should show small clones of cells producing antibody against levan as contrasted with clones of cells responding to Brucella abortus antigens for example.

Thymus helper effects and the differentiation of B lymphocytes.
When considering tolerance and other problems, it is important to know whether the helper effect of T lymphocytes occurs at the level of recognition of antigen by B lymphocytes with an ensuing stimulus to multiplication in the corresponding clones or on their differentiation into antibody-secreting cells. Evidence is accumulating that the helper effect of T lymphocytes is exerted on the last-named process. The evidence is of two kinds: one concerning the generation of B memory cells in animals deprived of T cells while the second concerns the mode of action of T cells and their products in vitro.

Roelants and Askonas (46) inoculated keyhole limpet hemocyanin into TXBM mice and found that although antibody formation was markedly impaired a population of B memory cells was built up, as shown by a considerable increase in cells binding specific antigen and adoptive transfer experiments. Askonas et al. (6) have shown that congenitally athymic (nu/nu) mice immunized with erythrocytes increase the number of B cells able to make antibody in vitro when cultivated with a T cell replacing factor.

Previously, Schimpl and Wecker (51) had shown that the T cell replacing factor (a supernatant of a mixed lymphocyte culture) allows formation of IgG in cultures of spleen cells from preimmunized T cell-deprived mice. The timing of the effect of the T cell-replacing factor suggests that it is required for the final stage of development of the B cell into an antibody-secreting cell.

In experiments performed in collaboration with Dr. J.L. Virelizier on antibody responses to influenza virus hemagglutinins, similar results have been obtained. In TXBM mice the population of memory lymphocytes built up following injection of this antigen is actually greater than in intact mice even though no antibody against specific determinants is demonstrable. It is, therefore, unlikely that small numbers of residual T cells in the TXBM mice can explain the observations.

The observations suggest that T cells do not help B lymphocytes to recognize antigen and multiply in response to antigen exposure, thereby generating a population of memory cells, but that the T cell helper effect facilitates the differentiation of cells of the B lineage into antibody-secreting cells. This interpretation which is illustrated in Fig. 9 has interesting implications for tolerance induction. In the absence of T cell helper effects, antigenic stimulation would build up a relatively large population of memory cells which are not diverted into the population of antibody-secreting cells with a finite life span (Fig. 10). However, if there were excessive help or the requirement for help were diminished, many of the cells in the clone would be diverted into the population of antibody-secreting cells. Particularly, if this were to occur early in the course of clonal expansion, the generation of memory cells would be severely impaired (Fig. 11). The result would be the production of a small amount of antibody (possibly so small as to be undetectable) followed by tolerance. This might occur following exposure to large doses of certain antigens which can overcome the requirement for T cell helper effects. Such a mechanism might be involved in high-dose tolerance. Paradoxically, too much helper effect might lead to hyperdiversion with the generation of only a small population of memory cells from the clone; the process would be manifested as a T cell suppressor effect on antibody formation. This is unlikely to be the only mechanism by which T cell suppressor effects are achieved, but it deserves investigation in certain models. Too much help (for example, by excessive sensitization to a carrier under conditions which favor a T cell response) might depress antibody formation especially the secondary response, to a hapten.

In general, the balance of proliferation and differentiation in lymphocytes is clearly of key importance both in the immune response and in the induction of tolerance.

REFERENCES

1. Ada, G.L. and Cooper, M.G., Ann. N.Y. Acad. Sci. 181: 96, 1971.

2. Allison, A.C., Proc. Roy. Soc. B. 177:23, 1971.

3. Allison, A.C., Lancet. 2:1401, 1971.

4. Allison, A.C., Ciba Foundation Symposium on Immunopotentiation ASP, Amsterdam, p. 73, 1971.

5. Allison, A.C., Denman, A.M. and Barnes, R.D., Lancet. 2:135, 1971.

6. Askonas, B.A., Schimpl, A. and Wecker, G., Eur. J. Immunol. 4:164, 1974.

7. Bankhurst, A.D., Torrigiani, G. and Allison, A.C., Lancet. 1:226, 1973.

8. Boyse, E.A., Bressler, E., Iritani, C.A. and Lardis, M., Transplantation. 9:339, 1970.

9. Burnet, F.M., The Clonal Selection Theory of Acquired Immunity, Cambridge University Press, Cambridge, 1959.

10. Burnet, F.M. and Fenner, F., The Production of Anti-bodies, Macmillan, Melbourne, 1949.

11. Busci, P.A. and Straussen, H.R., Experientia. 28:194, 1972.

12. Calder, E.A., Penhale, W.J., McLennan, D., Barnes, E.W. and Irvine, W.J., Clin. Exp. Immunol. 14:153, 1973.

13. Cannat, A. and Seligmann, M., Clin. Exp. Immunol. 3:99, 1968.

14. Cannat, A. and Varet, B., Biomedicine. 19:108, 1973.

15. Chiller, J., Habicht, G.S. and Weigle, W.O., Science. 171:813, 1971.

16. Clinton, B.A. and Weigle, W.O., J. Exp. Med. 130:1605, 1972.

17. Clagett, J. A. and Weigle, W.O., J. Exp. Med. 139:643, 1974.

18. Coutinho, A. and Möller, G., Eur. J. Immunol. 3:531, 1973.

19. Denman, A.M., Russell, A.S. and Denmann, E.J., Clin. Exp. Immunol. 5:567, 1969.

20. Denman, A.M., Russell, A.S. and Denman, E.J., Series Immunobiol. 16:253, 1970.

21. Dresser, D.W. and Mitchison, N.A., Advanc. Immunol. 8:129, 1968.

22. Ehrlich, P., Collected Studies on Immunity, 1906.

23. Feldmann, M. and Nossal, G.J.V., Transplant. Rev. 13:3, 1972.

24. Fialkow, P.J., Gilchrist, C. and Allison, A.C., Clin. Exp. Immunol. 13:479, 1973.

25. Harboe, A. and Haukenes, G., Acta Path. Microbiol. Scand. 68:98. 1966.

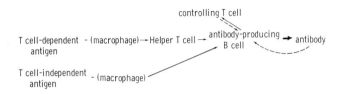

Fig. 3. The concept of T cell control of antibody formation by B cells. Stimulating interactions are shown by
thin arrows, inhibitory interactions by dotted arrows and
products by thick arrows.

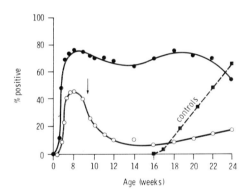

Fig. 4. Adoptive transfer of positive antiglobulin reactions to young NZB mice (Ref. 5).
    ●-● received 2 mg ALG four times intraperitoneally
        followed by 200-250 x 10⁶ spleen cells i.p. from
        old Coombs-positive NZB donors.

    o-o received normal rabbit IgG followed by similar
        injections of spleen cells.

    x-x received NRG only.

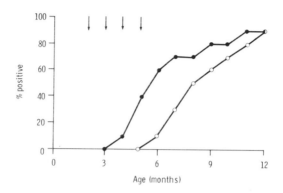

Fig. 5. Delay in the appearance of autoimmune hemolytic anaemia in NZB mice given repeated intravenous inoculations of thymus cells from syngeneic donors aged 2 weeks
(one thymus equivalent per recipient) at times shown by the
arrows.

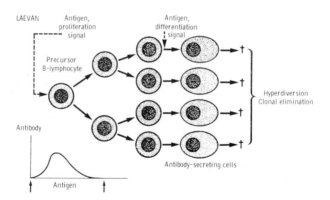

Fig. 6. Diagrammatic representation of the immune response to levan. B lymphocytes with receptors for levan
undergo clonal expansion, but since levan is also a powerful
stimulant of differentiation, a very high proportion of progeny cells differentiate into antibody-secreting cells
depleting the population of specific memory cells. The
antibody-secreting cells have a finite life span, and when
they have disappeared, there will be no further antibody
formation in response to a second challenge with antigen.

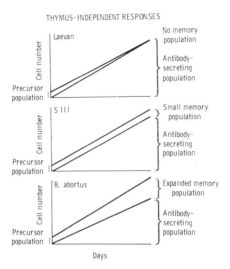

Fig. 7. Diagram showing the relationship of the specific precursor (B cell) population to the population of memory cells in the course of thymus-independent immune responses to representative antigens.

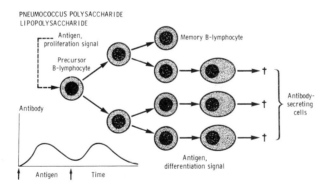

Fig. 8. Diagram of the response to thymus-independent antigens such as pneumococcus polysaccharide and lipopolysaccharide. Many of the cells in proliferating clones differentiate into antibody-secreting cells, but not all, so that a small (only slightly expanded or unexpanded) memory cell population remains. This gives a secondary immune response of the same order of magnitude as the primary.

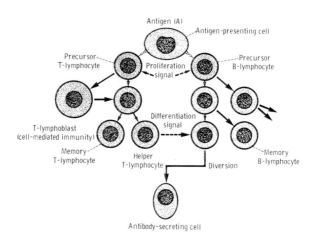

Fig. 9. Diagram showing the relationship between anti-
gen-presenting cells; T and B lymphocytes in the formation
of antibody against thymus-dependent antigens.

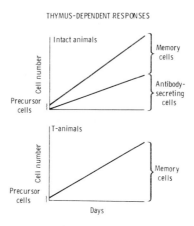

Fig. 10. Diagram contrasting the immune response to a
thymus-dependent antigen in a normal and a thymus-deprived
(T) animal. In the latter clonal expansion occurs, but
there is no diversion into the population of antibody-secreting cells; hence, a large memory cell population is built up.

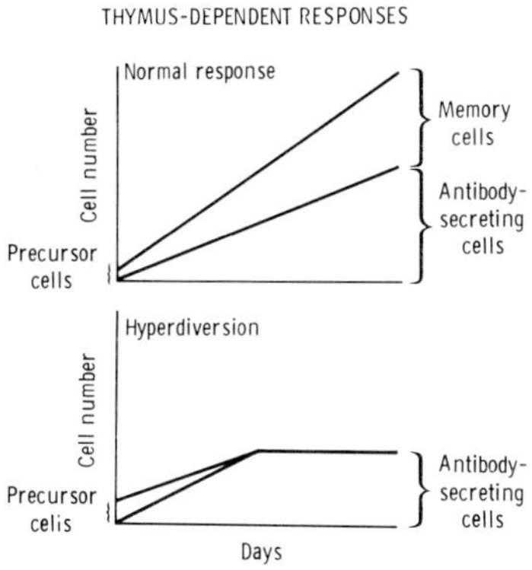

THYMUS-DEPENDENT RESPONSES

Fig. 11. Diagram showing hyperdiversion following exposure to high concentrations of antigen which overcome the need for T cell help or in the presence of a large number of T cells. The memory cell population is depleted.

DISCUSSION FOLLOWING ANTHONY ALLISON

BENACERRAF: Is there any evidence of an increase in the number of specific B cells in animals deprived of T cell function as a consequence of immunization?

ALLISON: Yes, Roelants has found an increase in cells binding antigen in T cell-deprived mice immunized with hemocyanin. Davie and Paul have similar results with DNP-hemocyanin and DNP-bovine serum albumin in thymectomized, irradiated, bone marrow reconstituted mice.

G. MÖLLER: If high dose tolerance affects both T and B cells and low dose only T cells, as suggested by your first point, how can you explain immunity?

ALLISON: Immunity to serum protein antigens in intermediate dosages may be experimental artifacts resulting from the presence of immunogenic forms of the antigens used. With soluble antigens the only important distinction appears to be that between low-dose unresponsiveness which selectively affects T cells and high-dose unresponsiveness which affects both B and T cells.

NOSSAL: I am doubtful whether the generally-held version of requirement for high antigen concentration will turn out to be correct for tolerogenesis of high affinity B cells. Therefore, I would like to ask whether the antibody formed against thyroglobulin was predominantly low affinity?

ALLISON: We have not measured the affinity of the anti-thyroglobulin antibodies. In the antigen-binding and suicide experiments very low concentrations of antigen were used (100 ng per ml which is the concentration in circulating blood); it is likely that we are dealing with high-affinity cells.

PAUL: The thesis that high dose tolerance to thymus-dependent antigens depends on a "hyper-activation" of T lymphocytes leads to the prediction that such tolerance in B cells should not be achievable in animals deprived of T lymphocytes. Have you tested the capacity of cells from thymus-deprived mice treated with a high dose of a T-dependent antigen to reconstitute responsiveness or irradiated syngeneic animals which have also been reconstituted with specifically activated T cells?

ALLISON: We have not studied this point. Roger Taylor has observations which will be presented later that T cells are required for the induction of unresponsiveness in B cells in mice exposed to sheep immunoglobulin.

WEIGLE: I would like to clarify the comments made on "high-low zone" tolerance. This phenomenon is a "red herring" and only occurs with a few antigens and under specific circumstances. We and others have not been able to show a "low-zone tolerance" with many antigens including heterologous thyroglobulins. The induction of tolerance in B cells with high doses of thyroglobulin results in tolerance in both T and B cells, while low doses of thyroglobulin results in tolerance in only the T cells. In answer to Göran Möller's question, immunity would not be involved since all doses result in tolerance in the intact animal.

ALLISON: I agree with your statement that low doses of thyroglobulin result in tolerance only of T cells. That is what I mean by low-dose unresponsiveness. The phenomenon does not necessarily require an immune response at intermediate dosages of antigen.

WAKSMAN: The Miller-Phillips group showed that, when mouse spleen cells were separated on discontinuous BSA gradients, one of the subpopulations (a) was capable of responding to antigen (SRBC, I think) in the absence of macrophages or T cells, i.e. even after treatment of the populations with anti-θ and C. This population was killed by hot thymidine and was therefore in the cell cycle. Another subpopulation (b) was not in the cell cycle, could not be killed with hot thymidine, and could be stimulated by antigen only in the presence of macrophages and T cells. This implies the exact opposite of what you're saying: that T cells promote B cell proliferation and that antigen provides the signal for B cell differentiation. How do we reconcile these diverse explanations?

ALLISON: It is difficult to extrapolate in vitro observations to the situation in vivo. The observations of Miller and Phillips show only that cells already multiplying are killed by hot thymidine. It is clear from the responses of cells from nude mice that B cells can be induced to synthesize DNA in the presence, at most, a small population of T cells.

HUMPHREY: I doubt whether TXBM mice can be regarded as sufficiently free from T cells to take the evidence of
Roelants and Askonas that B cells (protective memory
cells) binding haemocyanin, a T-dependent antigen, increase in the absence of T cells as proof that the latter are not required for generation of B memory cells.
Willcox and I have similar (unpublished) findings in
tetanus toxoid, but unless we could repeat them in nu/
nu mice, we would be very cautious of interpreting them
as you do.

ALLISON: The small residual population of T cells in TXBM
mice may well participate in the B memory phenomenon.
However, our TXBM mice develop better B memory following exposure to influenza hemagglutinin than normal
mice. When T cells are supplied they rapidly synthesize high levels of antibody. From these results, as
well as the in vitro studies of Schimpl, Wecker, and
Dutton, it is reasonable to suggest that the T cell
helper effect is exerted at the level of differentiation of B cells into antibody-secreting cells rather
than in the proliferation of the B cells. This idea
has interesting consequences which we believe deserve
discussion.

UNANUE: Do you have evidence for or against peripheral T
cells binding autologous thyroglobulin in normal individuals?

ALLISON: The thyroglobulin-binding cells were removed by
passage through anti-immunoglobulin columns, so they
appear to be B cells.

GERSHON: You listed B. abortus as representative of a class
of thymus-independent antigen. While this antigen does
yield a good antibody response in thymus-deprived mice,
it also elicits over and above that a thymus dependent
component of the antibody response when T cells are
present. Thus, one cannot attribute an effect produced
by B. abortus in intact mice as being B cell mediated.
This may have some bearing on your observation that B.
abortus yields a good memory response; this is probably
T cell mediated.

In regard to increased autoantibodies in thymectomized mice, it is possible that thymectomy allows viral
infection to break self-tolerance, which is one of the

mechanisms you proposed. Thus, it is possible that the
effects you reported are not due to a direct suppression of autoimmunity by T cells, but rather to an indirect suppression of viruses. It would be worthwhile
to see if thymectomy leads to autoimmunity in germ-free
animals.

ALLISON: Whether T cells are involved in memory in the immune response against B. abortus is not yet known.
There is no evidence that viruses are involved in the
genesis of autoimmune thyroiditis, although this possibility is difficult to exclude. Late transfer of T
lymphocytes prevents the development of the disease
and there are no overt signs of virus infection.

THE CELLULAR BASIS FOR ESTABLISHING TOLERANCE OR IMMUNITY TO BOVINE γ-GLOBULIN IN MICE

Carol Cowing, Ph.D., Miodrag Lukic, Ph.D. and
Sidney Leskowitz, Ph.D.

Department of Pathology
Tufts University School of Medicine
Boston, Massachusetts 02111

The studies I am going to describe represent the combined efforts of Drs. Carol Cowing and Miodrag Lukic working in my laboratory and have to do with a phenomenon which probably occurs before most of the events to be discussed at this meeting.

Inbred strains of mice exhibit impressive differences in ease of tolerance induction with γ-globulin antigens (1-3). One we have chosen to investigate involves the behavior of BALB/c and DBA/2 mice towards tolerance induction with bovine γ-globulin (BGG). The first strain is not rendered tolerant by even 20 mg of ultracentrifuged BGG, while the latter is uniformly tolerized by 0.2 mg.

In our first efforts to demonstrate the cellular basis for this difference in inducibility of tolerance (4), we were able to utilize a system involving cell transfers between these strains since they shared the same major histocompatibility locus ($H-2^d$). The test procedure consisted of injecting spleen cells from a normal donor into a lethally irradiated (900 rads) recipient. Four weeks later the reconstituted recipients were given various tolerizing doses of BGG, and a week later they were immunized with 100 μg BGG in complete Freund's adjuvant. One week following immunization, mice were tested for tolerance or immunity by injection with a test dose of about 2 μg ^{125}I-labelled BGG. Clearance of this test dose was followed by whole body scintillation counting over 3-5 days. Immune animals were regarded as those eliminating the tracer in 1-2 days, while tolerant animals cleared antigen at a rate little different from normal controls.

The results of these first experiments showed that when cells from BALB/c spleens were transferred to irradiated DBA/2 recipients, the animals behaved like normal DBA/2 mice, i.e. they were tolerizable by 0.2 mg doses of BGG. Furthermore, when DBA/2 spleen cells were transferred to lethally irradiated BALB/c recipients, the animals behaved like normal BALB/c mice, i.e. they could not be tolerized by even 2 mg doses of BGG. Although two independent tests showed that the irradiated reconstituted animals were true chimeras and contained lymphoid cells largely of allogeneic donor origin, they behaved like normal recipients in respect to tolerance induction by BGG.

This left the possibility that a radiation resistant cell of host origin was responsible for the residual property responsible for induction of tolerance or immunity. The most likely candidate was a phagocytic cell in the reticuloendothelial system responsible for processing antigen. Such a model had been proposed by Golub and Weigle (1) who suggested that BALB/c were so efficient in processing a small amount of aggregated human globulin present in most preparations that they became immunized before a competitive induction of tolerance of unaggregated HGG was complete.

We compared the capacity of the reticuloendothelial systems of BALB/c and DBA/2 mice to remove immunogenic material by studying biologic filtration in vivo. Large amounts of ^{125}I-trace labelled BGG were given to groups of mice of either strain. Two days later they were bled out and the amount of residual BGG in the serum estimated by scintillation counting. Various doses of this biologically-filtered BGG were given to normal BALB/c mice and their subsequent development of tolerance or immunity assessed in the usual way. As seen in Table I, the BGG passaged through BALB/c mice was able to induce tolerance in BALB/c mice down to a dose of 2.0 mg while 10 mg of DBA/2 filtered BGG was unable to induce tolerance.

TABLE I

TOLERANCE INDUCTION IN BALB/C MICE TREATED WITH BGG
PASSAGED THROUGH BALB/C OR DBA/2 MICE

Treatment	No. of Mice	Tolerant	Immune
Saline	3		3
10 mg BGG BALB/c passaged	3	3	
2.0 mg BGG BALB/c passaged	5	5	
10 mg BGG DBA/2 passaged	3		3

To see if, in fact, this ability to filter the immunogenic portion of BGG was radiation resistant, the same type
of experiment was performed using lethally irradiated (900 r)
BALB/c mice to filter the BGG. As seen in Table II, lethally
irradiated BALB/c mice still retained the ability to remove
the immunogenic fraction of BGG and 2.0 mg passaged through
irradiated or normal mice was sufficient to induce tolerance.

TABLE II

TOLERANCE INDUCTION IN BALB/C MICE TREATED WITH BGG
PASSAGED THROUGH IRRADIATED BALB/C MICE

Treatment	No. of Mice	Immune	Partially Tolerant	Tolerant
2.0 mg BGG BALB/c passaged	6			6
2.0 mg BGG passaged in lethally irra- diated BALB/c	6		1	5
2.0 mg BGG ultracentrifuged	4	4		

As an additional approach to evaluating the effectiveness of some component of the reticuloendothelial system in
establishing immunity in BALB/c mice, we studied the results
produced by treatment with carrageenan, a polysaccharide isolated from seaweed, which has been shown to be toxic for
macrophages (5). When BALB/c mice were injected intraperitoneally with 0.5 mg of carrageenan every other day for a
week, no apparent pathologic changes were noted, and the
mice cleared BGG at the normal rate. However, when BALB/c
mice were given an injection of 2 mg BGG immediately after
the carrageenan treatment, they became tolerant in sharp
contrast to untreated mice, thus demonstrating a role for
the carrageenan-sensitive cells in immune induction.

Since all in vivo evidence pointed to the macrophage
as the most likely cell responsible for the ease or difficulty in tolerance induction with the different strains of
mice, our next efforts were devoted to direct demonstration
in vitro of this effect. Spleens were removed from BALB/c
or DBA/2 mice and isolated spleen cell suspensions prepared
in RPM1 medium. These suspensions were then incubated in

culture media with BGG for 6 hours in a concentration of 10 mg BGG/2 x 10^7 cells. The supernatants were removed and measured quantities injected into normal BALB/c mice to see if tolerance could be induced. The results in Table III demonstrate that 10 or 2 mg of BGG subjected to in vitro biologic filtration by BALB/c cells was able to induce tolerance, while BGG filtered through DBA/2 cells was not. This process of filtration was shown to be an active metabolic process since cells held at 4° were unable to accomplish the removal of the immunogenic fraction.

TABLE III

TOLERANCE INDUCTION IN BALB/C MICE WITH BGG BIOLOGICALLY FILTERED IN VITRO BY BALB/C OR DBA/2 SPLEEN CELLS

Cells for Filtration	Amount of BGG + Administered	No. of Mice	Immune	Tolerant
None	2.0 mg	9	9	
	10.0 mg	9	9	
2 x 10^7 BALB/c spleen cells	2.0 mg	8	1	7
	10.0 mg	8	1	7
2 x 10^7 DBA/2 spleen cells	2.0 mg	6	5	1
	10.0 mg	6	5	1
2 x 10^7 BALB/c spleen cells a at 4°C	2.0 mg	9	9	
2 x 10^6 BALB/c adherent cells	2.0 mg	10		10
2 x 10^7 BALB/c non-adherent cells	2.0 mg	10	10	

In order to determine the cell type in BALB/c spleens responsible for their clearance of immunogen, the cells were separated into adherent and non-adherent components prior to culture with BGG. This was done by allowing them to settle on a glass petri dish and adhere. Non-adherent cells were purified further by allowing them to settle repeatedly on plastic petri dishes. The first adherent cell population was washed vigorously then eluted from the glass by EDTA treatment and found to comprise over 99% phagocytic cells. The final suspension of non-adherent cells was over 99% non-phagocytic as determined by neutral red uptake. When BGG was incubated with adherent cells in the ratio of 2 mg/2 x 10^6 cells, the supernatant was capable of inducing tolerance in normal BALB/c mice. Filtration of BGG by 10 times as many non-adherent cells was ineffective in removing immunogen (Table III).

To summarize, these results confirm previous impressions that the cell responsible for resistance to tolerance induction in BALB/c mice are especially capable of filtering out an immunogenic fraction of ultracentrifuged BGG; this ability is undiminished by lethal irradiation, is abrogated by a macrophage-toxic substance and resides in an adherent cell population. Some intriguing questions remain as to just why BALB/c mice, in contrast to many other strains, have this property of resistance to tolerance induction.

As a preliminary stage in answering some of them, we have undertaken a genetic analysis of the ability to resist tolerance induction. The F_1 cross of BALB/c x DBA/2 mice (CDF$_1$) all become tolerant just like the DBA/2 parental strain when treated with 2 mg of BGG. When backcrosses of CDF$_1$ to BALB/c mice were tested with the same regimen, approximately half (12) became tolerant and half (11) became immune. If further tests confirm this distribution, it would point to a single gene controlling the process of induction of immunity or tolerance with tolerance being the dominant allele. Since both parental strains are H-2^d, it is apparent that unlike Ir genes, there is no linkage to major histocompatibility loci. Moreover, the control seems to be exercised at the level of the macrophage rather than the T cell. There is at present no evidence to indicate what molecular structure is involved in this control mechanism.

REFERENCES

1. Golub, E.S. and Weigle, W.O., _J. Immunol._ 102:389,1969.

2. Kong, Y.M. and Wiger, D.L., _J. Immunol._ 105:370, 1970.

3. Das, S. and Leskowitz, S., _J. Immunol._ 105:938, 1970.

4. Das, S. and Leskowitz, S., J. Immunol. 112:107, 1974.

5. Allison, A.C., Harrington, J.S. and Birbeck, M., J. Exp. Med. 124:141, 1966.

THE ROLE OF ACCESSORY AND THYMUS-DERIVED CELLS IN RESISTANCE TO TOLERANCE INDUCTION

Bernhard Cinader and Michio Fujiwara

Institute of Immunology, Departments of Medical Genetics
Medical Biophysics and Clinical Biochemistry
Medical Sciences Building
University of Toronto, Toronto, Ontario Canada M5S 1A8

INTRODUCTION

Tolerance is attributable to unresponsiveness of bursal equivalent (B) and of thymus-derived (T) cell populations (1-4) and can be induced in each population without the obligatory participation of the other cell type (3). The relative difficulty of demonstrating unresponsiveness in the B cell population is due to recruitment of B cells from stem cells and to the accentuation of this process in the tolerogen-free reconstituted animal (4).

Accessory cells do not co-operate in the processes which result in B cell or T cell tolerance (3). Whether or not tolerance is induced depends on competition between a pathway of direct interactions between antigen and cells which leads to unresponsiveness and a pathway of antigen-cell and cell-cell interactions which leads to antibody formation. This second pathway becomes predominant when the antigen is in a form which directs it to accessory cells. In adult animals of some strains, a considerable resistance to tolerance induction has been observed (5-10). In BALB/c mice this resistance is attributable to the aggregate content of antigens (5) and the number or activity of accessory cells (11, 6). In at least one strain, SJL, a second factor appears to be involved; a polymorphism of the T cell population and interference with tolerance induction through an interaction between a sub-population of T and accessory cells. In this paper we shall examine the cellular basis of strain variations in tolerance inducibility.

Our procedures in the preparation of complete and incomplete Freund's adjuvant (CFA, IFA), of purified rabbit gamma globulin (RGG), of aggregate-freed lightly iodinated gamma globulin, of heat-aggregated RGG (6), of the target cell for plaque assays (12), and of cell suspensions have been provided in recent publications (3, 4 and 25). In these papers we have also given details for the performance of the liquid hemolytic plaque assay (PFC, Ref. 3, 13), and for the elimination test, based on whole body counts (3, 4). Here, it is only necessary to give some details of double transfer experiments and of the nomenclature we employ in this context. Three days after lethal irradiation animals lack functioning accessory cells (14). Lethally irradiated animals were injected with bone marrow (BM_n) and/or thymus (Th_n) cells immediately before or three days after irradiation. In some experiments donor bone marrow and thymus cells were passed over glass wool to remove accessory cells (Th_g, BM_g). In some cases the primary recipient was tolerized. In all cases spleen cells from the primary recipients were given to secondary, lethally irradiated recipients. Spleen cells from primary lethally irradiated recipients which had only received thymus cells are referred to as TDSC; those from animals which had only received bone marrow cells are referred to as BDSC, and those from animals which received both types of cells are referred to as BTDSC. Secondary recipients were immunized and their response was examined.

RESULTS

The metabolic life (T 1/2) of antigens, such as rabbit gamma globulin is strain dependent and is much shorter in SJL than in A mice. The immunological responsiveness to aggregates is also much greater in some strains than in others and is particularly large in BALB/c and SJL mice. In adult animals of these latter two strains, tolerance cannot be induced when aggregate-containing gamma globulin preparations are injected (6).

The molecular state of the antigen and the age of the animal determine tolerance in SJL mice and in hybrids.
Removal of aggregates by centrifugation yields antigen preparations to which BALB/c mice can be rendered tolerant but to which SJL mice cannot be rendered tolerant (Fig. 1). Biofiltration of rabbit gamma globulins appears to be particularly effective in removing aggregates. Preparations of RGG, obtained in this way, induced a moderate degree of tolerance in adult SJL mice (Table I).

The relative resistance of SJL mice to tolerance induction is an age-dependent phenomenon. In three week old animals, a fairly high degree of tolerance can be induced to aggregate-freed RGG while in twelve week old animals, this is no longer possible (Table II). The resistance to toler-

68

ance induction is found in hybrids between SJL and A or BALB/c mice and is thus inherited as a dominant trait. The rate of progression towards resistance against tolerance induction is slower than in the SJL parent (Figs. 1 and 2).

TABLE I

THE EFFECT OF BIOFILTERED RGG
ON RESPONSIVENESS TO RGG-CFA[a]

Group	Number of Mice	Preparation of RGG	Half-Life[b] (in days)
1	4	Centrifugation	1.1 ± 0.2
2	7	Biofiltration in SJL mice	3.7 ± 1.5
3	5	Biofiltration in A mice	3.1 ± 1.6

(a) Biofiltration of RGG was carried out on 12-14 weeks old A or SJL mice. SJL mice (female, 8 weeks old) were injected i.p. with 1.6 mg of either the biofiltered materials or aggregate-free RGG, obtained by centrifugation. Two weeks later the animals were injected (s.c.) with 0.25 mg RGG-CFA; three weeks later ^{131}I-RGG (10 µg) was injected i.p. and the elimination was followed.

(b) Comparison between groups:-
   1 and 2 $p < 0.0005$
   1 and 3 $p < 0.005$
   2 and 3 $p > 0.0005$

Cell types involved in tolerance induction.
   A double cell transfer experiment was carried out, and the number of plaque forming cells was determined when aggregate-freed tolerance-inducing antigen had been given to primary recipients, irradiated immediately before or three days before they received thymus and bone marrow cells (14). The ratio of plaque-forming cells (irradiation day 0/irradiation day -3) was 1.3 if tolerance-inducing antigen was not given to the primary recipient. If a tolerance-inducing antigen had been given, there was a 10-fold decrease in plaque number, if primary recipients were irradiated three days before the cell transfer, rather than on the day of cell transfer (Table III).

TABLE II

TOLERANCE INDUCTION AS A FUNCTION OF AGE[a]

Strain		Age of mice in weeks[b]			
		3	5	8	12
A	$T_{1/2}$[c]	12.7 ± 1.0	10.3 ± 0.7	9.1 ± 1.5	8.4 ± 0.9
	Ratio[d]	0.90 ± 0.08	0.95 ± 0.13	0.81 ± 0.18	0.83 ± 0.11
BALB/c	$T_{1/2}$	-	9.2 ± 0.8	8.2 ± 2.2	7.2 ± 1.6
	Ratio[d]	-	0.97 ± 0.20	0.85 ± 0.28	0.74 ± 0.23
SJL	$T_{1/2}$	6.7 ± 0.8	3.0 ± 2.5	1.7 ± 0.7	0.4 ± 0.3
	Ratio[d]	0.77 ± 0.14	0.35 ± 0.30	0.22 ± 0.09	0.06 ± 0.05

(a) Animals were injected i.p. with aggregate-free RGG (0.2 mg/g of body weight). Two weeks later they were given RGG-IFA (0.25 mg, s.c.). One week after this injection, ^{131}I-RGG 10 µg was administered i.p. and the half-life of elimination was determined.

(b) Age at which animals were given aggregate-free RGG; elimination tests were always carried out 3 weeks after this injection.

(c) Half life in days.

(d) Ratio = (half life of ^{131}I-RGG elimination from the body of animals injected with aggregate-free RGG) / (half life of animals not injected with aggregate free RGG).

TABLE III

THE EFFECT OF ACCESSORY CELLS (OPERATIONALLY DEFINED IN TERMS OF RADIATION RESISTANCE) ON TOLERANCE INDUCTION[a]

	PRIMARY RECIPIENTS		SECONDARY RECIPIENTS	
Group	Time of irradiation[b] in days	Dose of aggregate-Free RGG in mg	Number of recipients	$PFC_\ell/ 10^6$ spleen cells[c]
1	0	0	3	143.5 ± 12.5
2	0	5	3	11.6 ± 1.9
3	-3	0	4	107.0 ± 9.6
4	-3	5	5	1.2 ± 0.8

(a) Primary recipients were irradiated (950 rad) 3 days before or on the day of cell transfer when they received i.v. 1×10^8 thymus and 2×10^7 bone marrow cells. Some groups of animals were also given, at the same time, aggregate-free RGG (5 mg i.p.). Seven days later the primary recipients became spleen cell donors (5×10^7 cells/recipient) for lethally irradiated (850 rad) secondary recipients which were subsequently immunized with 0.5 mg aggregated RGG, at the time of cell transfer (i.v.) and again ten days later (i.p.). The animals were sacrificed two weeks after the cell transfer, and the number of $PFC_\ell/10^6$ spleen cells was determined.

(b) Zero time is the time of cell transfer to the primary recipient.

(c) The plaque number of animals in group 1 was compared with that in group 3 (p<0.005); PFC_ℓ from group 2 were compared with group 4 (p<0.005).

The accessory cell content of primary thymectomized recipients was maximally reduced by pre-irradiation of the recipients and by their reconstitution with thymus and bone marrow cells which had been passed over glasswool. Under these circumstances, a virtually complete state of tolerance was induced. The role of accessory cells in the resistance to tolerance induction was further examined by giving irradiated spleen cells to mice which were otherwise treated as indicated above; this resulted in a significant increase in plaque number (Table IV). It was apparent that resistance to tolerance depended on the intervention of accessory cells.

TABLE IV

THE EFFECT OF ACCESSORY CELLS (OPERATIONALLY DEFINED BY RADIATION RESISTANCE AND ADHERENCE TO GLASS) ON TOLERANCE INDUCTION IN THYMECTOMIZED MICE[a]

Group	Aggregate-free RGG in mg	Irradiated spleen cells	No. of mice	$PFC_\varrho/10^6$
1	0	-	3	$26.6 + 5.7$
2	0	+	4	$190.7 + 36.1$
3	5	-	2	0
4	5	+	4	$34.8 + 5.0$

(a) Female 5 week old SJL mice were thymectomized and were lethally irradiated (950 rad) when they were 7.5 weeks old. Three days after the irradiation all animals were injected i.v. with thymus cells and bone marrow cells which had been passed through glasswool (1×10^8 Thg and 2×10^7 BMg). Animals in groups 2 and 4 were additionally given i.v. 5×10^7 irradiated (1300 rad) spleen cells. At the same time animals in groups 3 and 4 received 5 mg aggregate-free RGG i.p. All animals were injected with 0.5 mg aggregated RGG i.v. on the 7th day, i.p. on the 17th day and were sacrificed on the 21st day after cell transfer (i.e. on the 24th day after whole body irradiation).

(b) A comparison was made between plaque-forming cell numbers. Groups 1 and 2: $p < 0.005$; groups 3 and 4: $p < 0.005$.

The responsiveness of thymus and bone marrow cells was next examined by a double transfer experiment in which pre-irradiated primary recipients were reconstituted with bone marrow and thymus cells; tolerance was induced in the cells of one group of the primary recipients. Secondary recipients of their spleen cells made only 1% of the response found in secondary recipients which had been reconstituted with spleen cells not exposed to aggregate-free RGG (Table V, groups 1 and 2). A corresponding comparison was made between secondary recipients which received normal thymus cells in addition to spleen cells from the primary recipient. Under these circumstances, the animals reconstituted with tolerized spleen cells had 40% of the plaque-forming cells of animals reconstituted with spleen cells from a primary donor which had not been rendered tolerant (Table V, expt. I). Normal thymus cell supplementation of recipients of normal spleen cells thus resulted in a 1.5-fold increase in plaque cells, where the same supplementation resulted in a 50-fold increase in recipients of tolerized spleen cells (Table V, expt. I). We turned to an experimental arrangement in which lethally irradiated primary recipients received only bone marrow or only thymus cells, and in each group some animals were injected with a tolerizing dose of RGG. Secondary recipients were given spleen cells from the primary recipient and, in addition, were given the complementary cell type from a normal donor.

There was a marked decrease in PFC, irrespective of whether bone marrow or thymus cells had been exposed to the tolerizing antigen. The relative effect of supplementation with bone marrow and thymus cells could be deduced from the recipients of non-tolerized spleen cells (TDSC or BDSC, respectively); the plaque ratio $\dfrac{\text{TDSC} + \text{BM}_n}{\text{BDSC} + \text{Th}_n}$ was 1.6; the corresponding ratio for the recipients of tolerized TDSC and BDSC was 0.078 (Table V).

Attempts to implicate accessory cells in age dependent changes to tolerance inducibility: As judged by the half life in ^{131}I-RGG elimination, eight weeks old hybrids between A and SJL animals (A x SJL) were intermediate ($T_{1/2}$ = 5.7 + 2.4) between A ($T_{1/2}$ = 9.1 + 1.5) and SJL ($T_{1/2}$ = 1.7 + 0.7) in their resistance to tolerance induction. Five week old hybrids ($T_{1/2}$ = 11.0 + 1.5) resemble their A parent ($T_{1/2}$ = 10.3 + 0.7) and not their SJL parent ($T_{1/2}$ = 3.0 + 2.5). We injected five week old A x SJL hybrids i.v. with 1 x 10^8 spleen cells from A or SJL donors which had been irradiated (950 rad) two hours before they became donors. The recipients were concurrently given 5 mg aggregate-free RGG and were immunized two weeks later

TABLE V TOLERANCE INDUCTION IN SPLEEN OF ANIMALS, RECONSTITUTED WITH THYMUS OR BONE MARROW CELLS OR WITH THYMUS AND BONE MARROW CELLS[a]

Experiment	Group	PRIMARY RECIPIENTS were given			SECONDARY RECIPIENTS were given spleen cells from primary recipients and in addition:			PFC_ℓ
		Thymus	Bone Marrow	Aggregate-free RGG	Thymus	Bone Marrow	Number of Recipients	
I	1	+	+	-	-	-	4	$107.0 +\!\!\!\mid\!\!\!+ 9.6$
	2	+	+	+	-	-	5	$1.2 +\!\!\!\mid\!\!\!+ 0.8$
	3	+	+	-	+	-	2	$154.2 +\!\!\!\mid\!\!\!+ 11.5$
	4	+	+	+	+	-	2	$68.2 +\!\!\!\mid\!\!\!+ 28.3$
II	5	+	-	-	-	+	2	$194.4 +\!\!\!\mid\!\!\!+ 12.3$
	6	+	-	+	-	+	3	$2.9 +\!\!\!\mid\!\!\!+ 0.9$
	7	-	+	-	+	-	3	$121.4 +\!\!\!\mid\!\!\!+ 11.3$
	8	-	+	+	+	-	4	$36.9 +\!\!\!\mid\!\!\!+ 19.9$
	9	-	-	-	-	-	3	0

(a) SJL female 8 week old mice were lethally irradiated (950 rad) and three days later were injected i.v. with a mixture of 1×10^8 thymus and with 2×10^7 bone marrow cells (expt. I). Other groups were injected only with 1×10^8 thymus cells or only with 2×10^7 bone marrow cells (expt. II). Some groups of mice were simultaneously injected i.p. with 5 mg aggregate-free RGG; appropriate controls were not injected with the tolerogen. Seven days later the reconstituted primary recipients became donors of BTDSC, TDSC or BDSC. The secondary recipients were lethally irradiated (850 rad) and received either only 5×10^7 BTDSC, TDSC or BDSC or, in addition, 1×10^8 thymus or 2×10^7 bone marrow cells. At the time of cell transfer and ten days later all mice received 0.5 mg aggregate RGG, i.v. and i.p., respectively. Mice were sacrificed, and the number spleen PFC_ℓ were determined four days after the last injection.

with RGG-IFA. The half life of ^{131}I-RGG in tolerized animals was 13.1 $\pm$ 2.3 days; in tolerized, immunized animals
$T_{1/2}$ was 11.8 $\pm$ 3.1 days; in tolerized, immunized SJL spleen
cell recipients $T_{1/2}$ was 12.3 $\pm$ 2.1;and in tolerized, immunized A spleen cell recipients $T_{1/2}$ was 11.7 $\pm$ 1.7 days.

The foregoing experiments had furnished evidence that
resistance to tolerance induction was due to a reaction which
involved accessory cells, but which did not appear to be exclusively dependent on the reactivity of the accessory cells.
It seemed possible that another cell population was the primary cause for resistance to tolerance induction. We pro-
ceeded to test B and T cells for age dependent changes.

The role of thymus derived cells in age dependent
changes in tolerance inducibility.
    Tolerance was induced in eight weeks old lethally irra-
diated mice which had been reconstituted with thymus and bone
marrow cells from three or twelve week old donors (Table VI).
The responsiveness of the spleen cells was determined after
transfer to a secondary lethally irradiated host which was
immunized. The indirect plaque-forming response of this host
was considerably greater (x5) when the primary host had received twelve week old thymus cells than when it received
thymus cells from a three week old donor. The ratio of
plaque-forming cells, made by tolerized and non-tolerized
animals, was independent of the age of the donors of thymus
and bone marrow cells (see Ratio[b] in Table VI).

We shall next consider the preceding data in terms of
the following questions: 1) Which cell types and which cell-
cell interactions are involved in the resistance to tolerance
induction of adult animals, and 2) can thymus and bursal
equivalent cell-populations attain tolerance without the cooperation of the other cell type?

We have previously demonstrated that accessory cells of
such strains as A and C3H do not participate in the cellular
interactions which result in the induction of tolerance nor
do they interfere with induction of tolerance to aggregate-
free gamma globulins (3). They do play a part in tolerance
induction of adult SJL and BALB/c mice which are relatively
resistant to tolerance induction. This resistance of BALB/c
mice ceases if the antigen is freed of aggregates by centrifugation (5). The same antigen preparation reduced responsiveness in SJL mice to a much lesser degree than in BALB/c
mice. Any maneuver which interfered with phagocytosis,

TABLE VI   TOLERANCE INDUCTION IN SJL MICE RECONSTITUTED WITH THYMUS AND BONE MARROW CELLS FROM 3 WEEK AND 12 WEEK OLD DONORS[a]

| Group | PRIMARY RECIPIENT | | | | | SECONDARY RECIPIENT | | |
| | Thymus Age of donors (in weeks) | | Bone Marrow Cells | | Aggregate-Free RGG | Number of Recipients | $PFC_\ell/10^6$ spleen cells | Ratio[b] |
	3	12	3	12				
1	+		+		−	4	29.0 ± 2.0	36.3 ± 22.8
2	+		+		+	5	0.8 ± 0.5	
3	+			+	−	3	35.4 ± 6.1	44.3 ± 11.42
4	+			+	+	4	0.8 ± 0.2	
5	+	+	+	+	−	3	160.9 ± 28.1	38.4 ± 14.4
6	+	+	+	+	+	4	4.2 ± 1.4	

(a) Primary recipients were irradiated (950 rad) three days before the cell transplants were given. Tolerance was examined in secondary recipients which were reconstituted with spleen cells from the primary recipients.

(b) Ratio between plaque numbers in secondary hosts when the primary host was not injected with aggregate-free RGG and when the primary host was injected with aggregate-free RGG.

Comparison between:
PFC_ℓ of groups

1 and 3	0.1>p>0.05	2 and 4	p>0.4
1 and 5	p<0.005	2 and 6	p<0.005
3 and 5	p<0.005	4 and 6	p<0.005

whether it rendered the antigen less subject to phagocytosis (removal of aggregates by biofiltration) or reduced phagocytic potency, resulted in a greater degree of tolerance in SJL mice (6). It was, therefore, reasonable to assume that the failure to induce tolerance in SJL mice may be connected with participation of the accessory cell in directing the response of some of the triggered cells to antibody formation. However, there remained some doubts that this was a full explanation for the exceptional features in the responsiveness of SJL mice, since neither aggregate removal nor blockade resulted in a tolerant state comparable to that of the other mice of this experiment series.

The involvement of accessory cells in SJL resistance to tolerance may, of course, not reflect unusual properties of these cells but a unique sensitivity of another cell, interacting with the accessory cell or its products. Wherever the primary SJL lesion may occur, it should be possible to induce SJL tolerance by interference with targets of accessory cell interaction. The alkylating agent, cyclophosphamide (CA), is a powerful immunosuppressant (15, 16) and can be employed to induce specific tolerance to foreign cells and to equine gammaglobulin (17-20).

Reconstitution experiments with CBA mice have led to the conclusion that cyclophosphamide tolerance could be attributed to thymus-derived cells in the recirculating lymphocytes outside the thymus (27). If this conclusion can be extended to other strains, it might be thought possible to render SJL tolerant by circumventing the interferring involvement of accessory cells. Using CA, tolerance to SRBC and to RGG could be induced in SJL animals (6). The effect of CA on the level of tolerance could be deduced from the ratio between the half lives of RGG in animals which had received combined treatment with CA and RGG and in animals tolerized with protein alone; the values for A and BALB/c were slightly above 1, but for SJL it was 3.5 (6). Though the level of tolerance observed in SJL mice was higher than that achieved by the other above-mentioned modes of tolerance induction, it was lower than in A or BALB/c animals. It thus appeared, that by a strategy which circumvented the accessory cell, a state of fairly profound tolerance could be induced in SJL mice. Still the level of tolerance was less profound than in other mice. This difference may reflect a lesion, in a cell type other than the accessory cell.

We used two approaches to test the effect of accessory cells on tolerance induction in SJL mice. In one series of experiments we used supplementation with accessory cells and in the other reconstitution so as to obtain an accessory cell deprived animal (6, 22).

Supplementation with accessory cells did not affect the capacity of animals to become tolerant while removal of accessory cells allowed tolerance induction in a normally tolerance-resistant animal. The greater magnitude of the change in tolerization than in immunization, and the low level of tolerance induction, leads us to the view that tolerizing antigen and accessory cell act through a common step; that accessory cells can prevent tolerance induction and that the competitive advantage at the target of antibody over tolerance induction must be considerable (22, 25).

Three day pre-irradiated (14, 23) T and B reconstituted mice produced less antibody and were much more effectively tolerized than were animals irradiated immediately before reconstitution. One methodological objection to the above experiment must be considered. Reconstitution of the pre-irradiated recipient with thymus and bone marrow cells may reintroduce a small number of accessory cells. To minimize this, accessory cells must be removed from the reconstituting B and T cells and this was done by removing glass adherent cells (24). So reconstituted pre-irradiated SJL mice made a very low plaque-forming response on immunization and ,no detectable response on tolerization followed by immunization. The role of the accessory cell, in both these processes, was established by comparing the responsiveness of animals which were reconstituted as before, but in addition, received irradiated spleen cells as a source of accessory cells. The plaque-forming response of immunized animals increased 7x and that of tolerized animals increased by a larger factor, i.e. from 0 to 35 $PFC_\ell/10^6$ spleen cells. It thus became evident that 3 day pre-irradiation was effective in reducing accessory cells but left a substantial number of accessory cells in a competent state and that SJL mice could be tolerized to the same level as other mice if accessory cells were reduced below the level achieved by pre-irradiation. We had thus obtained conclusive evidence that the accessory cell played a decisive role in preventing tolerance induction.

We can now turn to the status of the SJL thymus and bone marrow cell populations which were exposed to tolerizing antigen in pre-irradiated primary recipients and were tested

by spleen cell transfer in a secondary recipient of spleen cells. It became clear that both T and B cells could become tolerant and that tolerization of one cell type did not depend on the presence of the second partner of the two interacting cell types. The question of the relative unresponsiveness of the two cell types was more difficult to decide because it involved a number of uncontrolled factors. We did not know what proportion of the cells, injected into the primary recipient, reached the spleen cells and thus the secondary recipient, nor did we know the relative proportion of B and T cells in the spleen. Thus, any direct comparison between data from experiments, where both cell types or one cell type was tolerized in the spleen, depended on the number of cells transferred with the spleen and a comparison of that number (clearly a fraction of 5×10^7) with the 2×10^7 BM_n or 10^8 Th_n provided to the secondary host. It was necessary, therefore, to normalize the data from experiments in which the cells were not tolerized but which were, otherwise, identical. On this basis, thymus cells tolerized alone would give a plaque ratio of 0.015 ± 0.0005 (i.e. $\dfrac{2.9 + 0.9}{194.4 + 12.3}$)*,
bone marrow cells tolerized alone would give a plaque ratio of 0.304 ± 0.166 (i.e. $\dfrac{36.9 \pm 19.9}{121.4 - 11.3}$)*, while bone marrow and
thymus cells tolerized together would give 0.11 ± 0.008 (i.e. $\dfrac{1.2 \pm 0.8}{107.0 + 9.6}$)*. Thus it appeared as if the bone mar-
row cells were more effectively tolerized in the presence of thymus cells than in their absence. This could be tested by tolerizing bone marrow and thymus cells together and supplementing the secondary recipient with thymus cells. Under these circumstances the normalized value was 0.44 ± 0.19 (i.e. $\dfrac{68.2 \pm 28.3}{154.2 + 11.5}$)* and, thus, it was similar to the value
(0.304) obtained when bone marrow cells were tolerized alone. This was not compatible with the view, expressed above, that B cells were more effectively tolerized in the absence of T cells. It seemed that the tolerized T cells lost cooperative capacity; a sub-population of B cells did not (4) and tnat it was this sub-population which cooperated with the normal T cells, given to the secondary recipient. Before accepting this view, it was important to recognize that the effect of thymus supplementation of normal BTDSC reconstituted animals was 1.44 ± 0.17 (i.e. $\dfrac{154.2 \pm 11.5}{107.0 + \cdot 9.6}$)* and that the effect on
tolerant BTDSC-reconstituted animals was 56.9 ± 28.3 (*see Table V)

(i.e. $\dfrac{68.3 \pm 28.3}{1.2 \pm 0.8}$)[*] so that thymus supplementation has a much bigger effect on the response of tolerant than of normal BTDSC cells. It seemed clear from these results that T cells are not involved in tolerance induction of B cells, but it remains possible that inhibitory thymus cells were generated in tolerance induction, inhibited competent B cells, (i.e. prevented them from functional expression), but failed to do so in competition with thymus cells from normal donors. We now pursued this latter possibility in terms of the age difference in tolerance inducibility and identified the cellular basis of this change. We relied on reconstitution experiments in which the donors of thymus and bone marrow cells were either 3 or 12 weeks old. Animals, reconstituted with thymus cells from normal old donors and with bone marrow cells from normal young donors, gave a much higher response than did animals in which the ages of the donors were reversed. Thus, there appeared to occur a thymus cell dependent hyper-responsiveness with advancing age. Reconstitution experiments with cells from tolerant animals which were 3 and 12 weeks old showed that it was the thymus cell and not the bone marrow cell of the old animal which resulted in an incomplete state of tolerance (15). If the response of animals, reconstituted with tolerant cells, were normalized for the responses of corresponding animals, reconstituted with cells from donors which had not been rendered tolerant, there was no difference between animals reconstituted with thymus cells from old and with thymus cells from young animals. The failure to detect a difference might be connected with the high standard deviation of the normalized response of animals in group 6 of Table V. Thus, we could link the thymus cell with the age dependent resistance to tolerance induction but could not safely interpret it as a consequence of heightened responsiveness to antigen. We have found that passive transfer of accessory cells does not transfer the age dependent change in tolerance inducibility. However, we have demonstrated that the removal of accessory cells permitted induction of tolerance in eight week old SJL animals (6, 25). A synthesis of these apparently contradictory observations is possible. It seems conceivable that the accessory cell and its product acts on the T cell, or that participation of the accessory cell is dependent on the T cell; that there is some age dependent change in T cell function and that this change results in hyper-responsiveness to antigen, possibly competitive advantage of the interaction which results in antibody formation rather than in tolerance induction. Thus, the lesion would be in the thymus cell population but the manifestation would be dependent on the presence of accessory cells. It would be attractive to attribute the lesion to a progressive loss of inhibitory T cells (27-29) or to a disturbance in the equilibrium between inhibitory and cooperating T cells (26, 29-33), but a decision on the validity of this proposal must await appropriate experimentation.

Of the four mouse strains, SJL, NZB, BALB/c, BW, which have proven relatively resistant to tolerance induction, all but B/W are predisposed to either Hodgkin's like reticulum cell neoplasm (33-36), lymphomas (37-40) or plasmacytomas (41). The alteration in immunological mechanism, which we have analysed in the preceding pages, may involve failure of T cell function which may be responsible for the development of lymphoid malignancies. Indeed, it is quite possible that the same virus may play a part in the development of the immunological abnormality and, directly or indirectly, in the development of neoplastic change (42044).

ACKNOWLEDGMENTS

This manuscript is supported by the Medical Research Council, the National Cancer Institute and the Ontario Heart Foundation. Dr. Michio Fujiwara's present address is The Department of Immunology, Institute of Medical Science, University of Tokyo, Tokyo, Japan.

REFERENCES

1. Chiller, J.M., Habicht, G.S. and Weigle, W.O., _Science_. 171:813, 1971.

2. Weigle, W.O., Chiller, J.M. and Habicht, G.S., _Transplant. Rev_. 8:3, 1972.

3. Kaplan, A.M. and Cinader, B., _Cellular Immunology_. 6: 429, 1973.

4. Kaplan, A.M. and Cinader, B., _Cellular Immunology_. 6: 442, 1973.

5. Golub, E.S. and Weigle, W.O., _J. Immunol_. 102:389, 1969.

6. Fujiwara, M. and Cinader, B., _Cellular Immunology_. 12: 11, 1974.

7. Cerottini, J.C., Lambert, P.H. and Dixon, F.J., _J. Exp. Med_. 130:1093, 1969.

8. Staples, P.J. and Talal, N., _J. Exp. Med_. 129:123, 1969.

9. Staples, P.J., Steinberg, A.D. and Talal, N., J. Exp. Med. 131:1223, 1970.

10. Playfair, J.H.L., Immunology. 21:1037, 1971.

11. Das, S., Leskowitz, S.J., J. of Immunol. 112:107, 1974.

12. Kaplan, A.M. and Freeman, M.J., Proc. Soc. Exp. Biol. Med. 127:574, 1968.

13. Cunningham, A.J. and Szenberg, A., Immunology. 14:599, 1968.

14. Gorczynski, R.M., Miller, R.G. and Phillips, R.A., Jr., J. Exp. Med. 134:1201, 1971.

15. Santos, G.W., Burke, P.J., Sensenbrenner, L.L. and Owens, A.H., Jr., In Pharmacologic Treatment in Organ and Tissue Transplantation , Milan, Italy, 1969, edited by A. Bertelli and A.P. Monaco. Proc. International Symposium, pp. 24-31, Excerpta Medica Foundation, Amsterdam, 1970.

16. Makinodan, T., Santos, G.W. and Quinn, R.P., Pharm. Rev. 22:189, 1970.

17. Santos, G.W. and Owens, A.H., Jr., Fed. Proc. 27:506, 1968.

18. Aisenberg, A.C. and Davis, C., J. Exp. Med. 128:35, 1968.

19. Playfair, J.H., Nature (London). 222:1882, 1969.

20. Stockman, G.D. and Trentin, J.J., J. Immunol. 108:112, 1972.

21. Miller, J.F.A.P. and Mitchell, G.F., J. Exp. Med. 131:675, 1970.

22. Fujiwara, M. and Cinader, B., Cellular Immunology. 12:194, 1974.

23. Shortman, K., Diener, E., Russell, P. and Armstrong, W.D., J. Exp. Med. 131:461, 1970.

24. Mosier, D.E., Science (Washington). 158:1573, 1967.

25. Fujiwara, M. and Cinader, B., *Cellular Immunology*. <u>12</u>: 214, 1974.

26. Fujiwara, M. and Cinader, B., *Cellular Immunology*. <u>12</u>: 205, 1974.

27. Gershon, R.K. and Kondo, K., *Immunology*. <u>21</u>:903, 1971.

28. Jacobson, E.B., Herzenberg, L.A., Riblet, R. and Herzenberg, L.A., *J. Exp. Med*. <u>135</u>:1163, 1972.

29. Cinader, B., Koh, S.W. and Kuskin, P., *Cellular Immunology*. <u>11</u>:170, 1974.

30. Dutton, R.W., Falkoff, R., Hirst, J.A., Hoffman, M., Kappler, J.W., Kettman, J.R., Lesley, J.F. and Vann, D., In *Progress in Immunology*, Proceedings of the 1st International Congress of Immunology, Washington, D.C., 1971, edited by B. Amos, Academic Press, New York, 1971.

31. Sjöberg, O., Andersson, J. and Möller, G., *J. Immunol*. <u>109</u>:1379, 1972.

32. Blaese, R.M., Martinez, C. and Good, R.A., *J. Exp. Med*. <u>119</u>:211, 1964.

33. Lapp, W.S. and Möller, G., *Immunology*. <u>17</u>:339, 1969.

34. Murphy, E.D., *J. Nat. Cancer Inst., U.S.A*. <u>42</u>:797, 1969.

35. McIntire, K.R. and Law, L.W., *J. Nat. Cancer Inst., U. S.A*. <u>39</u>:1197, 1967.

36. Wanebo, H.J., Gallmeier, W.M., Boyse, E.A. and Old, L.J., *Science*, Washington. <u>154</u>:901, 1966.

37. Mellors, R.C., *Blood*. <u>27</u>:435, 1966.

38. Staples, P.J., Steinberg, A.D. and Talal, N., *J. Exp. Med*. <u>131</u>:1223, 1970.

39. Chused, T.M., Steinberg, A.D. and Parker, L.M., *J. Immunol*. <u>111</u>:52, 1973.

40. Steinberg, A.D., private communication.

41. Potter, M. and Robertson, C.L., <u>J. Nat. Cancer Inst.</u>, U.S.A. <u>25</u>:847, 1960.

42. Mellors, R.C. and Huang, C.Y., <u>J. Exp. Med.</u> <u>126</u>:53, 1967.

43. Thivolet, J., Morrier, J.C., Ruel, J.P. and Richard, M.H., <u>Nature</u>, London. <u>204</u>:1134, 1967.

44. Oldstone, M.B.A., Tishon, A., Chiller, J.M., Weigle, W.O. and Dixon, F.J., <u>J. Immunol.</u> <u>110</u>:1268, 1973.

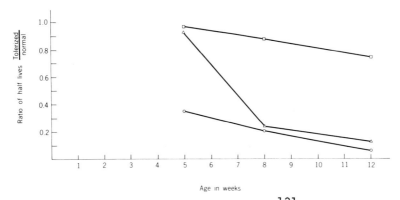

Fig. 1. The relative half life of ^{131}I-RGG in tolerized and immunized A, BALB/c, SJL mice and in hybrids
between them. Inbred mice and hybrids BALB/c (□), SJL (0)
and BALB/c x SJL (△) were injected i.p. with 0.2 mg/g body
weight of aggregate-freed RGG at the age indicated on the
horizontal axis. Two weeks later these mice were immunized
subcutaneously with 0.25 mg RGG-IFA. One week after this
immunization they received 10 μg ^{131}I-RGG. Normal animals
received 10 μg ^{131}I-RGG at the same age. The average $T_{1/2}$
of the antigen in animals tolerized and immunized are shown
as a fraction of the average $T_{1/2}$ in normal animals of the
same age.

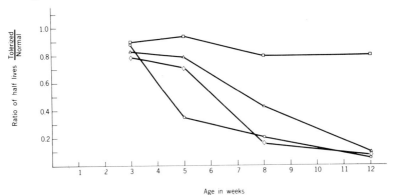

Fig. 2. The relative half life of ^{131}I-RGG in tolerized and immunized A, SJL mice and hybrids between them.
Inbred mice and hybrids A (□), A x SJL (△), SJL x A (◊) and
SJL (0) were injected i.p. with 0.2 mg/g body weight of
aggregate free RGG at the age indicated on the horizontal
axis. Two weeks later these mice were immunized subcutaneously with 0.25 mg RGG-IFA. One week after this immunization they received 10 μg ^{131}I-RGG. Normal animals received
10 μg ^{131}I-RGG at the same time. The average $T_{1/2}$ of the
antigen in animals tolerized and immunized are shown as a
fraction of the average $T_{1/2}$ of normal animals of the same
age.

SUPPRESSOR ACTIVITY IN MICE TOLERANT OF HEMOCYANIN

G.L. Ada and M.G. Cooper

Department of Microbiology
The John Curtin School of Medical Research
The Australian National University
P.O. Box 334, Canberra, A.C.T. 2601. Australia

ABBREVIATIONS

B cells, thymus-independent lymphocytes; T cells, thymus-dependent lymphocytes; BSA, bovine serum albumin; HCY, hemocyanin; MON, monomeric flagellin; POL, polymerized flagellin; FCA, Freund's complete adjuvant; ABC, antigen-binding cell(s); DTH, delayed-type hypersensitivity; SRBC, sheep erythrocytes; WBC, white blood cells; NRS, normal rabbit serum; and ATS, rabbit anti-thymocyte serum.

INTRODUCTION

Immunological tolerance to protein antigens can be a property of either B or T lymphocytes. There are several examples of tolerance involving B cells, viz. the induction of tolerance in vitro to flagellar antigens (1, 2) and in vivo to pneumococcal polysaccharide (3), E. coli lipopolysaccharide (4), and to a hapten substituted polypeptide, DNP-D-GL (5, 6). On the other hand, tolerance to histocompatibility antigens has been induced in bursectomized chickens (7), indicating that tolerance can be a function solely of T cells without the intervention of B cells. Low zone tolerance to BSA in mice can be briefly abrogated by the injection of T cells activated to this antigen, whereas high zone tolerance is refractory (8, 9). These and other findings led to the hypothesis that low zone tolerance was a function of T cells, whereas high zone tolerance was a function of both T and B cells (9).

Tolerance in the B cell population can be induced either directly by the tolerogen or indirectly by the tolerogen and the B cell product, antibody, acting in concert on the B cell (1, 10). The situation regarding the induction of tolerance in T cells is not so clear cut. Until recently, it might have been thought that T cells were also directly inactivated by the tolerogen. To our knowledge, there are no experiments reported which unequivocally show this. On the other hand, Gershon and Kondo (11, 12) have described a form of tolerance - "infectious" tolerance - in which it seems that T cells may be converted by the tolerogen to suppressor cells, and these, in turn, perhaps liberate a specific suppressor substance, IgY, which acts on other T cells. In addition, there are now increasing numbers of reports that T cells can exhibit suppressor activity during the immune response (e.g. 13-17).

In this paper we report the induction of high zone tolerance to hemocyanin in neonatal mice and evidence which suggests that in this model: 1) The B cells are affected but probably not deleted, and 2) there are suppressor effects which are a property of the T cells.

MATERIALS AND METHODS

Animals.
Three inbred strains of mice were used. CBA and C57B1 mice, maintained at the John Curtin School of Medical Research and AKR mice purchased from the Jackson Laboratory Bar Harbor, Maine.

Irradiation.
Mice were given 750 rads whole body gamma radiation at 40-42 rads per minute from a ^{60}Co source as described earlier (18).

Antigens.
Hemocyanin (HCY), molecular weight 450,000, was obtained from the hemolymph of the South Australian crayfish, Jasus lalandii (19), and aggregated with 1% chromic chloride (20). Monomeric flagellin (MON), molecular weight 40,000, and its particulate derivative, polymerized flagellin (POL), were prepared from the flagella of different Salmonella strains (SW 1338, SL 870) as described by Nossal and Ada (21). Antigen solutions were made up in Dulbecco's medium (22) or saline and, where indicated, emulsified in Freund's complete adjuvant (FCA) (Difco) or added to a suspension of killed Bordetella pertussis organisms (Commonwealth Serum Laboratories, Melbourne). Endotoxin (lipopolysaccharide B) from E. coli was purchased from Difco Laboratories, Detroit, Michigan.

Radioiodination.
Antigens were radioiodinated with carrier-free iodide-125 (IMS. 3, Radiochemical Centre, Amersham, U.K.) by the

88

chloramine T oxidation procedure (23). Preparations of ^{125}I-HCY (about 30 μC/μg) and ^{125}I-POL (27.0 μC/μg) were used for antigen-binding cell (ABC) assays.

Induction of tolerance.
Mice were injected intraperitoneally on the day of birth and three times per week thereafter for 8-14 weeks with 5 mg HCY in 0.05 ml Dulbecco's medium.

Preparation of cell suspensions.
Mouse thymus, spleen or lymph node cell suspensions were prepared by cutting these organs into small pieces with a pair of scissors and gently teasing the pieces through a stainless steel sieve into cold medium, viz. Dulbecco's medium containing 10% fetal calf serum, 4 I.U. per ml heparin (Evans Medical Australia Pty. Ltd.) and 15 mM sodium azide.

Activated T cells.
These were prepared as described elsewhere (24).

AKR mouse anti-θC3H serum and ascites fluid.
These were prepared as described elsewhere (25). The pooled serum had a cytotoxic titre for normal CBA thymocytes of 1 in 50, i.e. 0.2 ml of a 1 in 50 dilution of serum was cytotoxic for 50% of 7×10^6 thymocytes.

Anti-thymocyte serum (ATS).
This was a gift from Dr. R.V. Blanden. Its preparation and properties have been described elsewhere (26).

Treatment of cell suspensions with anti-θ serum and complement.
CBA mouse spleen cells or thymocytes for treatment with normal CBA mouse serum (NMS) or AKR anti-θ serum and complement were incubated at concentrations of 3.5×10^7 to 1.0×10^8 cells/ml in undiluted serum for 30 minutes at 37°C, washed once in Dulbecco's medium and incubated in complement (undiluted guinea pig serum) in the same way.

Treatment of cell suspensions with radiolabelled antigens.
Cells were incubated with ^{125}I-labelled antigen as described previously (23).

Incubation of cell suspensions in vitro.

Mouse lymphoid cell suspensions were prepared under aseptic conditions in sterile Eagle's minimum essential medium (Grand Island Biological Co., New York) containing 10% fetal calf serum and adjusted to pH 7.0. The sterile cell suspensions (5×10^7 cells/nl) were incubated for 9 hours either: 1) at $37^\circ C$ in a warm air incubator containing 5% CO_2, or 2) at $4^\circ C$ in the refrigerator.

Titration of serum antibody.

Serum anti-HCY and anti-POL titres were estimated by the passive hemagglutination assay (20). All serum antibody titres were expressed in $\log_2$ units where 1.0 = 50% agglutination by an initial serum dilution of 1 in 10.

Assay of delayed-type hypersensitivity.

This was measured as described previously (24).

RESULTS

Induction of tolerance to hemocyanin.

In the experiments reported in this paper, both CBA and C57Bl mice were given the neonatal course of injections of 5 mg fluid HCY. All mice used contained no detectable anti-HCY antibody in their sera 1-2 days after the last injection of tolerogen. They failed to produce primary or secondary antibody responses to HCY (Fig. 1a) but produced normal responses to POL (Fig. 1b). Thus, the tolerance produced was complete and specific.

State of specific B lymphocytes in the tolerant mouse.

Three types of experiments were carried out to investigate B cells in tolerant mice.

Antigen binding cells.

If allowance was made for the variation in the number of B cells in different samples (e.g. in spleen, they can vary from 35-55%), by estimating the number of cells binding either labelled anti-Ig or a labelled unrelated antigen, and using conditions where only B and not T cells bound antigen, then no difference was found in the number of binding cells in tolerant v normal mice (Table I).

TABLE I

INCIDENCE OF ^{125}I-HCY AND ^{125}I-POL BINDING CELLS
IN SPLEEN CELL SUSPENSIONS PREPARED FROM
NORMAL OR HCY-TOLERANT CBA MICE

Mouse Status	Labelled Antigen*	Cells Scanned $(\times 10^{-5})$	ABC Per 10^5 Cells
Normal	HCY	1.18	275
Tolerant	HCY	0.67	229
Normal	POL	0.98	159
Tolerant	POL	1.10	129

*HCY = 5 ng ^{125}I-HCY (29.8 μC/μg)

 POL = 100 ng ^{125}I-HCY (27.0 μC/μg)

Exposure to a B cell mitogen.
Experiments of Chiller and Weigle (27, 28) suggest that if, in tolerant mice, the T cells are tolerant and the B cells normal, injection of the tolerogen with a B cell mitogen, such as endotoxin, will cause a specific antibody response to a T-dependent antigen because the need for T cells is by-passed.

In this case the protocol of Chiller and Weigle (27,28) was followed. Normal and tolerant mice were injected with hemocyanin and endotoxin at times up to 5 weeks later than the time of the last injection of tolerogen. If carried out within the first two weeks of cessation of tolerogen,injections failed to break tolerance and only caused partial breakage of tolerance if carried out within the next three weeks (Fig. 2).

Injection of allogeneic cells.
McCullagh (29) has reported the abrogation of tolerance to SRBC in rats following the transfer of allogeneic lymphocytes. In the following experiments irradiated CBA mice were reconstituted with spleen and lymph node cells from

HCY - tolerant CBA donors within 2-4 hours of irradiation and with similar cells from HCY - tolerant C57Bl donors 24 hours later. The irradiated recipients were challenged with HCY 0-10 minutes after the transfer of the allogeneic C57Bl cells and their serum anti-HCY responses determined 4-14 days later (Table II). Abrogation of tolerance was not observed on this occasion, nor in a subsequent experiment when cells from tolerant mice were transferred to allogeneic HCY - tolerant recipients. These three observations were consistent with the concept that inactivated, specific B cells were present in these tolerant mice.

The state of T cells in tolerant mice.
(1) Mice which were neonatally thymectomized were unable to produce a primary antibody response to HCY (Table III). (2) DTH reactivity to protein antigens has been shown to be a T cell function in mice (26); there is little evidence that B lymphocytes play a role in this reaction. Mice tolerant of HCY did not give a DTH reaction to this antigen but responded normally to POL (Table IV).

Transfer experiments.
(a) Into normal mice:
Mice injected with 10^8 spleen and lymph node cells from tolerant mice responded better to hemocyanin than did mice injected with the same number of cells from normal mice. We have not injected larger numbers of cells.
(b) Into X-irradiated normal mice:
(1) Three groups of X-irradiated mice were given spleen and lymph node cells as follows: 1) 5×10^7 cells from normal mice; 2) 5×10^7 cells from tolerant mice; and 3) mixtures of these cells (i.e. 10^8 cells/mouse). They were then injected with HCY, MON and B. pertussis organisms (Fig. 3). There was a specific suppression of antibody production to HCY but not to MON in mice receiving cells from both normal and tolerant donors.

(2) Groups of X-irradiated mice received 4 or 5 x 10^7 spleen and lymph node cells from normal mice together with cells from tolerant mice varying in numbers from 1×10^7 to 2×10^5. They were then injected (as above) with HCY and MON. All mice responded equally well to MON. Mice receiving 1×10^7, 2.5×10^6 or 1×10^6 cells from tolerant mice plus 4×10^7 cells from normal mice showed a significantly suppressed response to hemocyanin (Fig. 4).

(3) Groups of X-irradiated mice received mixtures of cells from normal and tolerant mice (5×10^7 cells/each). The cells from tolerant mice were harvested at different times (1, 2, 3, 4, 7, 10 and 14 days) after the last injection of tolerogen. The recipient mice were then injected with HCY and MON with the following results. Cells removed from tolerant mice up to 3 days after the last injection of tolerogen demonstrated suppressor activity. Cells removed at 4-7 days did not demonstrate either suppressor or enhancing activity. Cells harvested from tolerant mice 10-14 days later considerably enhanced the response of cells from normal mice (Fig. 5).

The cellular basis of suppressor activity.
Two experiments suggest that T lymphocytes in the tolerant mice were involved in suppressor activity.
1) Cells from tolerant mice, after treatment with anti-Θ and complement, no longer suppressed cells from normal mice, when both were injected into X-irradiated mice (Fig. 6).
2) It was argued that if T cells in tolerant mice had suppressor activity, then their destruction and replacement by other T cells might allow an antibody response to be expressed if some intact B cells were present. A group of normal mice (A) and a group of tolerant mice (B) were given two injections of ATS (0.2 ml) i.v. 4 and 2 days prior to removal of their spleens. Another group of tolerant mice (C) were given two injections of NRS. The spleens of mice in each group were then removed and cell suspensions prepared. Cells from groups A and B were treated with anti-Θ serum and complement; cells from group C with normal mouse serum and complement. Three groups of normal mice were then irradiated. Each group received 10^8-treated spleen cells (from either groups A, B or C) together with 10^7-activated T cells. The antibody responses are shown in Fig. 6. Recipients of group A cells and activated T cells responded in a linear fashion, reaching peak titres at day 28 and then declining. Recipients of group C cells and activated T cells showed a slight but significant titre at day 20, which did not increase further until after day 23. In contrast, recipients of group B cells and activated T cells responded as did recipients of normal (A) cells until day 20. Titres then plateaued until day 31. The titres of recipients of group B cells were significantly higher than those of recipients of group C cells at days 20 and 23 and significantly less than those of recipients of group A cells at days 23, 28 and 31.

TABLE II

SERUM ANTI-HCY RESPONSES OF LETHALLY IRRADIATED CBA MICE RECONSTITUTED WITH LYMPHOID CELLS FROM HCY-TOLERANT CBA AND/OR HCY-TOLERANT C57BL MICE

Cells Transferred*		Mean Log_2 Anti-HCY Titres**			
Day 0	Day 1	Day 5	Day 8	Day 11	Day 15
-	-	<0.3 (5)	<0.3 (5)	<0.3 (5)	<0.3 (4)
Tolerant CBA (2×10^8)	-	<0.3 (5)	<0.3 (5)	<0.3 (5)	<0.3 (5)
-	Tolerant C57BL (2×10^8)	<0.3 (5)	<0.3 (4)	<0.3 (1)	-
Tolerant CBA (1×10^8)	Tolerant C57BL (1×10^8)		<0.3 (5)	<0.3 (3)	<0.3 (1)
Normal CBA (1×10^8)	Normal C57BL (1×10^8)	0.9 ± 0.3 (5)	3.4 ± 0.2 (5)	4.1 ± 0.3 (5)	2.9 ± 0.5 (2)

*Spleen and mesenteric lymph node cells

**All recipients challenged i.v. on Day 1 with 10 mg HCY and 10^9 B. pertussis. Number of mice per group in brackets.

94

TABLE III

SERUM ANTI-HCY RESPONSES OF NORMAL
AND NEONATALLY-THYMECTOMIZED CBA MICE

Mouse	Mean Log$_2$ Anti-HCY Titres**		
Status*	Day 7	Day 14	Day 21
Normal	4.4 $\pm$ 0.8 (5)	6.8 $\pm$ 0.6 (5)	8.1 $\pm$ 0.6 (5)
NNTx	<0.3 $\pm$ 0.0 (7)	<0.3 $\pm$ 0.0 (7)	<0.3 $\pm$ 0.0 (7)

*NNTx = neonatally thymectomized mice kindly supplied by
Dr. R.E. Langman.

**All mice challenged i.v. with 1 mg aggregated HCY.
Number of mice per group in brackets.

DISCUSSION

The main findings of these experiments were that a state
of tolerance to HCY could be induced in neonatal mice with
injections beginning on the day of birth. The tolerance induced was both specific and complete and was stable on adoptive transfer to lethally irradiated recipients. The existence of a specific suppressive mechanism was demonstrated
by showing that addition of cells from tolerant animals
interfered with the ability of cells from normal mice to respond to the tolerogen.

Injection of tolerant mice with tolerogen and either
tolerant allogeneic cells or a B cell mitogen failed to break
the tolerant state. This would suggest that specific B cells
were either deleted or, if present, non functional. Two additional results favor the latter interpretation. First, on
the several occasions examined, no decrease in the number of
specific-binding cells has been observed in contrast to reports on several other systems where a substantial decrease
in the number of specific-binding cells in tolerant animals
has been observed (30, 5, 31). Secondly, destruction of T
cells from tolerant mice and their replacement by specifically activated T cells allowed a partial production of antibody. The possibility that a very small proportion only of

specific B cells was deleted is, however, difficult to exclude.

The suppressor activity observed seemed to be a property of the T cells. It has been shown clearly elsewhere (32) that suppressor T cells can interfere with the activity of other T cells which normally would be sensitized by antigen and participate in a DTH reaction. The results in the present report are entirely consistent with this finding, though they do not directly suggest a mechanism. Adding as few as one fortieth the number of cells from tolerant mice to cells from normal mice showed some suppressive effect. As the X-irradiated recipients of these cells were injected immediately with antigen, it is unlikely that the small amount of free antigen which might have been carried over contributed to the result unless this antigen was in a changed ("suppressor") form. It is most likely that transferred T cells were responsible. The other important finding was that the suppressor effect was relatively short lived (some 3 or 4 days) and was succeeded by an enhancing effect. This suggested that suppression occurred either as a result of too much help and that these cells had a short half life or because there were two populations of T cells, one suppressor, the other helper, with different half lives.

At one stage during the carrying out of the experiments reported here, some mice showed a pattern of tolerance which differed in one major respect from that described in the report. Although the tolerant mice were unresponsive upon challenge with antigen and adjuvant, the tolerance was not stable upon transfer to X-irradiated recipients so that suppressor activity, if present, could not be demonstrated. The only known factor which may have contributed to this different result was the presence in the antigen preparation of a small proportion of oligomers with changed conformation. The results highlight two aspects: 1) The physical state of the tolerogen injected may determine the characteristics of the tolerance pattern seen; and 2) Where T cells are involved, is the tolerant state observed always a balance between activation towards help and suppression?

TABLE IV

DTH RESPONSES OF HCY-TOLERANT CBA MICE TO HCY AND POL

Mouse status*	Mean % increase in footpad thickness 24 hours after challenge with:**	
	HCY	POL
HCY-tolerant	0.0 ± 0.7 (6)	16.6 ± 1.4 (6)
Immune control	20.6 ± 4.6 (5)	14.1 ± 2.8 (5)

*HCY-tolerant and normal mice which had been challenged 8 days prior to footpad assay with: 1) 1 mg aggregated HCY in 0.1 ml Dulbecco's medium (i.p.); 2) 0.5 mg fluid HCY in 0.1 ml FCA (sub.cut.), and 3) 10 μg POL in 0.1 ml Dulbecco's medium (sub.cut.).

**All mice injected sub. cut. in left hind footpad with 1 mg fluid HCY in 10 μl saline and in right hind footpad with 10 μg POL in 10 μl saline. Number of mice per group in brackets.

ACKNOWLEDGMENT

The present address for Dr. M.G. Cooper is Wallaceville Animal Research Centre, Upper Hutt, New Zealand.

REFERENCES

1. Diener, E. and Feldmann, M., Transplant. Rev. 8:76, 1972.

2. Feldmann, M., J. Exp. Med. 136:532, 1972.

3. Howard, J.G., Transplant. Rev. 8:50, 1972.

4. Sjöberg, O., J. Exp. Med. 135:850, 1972.

5. Katz, D.H., Davie, J.M., Paul, W.E. and Benacerraf, B. J. Exp. Med. 134:201, 1971.

6. Katz, D.H., Hamaoka, T. and Benacerraf, B. J. Exp. Med. 136:1404, 1972.

7. Rouse, B.T. and Warner, N.L. Eur. J. Immunol. 2:102, 1972.

8. Mitchison, N.A. In Cell Interactions and Receptor Antibodies in Immune Responses, edited by O. Makela, A. Cross and T.U. Kosunen, Academic Press, London, p. 249, 1971.

9. Rajewsky, K., Proc. Roy. Soc. Lond. B. 176:385, 1971.

10. Ada, G.L. and Ey, P.L., In The Antigens, edited by M. Sela, Academic Press, London, Vol. 4. In press.

11. Gershon, R.K. and Kondo, K, Immunology. 18:723, 1970.

12. Gershon, R.K. and Kondo, K, Immunology. 21:903, 1971.

13. Baker, P.J., Stashak, P.W., Amsbaugh, D.F., Prescott, B. and Barth, R.F., J. Immunol. 105:1581, 1970.

14. Allison, A.C., Denman, A.M. and Barnes, R.D., Lancet. 2:135, 1971.

15. Okumura, K. and Tada, T., J. Immunol. 107:1682, 1971.

16. Eidinger, D. and Pross, H., Scand. J. Immunol. 1:193, 1972.

17. Haskill, J.S. and Axelrad, M.A., Nature New Biol. 237:251, 1972.

18. Cooper, M.G., Scand. J. Immunol. 1:237, 1972.

19. Moore, C.H., Henderson, R.W. and Nichol, L.W., Biochemistry. 7:4075, 1968.

20. Cooper, M.G., Ada, G.L. and Langman, R.E., Cell. Immunol. 4:289, 1972.

21. Nossal, G.J.V. and Ada, G.L., Antigens, Lymphoid Cells and the Immune Response, Academic Press, New York, 1971.

22. Dulbecco, R. and Vogt, M., J. Exp. Med. 99:167, 1954.

23. Byrt, P. and Ada, G.L., Immunology. 17:503, 1969.

24. Cooper, M.G., Scand. J. Immunol. 1:167, 1972.

25. Cooper, M.G. and Ada, G.L., Scand. J. Immunol. 1:247, 1972.

26. Blanden, R.V., J. Exp. Med. 132:1035, 1970.

27. Chiller, J.M. and Weigle, W.O., J. Immunol. 110:1051, 1973.

28. Chiller, J.M. and Weigle, W.O., J. Exp. Med. 137:720, 1973.

29. McCullagh, P.J., J. Exp. Med. 132:916, 1970.

30. Naor, D. and Sulitzeanu, D., Int. Arch. Allergy. 36: 112, 1969.

31. Louis, J., Chiller, J.M. and Weigle, W.O., J. Exp. Med. 137:461, 1973.

32. Zembala, M. and Asherson, G.L., Nature. 244:227, 1973.

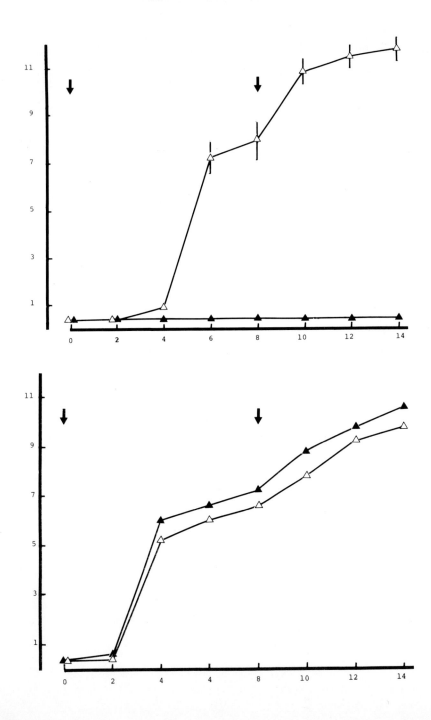

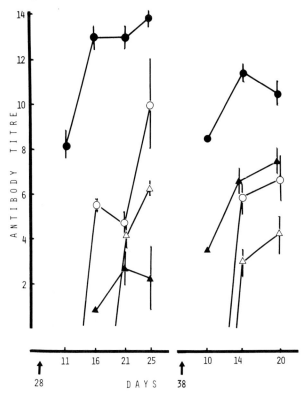

Fig. 2. Mean serum anti-HCY titers ($\log_2$) of normal or tolerant mice injected with HCY with or without endotoxin. Groups of normal and tolerant mice were injected i.p. on days 1 and 5 with HCY (1 mg) with or without endotoxin (50 µg) and on day 11 bled before injecting with 1 mg HCY and 10^9 B. pertussis. Normal (●) and tolerant (▲) receiving HCY and endotoxin. Normal (○) and tolerant (△) not receiving endotoxin. Experiments started 28 and 38 days after last injection of tolerogen into tolerant mice. Vertical bars indicate two SEM; abscissa, time (in days).

Fig. 1a and 1b. Mean serum anti-HCY (1a) and anti-POL (1b) titers of normal control mice (△) and HCY tolerant mice (▲) following antigenic challenge (indicated by arrows). First challenge; 1 mg aggregated HCY (i.p.), 0.5 mg HCY in FCA (sub.cut.) and 10 mg POL 1338 (sub.cut.). Second challenge; 1 mg HCY (sub.cut.) and 10 mg POL 1338 (sub.cut.). Six mice per group. Vertical bars on Fig. 1a indicate two standard errors of the mean (SEM). In Fig. 1b the SEM values are not shown as the anti-POL titers of the two groups were not significantly different. Ordinate, $\log_2$ anti-HCY titer. Abscissa, days after first injection of antigen.

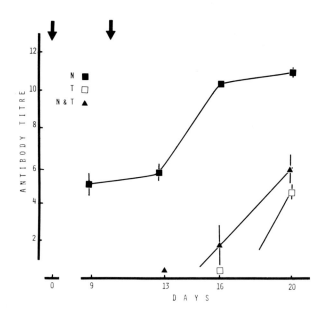

Fig. 3. Mean serum anti-HCY titers ($\log_2$) of X-irradiated mice which received 5 x 10^7 cells from normal mice
(■), 5 x 10^7 cells from tolerant mice (□) or both (▲).
Vertical arrows indicate times of challenge with antigen.
Day 1, 1 mg HCY, 1 ug MON (SW1338) and 10^9 B. pertussis.
Day 9, 1 mg HCY, 10^9 B. pertussis. Vertical bars, two SEM.
At each time point the anti-MON titers were not significantly
different from each other. Abscissa, time (in days) after
first injection of antigen.

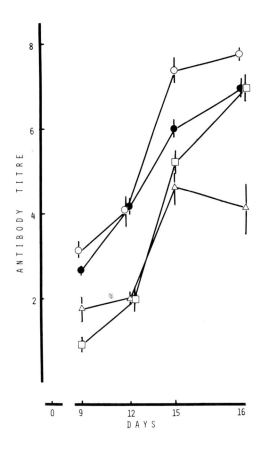

<u>Fig. 4</u>. Mean serum anti-HCY titers ($\log_2$) of X-irra-
diated mice which received 5 x 10^7 cells from normal mice
alone ($\bigcirc$); 4 x 10^7 cells from normal mice alone ($\bullet$) or
with either 2.5 x 10^6 cells from tolerant mice ($\triangle$) or 1 x 10^6
cells from tolerant mice ($\square$). Injection of antigens was as
in Fig. 3. Vertical bars are two SEM. All points on curve
$\triangle$ and first 2 points on curve $\square$ are significantly (p< 0.05)
lower than points on curves $\bigcirc$ and $\bullet$. At each time point
anti-MON titers were not significantly different from each
other. Abscissa, time (in days) after first injection of
antigen.

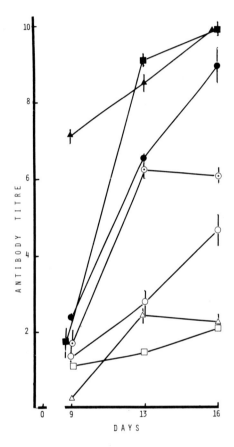

Fig. 5. Mean serum anti-HCY titers ($\log_2$) of X-irradiated mice (6 per group) which received 5 x 10^7 spleen and
lymph node cells from normal mice alone (●) or with 5 x 10^7
spleen and lymph node cells from tolerant mice which had
been killed 1 day (O) 2 days (□) 3 days (△) 4 days (⊙)
10 days (■) or 14 days (▲) after the last injection of
tolerogen. Injection of antigen was as in Fig. 3. Values
at days 13 and 16 for curves □ , △ and O are significantly
lower than the control (●) values. Values at days 9 and 13
for curve ▲ and at day 13 for curve ■ are significantly
higher than control (●) values. Abscissa, time (in days)
after first injection of antigen.

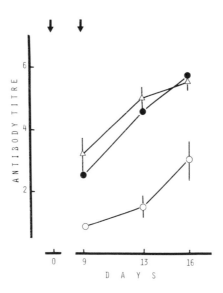

Fig. 6. Mean serum anti-HCY titers ($\log_2$) of X-irradiated mice (5 per group) which received 4×10^7 spleen and
lymph node cells from normal mice alone (Δ) or these cells
together with 1×10^4 tolerant spleen and lymph node cells
which had been pretreated with either mouse anti-θ ascites
fluid and complement (○) or mouse ascites fluid and complement (●). Injection of antigen was as in Fig. 3. All
values for curve ● are significantly lower than those of
curves Δ or ○ . Abscissa, time (in days) after first injection of antigen.

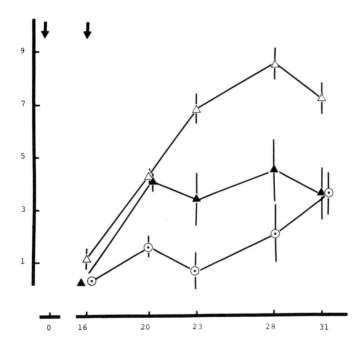

Fig. 7. Mean serum anti-HCY titers of irradiated mice reconstituted with HCY-activated T cells and:(1) ATS and anti-θ treated spleen cells from normal donors (△);(2) ATS and anti-θ treated spleen cells from HCY-tolerant donors (▲), or (3) normal serum treated spleen cells from HCY-tolerant donors (⊙). Five recipients per group. Arrows indicate HCY challenge, (day 1, 1 mg HCY plus 10^9 B. pertussis i.p., day 16, 1 mg HCY i.p.), and vertical bars indicate two standard errors of the mean. Ordinate, $\log_2$ anti-HCY titer; Abscissa, days after first injection of antigen.

SPECIFIC SUPPRESSION OF THE IMMUNE RESPONSE BY T CELLS

Antony Basten

The Departments of Bacteriology & Medicine
University of Sydney
Sydney, Australia 2006

The purpose of this contribution is to present two groups of experiments designed to study the mechanism of T cell tolerance. In the first group (carried out in colla-boration with Drs. Miller, Sprent and Cheers (1)), tolerance was induced in CBA mice to the soluble protein antigen fowl gammaglobulin (FγG) by an injection of 15 mg of deaggregated material per mouse. A tolerant state was detectable 6-10 days after innoculation. It was stable on adoptive transfer into irradiated mice (see Table I below) and predominantly affected IgG production (as measured by indirect PFC). Specificity was established by demonstrating an unimpaired response of the same recipients of tolerant cells to an un-related antigen, donkey red cells (DRC) or horse red cells (HRC). Trace-labelling studies with ^{125}I-labelled deaggre-gated FγG excluded transfer of significant amounts of non-cell-associated tolerogen.

The stability of tolerance in adoptive transfer enabled us to utilize this system in an in vivo analysis of the site and mechanism of the unresponsive state. Spleen cells from tolerant and normal mice were transferred alone or in com-bination into irradiated recipients, together with FγG, in immunogenic form, and a control antigen, DRC. As shown in Table I, normal spleen cells alone produced an appreciable indirect (7S) PFC response to FγG and DRC. However, when a similar number of tolerant cells were added, a significant decrease in indirect FγG-PFC but not in DRC-PFC was observed. No appreciable reduction in direct FγG-PFC occurred.

The inhibitory effect of the cells from tolerant mice was reversible by treatment with anti-θ C3H serum and comple-ment. Furthermore, normal T cells (purified on anti-immuno-globulin coated columns) proved capable of restoring the adoptive primary response of previously tolerant cells pro-vided they were pretreated with anti-θ C3H serum and comple-ment (Table II). Normal B cells had no such effect. Taken together these results implied that tolerance of this kind: (a) had been induced at the level of the T cell not the B cell;(b) was not due to clonal deletion;and (c) was mediated

TABLE I

CAPACITY OF FγG TOLERANT SPLEEN CELLS TO SUPPRESS THE PRIMARY ADOPTIVE RESPONSE TO FγG. DEPENDENCE OF THE SUPPRESSOR EFFECT ON A Θ-SENSITIVE CELL POPULATION

Group	Number and source of cells given	Number of irradiated recipients[a]	PFC/spleen at 7 days			
			anti-FγG		anti-DRC	
			19S	7S	19S	7S
1	1.5 x 10^7 FγG tolerant spleen cells	7	875 + 260[b]	350 + 140	1680 + 450	3405 + 450
2	1.5 x 10^7 normal spleen cells	7	970 + 495	1945 + 495	415 + 165	4075 + 1055
3	1.5 x 10^7 FγG tolerant spleen cells + 1.5 x 10^7 normal spleen cells	8	2165 + 1055	150 + 105	2615 + 775	7225 + 1985
4	1.5 x 10^7 FγG tolerant spleen cells treated with anti-Θ serum + 1.5 x 10^7 normal spleen cells	8	520 + 170	5180 + 965	2230 + 760	8630 + 2000
5	3 x 10^7 normal spleen cells	9	865 + 370	3675 + 1350	2565 + 240	7730 + 800
6	3 x 10^7 tolerant spleen cells	8	1565 + 685	670 + 320	1740 + 395	6005 + 730

a - Each recipient given 500 µg FγGA, i.p. and 5 x 10^8 DRC, i.v.

b - Arithmetic mean + SE

by a positive thymus dependent suppressor influence.

The duration of the suppressor effect was assessed in a second series of experiments in which spleen cells from normal donors were transferred alone or in combination with tolerant cells into irradiated hosts together with FɣG and HRC. Groups of recipients were killed at days 4, 7, 10 and 15. On each occasion spleens were collected for PFC assay and blood for serum antibody levels. As shown in Fig. 1, specific inhibition by tolerant spleen cells of indirect PFC production persisted, being more pronounced at days 10 and 15 than at day 7. No reduction in direct PFC occurred. Serum antibody levels displayed a similar trend to the indirect PFC (Fig. 2). In other words the suppressor effect of tolerant spleen cells does not appear to be due to antibody production in other sites than spleen, nor does it represent a delay in differentiation of antibody-forming cells. Furthermore, the reduction in serum antibody levels makes a T cell-mediated switch in antibody production or allotype expression an unlikely explanation.

A number of predictions can be made from these findings. First, one would expect no decrease in the number of antigen binding (B) cells to FɣG detectable in tolerant cell populations. This, indeed, proved to be the case in both spleen and thoracic duct lymph. Secondly, the tolerant state ought to be "infectious" (2). If large enough numbers of cells $(2.5 \times 10^8 - 10 \times 10^8)$ from tolerant mice were injected into normal (non-irradiated) recipients, specific abrogation of antibody production occurred on subsequent challenge with immunogenic FɣG (1). Thirdly, the demonstration of a positive suppressor influence implied that tolerant cells had not been deleted. The most direct functional assay for this was to test whether suppression was reversible by the antigen "suicide" technique. Spleen cells from tolerant mice were, therefore, treated with highly substituted ^{125}I-FɣG under conditions known to interfere with helper function of T cells (3). When this was performed, the inhibitory effect of tolerant cells on a primary adoptive immune response was specifically abrogated (Table III). Furthermore, ^{125}I-treated tolerant cells injected alone were ineffective in transferring an FɣG response although they were capable of inducing normal antibody production to the control antigen, HRC. These findings implied that the "suppressor" T cell population in tolerant spleen:(a) was able to bind antigen specifically and (b) was radiosensitive.

TABLE II

CAPACITY OF FγG TOLERANT SPLEEN CELLS TO SUPPRESS THE PRIMARY ADOPTIVE RESPONSE TO FγG. REVERSAL OF THE Θ-SENSITIVE SUPPRESSOR EFFECT WITH PURIFIED T CELLS

Group	Number and source of cells given[a]	Number of irradiated recipients[b]	PFC/spleen at 7 days			
			anti-FγG		anti-DRC	
			19S	7S	19S	7S
1	1.5 x 10^7 normal T cells	8	200 ± 65[c]	80 ± 45	120 ± 35	140 ± 100
2	1.5 x 10^7 normal B cells	8	45 ± 25	270 ± 220	135 ± 65	285 ± 170
3	1.5 x 10^7 normal T cells and 1.5 x 10^7 normal B cells	9	710 ± 225	4225 ± 1530	1205 ± 345	4930 ± 1200
4	1.5 x 10^7 FγG tolerant spleen cells + 1.5 x 10^7 normal T cells	7	1095 ± 685	35 ± 20	1740 ± 430	4310 ± 880
5	1.5 x 10^7 FγG tolerant spleen cells treated with anti-Θ serum + 1.5 x 10^7 normal T cells	10	70 ± 30	4885 ± 1110	1275 ± 380	6760 ± 1850
6	1.5 x 10^7 FγG tolerant spleen cells + 1.5 x 10^7 normal B cells	7	820 ± 615	315 ± 195	1095 ± 280	5925 ± 2090

a - T cells obtained by column treatment of spleen cell suspension; B cells obtained by treatment of spleen cells with anti-Θ serum and complement.

b - Each recipient given 500 µg FγGA intraperitoneally (i.p.) and 5 x 10^8 DRC intravenously (i.v.).

c - Arithmetic mean ± SE

TABLE III

ABROGATION OF THE SUPPRESSOR EFFECT OF FγG-TOLERANT
SPLEEN CELLS BY PRETREATMENT WITH ^{125}I-FγG

Group	Number and type of cells given	Number of irradiated recipients[a]	7S PFC/spleen at 7 days anti-FγG	anti-HRC
1	1.5 x 10^7 tolerant spleen cells preincubated with ^{127}I-FγG	7	555 + 165	21,430 + 1800
2	1.5 x 10^7 normal spleen cells	7	9200 + 790	20,355 + 1610
3	1.5 x 10^7 normal spleen cells + 1.5 x 10^7 tolerant spleen cells preincubated with ^{127}I-FγG	8	800 + 130	60,690 + 3955
4	1.5 x 10^7 normal spleen cells + 1.5 x 10^7 tolerant spleen cells preincubated with ^{125}I-FγG	7	11,115 + 1315	63,785 + 5140
5	1.5 x 10^7 tolerant spleen cells preincubated with ^{125}I-FγG	6	950 + 185	18,750 + 2070

a – Each recipient given 500 μg FγGA i.p. and 5 x 10^8 HRC i.v.

b – Arithmetic mean + SE

Several mechanisms may be envisaged for T cell tolerance of this kind (Table IV). The experiments described to date tend to exclude the first three possibilities. To examine the other alternatives, a study of tolerance induction to human IgG (HGG) was initiated. HGG tolerance was selected since much is known about its kinetics from the work of Weigle and his colleagues (4) and a Θ-sensitive suppressor effect analogous to that described for FγG has been reported by Huchet and Feldmann (5). These experiments were carried out in collaboration with my colleagues P. Johnson and E. Chia. CBA or (CBA x C57BL/6J)Fl mice were given a single injection of 2.5 mg deaggregated HGG. For most experiments the mice were used 5-10 days later. The unresponsive state was assessed in adoptive transfer to irradiated hosts by demonstrating a lack of help in a hapten (DNP) carrier collaborative system. To test whether a suppressor effect was present, HGG tolerant cells were injected together with cells from HGG and DNP-flagellin (Fla)-primed mice and DNP-HGG. As shown in Table V, significant inhibition particularly of the indirect DNP PFC response was observed if at least 25 x 10^6 tolerant cells were used. The specificity of suppression was established by demonstrating: a) abrogation of the DNP response of recipients given tolerant cells plus HGG-primed cells and DNP-HGG but not of recipients given KLH-primed cells and DNP-KLH plus HGG; b) a comparable HRC response in recipients of tolerant cells whether they received HGG or KLH-primed cells; and c) no significant reduction in DNP response to DNP-KLH of recipients given normal rather than tolerant cells plus KLH-primed cells. These data shed some light on the site of action of the suppressor influence in that the target appears to be the corresponding carrier reactive (T) not the hapten sensitive (B) cell population. In other words, suppression appears to require the presence of specific helper cells for its expression, a finding which is consistent with the previous in vitro results reported by Feldmann (6).

In a similar experiment FγG-primed spleen cells were used instead of KLH-primed cells as a specificity control. When they were transferred into irradiated recipients with spleen cells from HGG tolerant and DNP-Fla-primed donors, a highly significant reduction in DNP response to DNP-FγG occurred whether or not HGG was given as well. This was at first sight surprising since FγG and HGG do not appear to cross react in the normal animal (7). Presumably, the phenomenon represents another example of increased cross reactivity at the level of the T cell consequent on priming.

The demonstration of cross tolerance in a suppressor system has important implications in regulation of the immune response, particularly to self antigens (Table VI).

TABLE IV

POSSIBLE MECHANISMS OF T CELL DEPENDENT SUPPRESSION
OF THE IMMUNE RESPONSE

1. Delay in differentiation of antibody-forming cell precursors (AFCP)

2. Redistribution of AFCP to sites other than spleen

3. T cell-mediated switch in antibody production or allotype expression

4. Mediation by T cells coated with immune complexes

5. Too much "help"

6. Mediation by a distinct clone of suppressor cells

The duration of suppression was examined by testing the inhibitory capacity of spleen cells collected at intervals following tolerance induction. As in the FγG system, the effect was demonstrable for only a brief period, from approximately 3-15 days. This is in marked contrast to the much longer duration of HGG tolerance reported both at the level of the whole animal and in thymus and bone marrow cells (4). It does, however, coincide with the time at which antigen binding cells to HGG are reported to be undetectable in the spleen (4). Although the association of the two phenomena may be fortuitous, it is tempting to suggest that suppressor T cells may play a role in induction of B cell tolerance by "diversion" of carrier reactive cells, thereby permitting receptor "blockade" on B cells by haptenic determinants. The lack of antigen-binding cells to HGG, but not to FγG, could be a reflection of the tolerogenic potential of the two antigens. Thus, the duration of tolerance to FγG in intact mice is less than three weeks (see above) whereas, in the case of HGG, it exceeds 100 days (4).

TABLE V

CAPACITY OF HGG TOLERANT SPLEEN CELLS TO INHIBIT A SECONDARY ADOPTIVE RESPONSE TO DNP. SPECIFIC SUPPRESSION OF HGG-PRIMED CELLS.

Group	HGG tolerant spleen cells (2.5×10^7)[a]	Source of carrier-primed cells given (5×10^6)	Antigens[b]	Number of irradiated recipients[c]	19S anti-DNP	7S anti-DNP	7S anti-HRC
1	+	-	DNP-HGG	8	445± 90[d]	910± 725	-
2	-	HGG-primed spleen	DNP-HGG	8	7255± 890	60370+6705	-
3	+	HGG-primed spleen	DNP-HGG	8	650+ 150	2545+ 775	126515+11390
4	-[e]	KLH-primed spleen	DNP-KLH + HGG	8	4250±1085	15400+5855	-
5	+	KLH-primed spleen	DNP-KLH + HGG	8	4730±1460	22065+3450	159840+44445

a - Preliminary experiments showed that lower doses of tolerant cells, e.g. 5×10^6 and 1×10^6 were progressively less inhibitory.

b - Doses of antigens/recipient: 200 μg HGG, 200 μg DNP-HGG or 100 μg DNP-KLH i.v. and 5×10^8 HRC i.v.

c - Each recipient given 5×10^6 DNP-Fla-primed cells i.v.

d - Arithmetic mean± SE

e - 25×10^6 normal spleen cells substituted for HGG tolerant spleen cells

TABLE VI

CAPACITY OF HGG TOLERANT SPLEEN CELLS TO INHIBIT A SECONDARY ADOPTIVE RESPONSE TO DNP. SUPPRESSION OF FγG-PRIMED SPLEEN CELLS.

Group	Number of tolerant spleen cells	Source of carrier-primed cells (5 x 10^6)	Antigens	Number of irradiated recipients[a]	Anti DNP-PFC/spleen at 7 days 19S	7S
1	–	HGG-primed spleen	DNP-HGG	8	465 + 90[b]	75,800 + 16,985
2	25 x 10^6	HGG-primed spleen	DNP-HGG	6	400 + 95	3,385 + 440
3	–	FγG-primed spleen	DNP-FγG + HGG	8	1940 + 340	22,840 + 7,690
4	25 x 10^6	FγG-primed spleen	DNP-FγG + HGG	8	270 + 75	3,945 + 900
5	25 x 10^6	FγG-primed spleen	DNP-FγG	8	700 + 160	1,625 + 955

a - Each recipient given 5 x 10^6 DNP-Fla-primed spleen cells i.v.

b - Arithmetic mean + SE

The θ sensitivity of the suppressor effect demonstrated by us with FγG and by Huchet and Feldmann (5) with HGG made it important to test whether a purified population of T cells from HGG tolerant mice could inhibit a specific anti-DNP response as effectively as the equivalent number of intact spleen cells from tolerant mice. As shown in Table VII, this indeed proved to be the case, implying that the tolerant T cell itself may initiate the suppressor signal.

The previous studies with FγG, although tending to exclude the first three possible mechanisms summarized in Table IV, do not shed much light on the other alternatives. If suppression is due to suprapriming of T cells, for example, one would predict that small numbers of tolerant cells might help rather than inhibit an anti-DNP response. Graded numbers of cells from HGG tolerant mice were injected into irradiated hosts either alone or with HGG-primed cells plus DNP-Fla-primed cells and DNP-HGG. Even when as few as 10^5 tolerant cells were used, no augmentation in anti-DNP antibody production was observed (Table VIII). Before suprapriming can be convincingly excluded, however, it is essential to test whether high doses of primed T cells:(a) might suppress rather than help and (b) might reinforce the suppressor effect of tolerant T cells.

Tolerance induction could, alternatively, be associated with the formation of immune complexes which might coat antigen sensitive T cells. T cells with receptors covered by antigen in this form might exert a suppressor rather than a helper effect. This possibility is currently under investigation by incubating tolerant cells overnight in the presence of antigen and by treating them with chymotrypsin before transfer. If both of the last two hypotheses are excluded, it will then be difficult not to accept the possible existence of two distinct types of T cells, one suppressor and the other helper reacting to similar carrier determinants. The data presented in this symposium by Drs. Benacerraf and McDevitt would be consistent with this hypothesis.

Taken together, the data from the two systems studied lead to the following conclusions:

1) Tolerance induction to protein antigens at the level of the T cell is manifest by a suppressor effect;
2) The suppressor effect is exerted directly by T cells;

116

TABLE VII

CAPACITY OF PURIFIED T CELLS FROM HGG TOLERANT MICE
TO SUPPRESS THE SECONDARY ADOPTIVE RESPONSE TO DNP.

Group	Source and number of cells	Number of HGG-primed spleen cells	Number of DNP-Fla-primed spleen cells	Number of irradiated recipients[a]	Anti-DNP PFC/spleen at 7 days 19S	7S
1	25×10^6 normal spleen cells	5×10^6	5×10^6	8	1065 ± 470[b]	4975 ± 1165
2	25×10^6 tolerant spleen cells	5×10^6	5×10^6	8	225 ± 50	675 ± 230
3	15×10^6 tolerant spleen cells after passage through anti-Ig coated column	5×10^6	5×10^6	8	1050 ± 260	995 ± 300
4	25×10^6 tolerant spleen cells	-	5×10^6	8	535 ± 140	285 ± 355

a - Each recipient given 100 μg DNP-HGG i.p.

b - Arithmetic mean $\pm$ SE

117

TABLE VIII

CAPACITY OF VARYING NUMBERS OF HGG TOLERANT SPLEEN CELLS GIVEN ALONE OR WITH HGG-PRIMED SPLEEN CELLS TO AFFECT THE ADOPTIVE SECONDARY RESPONSE TO DNP.

Group	Number of tolerant Spleen cells	Number of HGG-primed spleen cells	Number of irradiated recipients[a]	7S Anti-DNP PFC/spleen at 7 days
1	-	5×10^6	8	$64,740 \pm 9835$[b]
2	25×10^6	5×10^6	6	$3,685 \pm 520$
3	1×10^6	5×10^6	6	$31,685 \pm 9035$
4	1×10^6	-	8	670 ± 120
5	1×10^5	-	8	345 ± 115

a - Each recipient given 5×10^6 DNP-Fla-primed spleen cells i.v. + 200 μg DNP-HGG i.p.

b - Arithmetic mean $\pm$ SE

3) Suppression abrogates antibody production, not by a direct effect on AFCP (hapten sensitive cells) but via non-tolerant carrier reactive (T) cells of appropriate specificity;

4) T cell cross reactivity is manifest in the suppressor system; and

5) Suppressor activity in the HGG system is found in the spleen for only a short period which coincides with the time when antigen binding cells are undetectable.

REFERENCES

1. Basten, A., Miller, J.F.A.P., Sprent, J. and Cheers, C., submitted in 1974.

2. Gershon, R.K. and Kondo, K., Immunology. 18:723, 1971.

3. Basten, A., Miller, J.F.A.P., Warner, N.L. and Pye, J., Nat. New. Biol. 231:104, 1971.

4. Weigle, W.O., Chiller, J.M. and Habicht, G.S., Transplant. Rev. 8:3, 1972.

5. Huchet, R. and Feldmann, M., Europ. J. Immunol. In press.

6. Feldmann, M., In Proceedings of the Eighth Leucocyte Culture Conference, edited by Roy Schwarz, Academic Press, New York, 1973.

7. Ruben, T.J., Chiller, J.M. and Weigle, W.O., J. Immunol. 111:805, 1973.

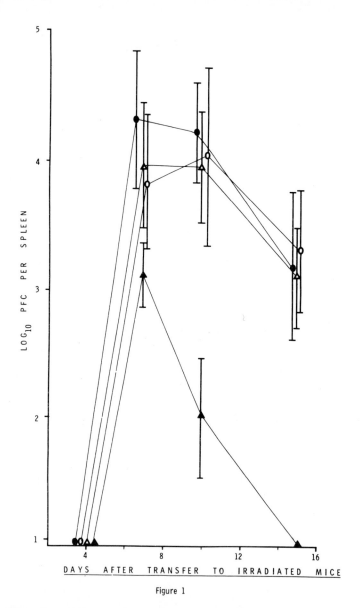

Figure 1

<u>Fig. 1</u>. Time response curve of the inhibitory effect
of tolerant spleen cells on the primary adoptive 7S PFC
response to FγG in irradiated hosts: 15 x 10^6 normal spleen
cells were given intravenously alone or together with 15 x
10^6 FγG tolerant spleen cells. Irradiated recipients were
challenged with 500 μg FγGA and 5 x 10^8 HRC. △ 7S anti-FγG
PFC in recipients of normal spleen cells; ▲ 7S anti-FγG PFC
in recipients of normal and tolerant spleen cells: ○ 7S
anti-HRC PFC in recipients of normal spleen cells: ● 7S
anti-HRC PFC in recipients of normal and tolerant spleen
cells. The vertical bars represent the 95% confidence
limits. 7-8 mice per group.

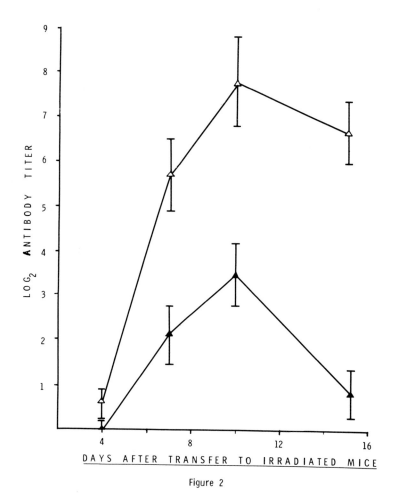

Figure 2

Fig. 2.   Time response curve of the inhibitory effect
of tolerant spleen cells on the primary adoptive serum antibody response to FɣG in irradiated hosts. 15 x 10[6] normal
spleen cells were given intravenously alone or together with
15 x 10[6] FɣG tolerant spleen cells.   Irradiated recipients
were challenged with 500 µg FɣGA and 5 x 10[8] HRC.   Δ anti-
FɣG antibody titer in recipients of normal cells; ▲ anti-FɣG
antibody titer in recipients of normal and FɣG tolerant
cells.   The vertical bars represent the 95% confidence
limits.   7-8 mice per group.

TOLERANCE TO CONTACT SENSITIVITY--
A ROLE FOR SUPPRESSOR T CELLS?

Henry N. Claman, M.D.
Praphan Phanuphak, M.D.
John W. Moorhead, Ph.D.

Division of Clinical Immunology, Departments of Medicine
and Microbiology, University of Colorado Medical School,
Denver, Colorado 80220

We will attempt to do three things. First, to describe
criteria which may be helpful in defining systems for
showing specific immunologic suppression via T cells.
Second, to see how the model of contact sensitivity in the
mouse can fit these criteria. Third, to discuss how
specific immunologic suppression via T cells might work in
this model.

   A. Criteria for a model system to show suppressor T
   phenomena.
      1. An immunologically specific positive response
must be demonstrable, i.e., one must have something to
suppress.
         a. One should know the components of the
response--in cellular terms, whether it involves T cells
only, B cells only, or T and B cells. If it is a T cell
response, it's nice to measure it by looking at T cell
function rather than solely by looking at a B cell product.
One should know what role accessory cells play, e.g. macrophages.
         b. One should know whether antibody is
produced and whether it regulates the response.
         c. Ideally, this response should be seen in
vivo and in vitro.
      2. Suppression of this positive response must be
demonstrable.
         a. The suppression must be antigen-specific.
(If it is not, we are looking at another phenomenon.)
         b. Suppression must require the presence of
T lymphocytes (regardless of whatever else is required).
         c. Ideally, suppression should be shown in
vivo and in vitro.

   B. How does contact sensitivity in the mouse fit these
criteria?
         Credit for developing and popularizing this model

should go to Geoffrey Asherson, who, with his colleagues, has shown that mice can be specifically contact sensitized to such antigens as picryl chloride (PiCl) and oxazolone(1). This work builds on previous experiments of Chase (2) and de Weck (3) to mention only a few. Sensitization occurs after the skin is painted with a contact sensitizer and elicitation is seen most easily by painting the ears with a dilute solution of the contactant and measuring ear swelling with an engineer's micrometer. Tolerance to PiCl can be specifically produced by prior injection of picryl sulfonic acid, and it can be transferred to normal recipients via T cells.

We have repeated and extended Asherson's work using DNFB as a sensitizer. We have also shown that elicitation can be shown in vitro as well as in vivo (4,5,6). In the light of our experiments, how does this model measure up to the criteria for showing suppressor T cell phenomena?

1. Sensitization.
Mice can be sensitized with 0.5% DNFB by two paintings on the abdomen. Four days later, they are challenged by painting the ears with 0.5% DNFB. Ear swelling is maximal at 24 hours. Histologically, there is no evidence of cutaneous basophil hypersensitivity. Sensitization is specific. After two paintings antibody is not seen free in the circulation. Sensitivity can be transferred to normal mice with sensitized cells but not with serum from sensitized mice.

The contact response is T cell dependent. It is not seen in nude mice nor in neonatally-thymectomized mice.

Elicitation can be seen in vitro. If draining lymph node cells from sensitized mice are cultured for three days and stimulated with $DNBSO_3$, they proliferate, as shown by ^{3}H-T uptake. This is not seen with cells from normal mice or oxazolone treated mice. This in vitro antigen-driven DNA synthesis is T cell dependent since it is eliminated if the sensitized cells are treated with anti-Θ + C. Nevertheless, although the response is T cell dependent, B cells are also proliferating in vitro. This is shown by the fact that from 10 - 50% of the in vitro ^{3}H-T uptake can be abolished by anti-Ig + C.

2. Specific immunologic tolerance.

This contact sensitivity can be specifically prevented if the mice are previously treated with $DNBSO_3$. Mice thus pretreated and then sensitized with DNFB show no contact sensitivity when challenged on the ears, nor do their lymph nodes respond to $DNBSO_3$ in vitro. Tolerance is better established 1-2 weeks after $DNBSO_3$ treatment.

Tolerance can be transferred to normal mice, but transfer of tolerance is easier to see if the recipients have been lightly irradiated (250 R ^{60}Co--this does not interfere with sensitization and ear challenge of "positive controls"). Tolerance cannot be tranferred with tolerant serum, only with tolerant LN (100×10^6) or tolerant spleen cells (160×10^6). This is shown in Fig. 1. The transfer of tolerance with cells depends on T cells in the suspension; if the cells are passed over an anti-Ig column (to deplete them of B cells), they can still transfer tolerance. If, however, they are treated with anti-Θ + C, they lose their ability to transfer tolerance (6,7).

In general, this simple system may serve as a good experimental model for the study of "suppressor T cells", if that is what one calls the T cells in the tolerant spleen or LN suspensions which are responsible for tolerance transfer.

C. What do these "suppressor T cells" do?

A number of mechanisms have been implicated in specific immunologic tolerance. It is quite likely that there is more than one mechanism of tolerance. In fact, more than one mechanism may be operating in a single system.

1. Clone loss or clone inhibition.

A prediction of this theory is that tolerance should not be transferred with cells. Since tolerance can be transferred with cells, this seems to eliminate clone loss as a mechanism for this tolerance.

2. Antibody-mediated tolerance (enhancement).

If some kind of blocking antibody is responsible for this tolerance, it appears not to be free in the serum. We cannot transfer tolerance with serum, although it has been done by others (8). Cytophilic antibody has been reported to be responsible for transfer of contact sensitivity to some antigens (9). Could a different antibody be responsible for transfer of tolerance? In addition, if cytophilic antibody were responsible for transfer of tolerance, we might expect the responsible cells to be removed on an anti-Ig column, which they are not.

     3. "Super-tolerogen" (transfer of antigen).
Since it requires 10 mg of $DNBSO_3$ to tolerize an intact mouse, it seems unlikely that enough antigen to tolerize a recipient could be transferred even on 100×10^6 cells. Nevertheless, it could be argued that small amounts of highly tolerogenic antigen ("super-tolerogen") could be present on the transferred T cells, which, by virtue of being T cells, could home to T dependent regions in the recipient and prevent sensitization.

     4. A specific suppressor T cell product.
Just what this could be is not clear to us unless it were IgT + antigen.

    D. Where do these "suppressor T cells" work?
Our experiments do not tell us which, if any, of the above mechanisms might be in play. Can we gain any insight from finding out whether tolerant T cells exert their suppressive action by preventing induction of sensitization (afferent limb) or by preventing expression of sensitization (efferent limb)? Our results differ somewhat from those of Asherson in that we find that tolerant cells seem capable of inhibiting only the afferent limb, not the efferent limb. The experiments show the following: a) Tolerant LN cells incubated with or pre-incubated with sensitized cells do not prevent the sensitized cells from responding to $DNBSO_3$ in vitro with enhanced ^{3}H-T uptake; b) In vivo tolerant cells transferred to an irradiated recipient do not inhibit the ability of similarly transferred sensitized cells to express their sensitivity by ear swelling; and c) Sensitive cells transferred to tolerant donors can still express sensitivity when the recipients are challenged on the ear.

SUMMARY

The model of contact sensitivity in the mouse provides a simple system where specific sensitization and tolerance to a defined hapten can be measured in vivo and in vitro. Tolerance can be transferred with T cells from tolerant donors and these may then qualify for the title of "suppressor T cells". The mechanism(s) of this tolerance is obscure, but it appears to act on the afferent limb of sensitization.

ACKNOWLEDGMENTS

This work was supported in part by U.S.P.H.S. Grant number AM-10145, Anandhamahidol Foundation of Thailand and the Leukemia Society.

REFERENCES

1. Asherson, G.L. and Ptak, W., Immunology. 15:405, 1968.

2. Chase, M.W., Harvey Lectures. 61:169, 1967.

3. de Weck, A. and Frey, J.R., In Immunotolerance to Simple Chemicals, American Elsevier Co., N.Y., 1966.

4. Phanuphak, P., Moorhead, J.W. and Claman, H.N., J. Immunol. 112:115, 1974.

5. Phanuphak, P., Moorhead, J.W. and Claman, H.N., J. Immunol. 112:849, 1974.

6. Phanuphak, P., Moorhead, J.W. and Claman, H.N., submitted to J. Immunol.

7. Zembala, M. and Asherson, G.L., Nature. 244:227, 1973.

8. Halliday, W.J. and Walters, B.A.J., Clin. Exp. Immunol. 16:203, 1974.

9. Zembala, M. and Asherson, G.L., Cell. Immunol. 1:276, 1970.

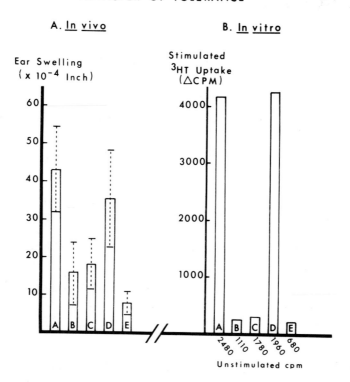

TRANSFER OF TOLERANCE

A. In vivo   B. In vitro

Fig. 1. BALB/c mice were tolerized by i.v. injection of DNBSO3. Seven days later, LN, spleen or serum were transferred to lightly irradiated recipients (6 recipients/ group). Recipients were then sensitized with DNFB, ear challenged five days later and draining LN cell cultured with and without antigen. Mean, with 95% confidence limits, are shown for 24-hour ear swelling results. The mean of triplicate cultures are shown for antigen stimulation in vitro. A - no cells transferred, positive control; B - tolerant LN cells transferred; C - tolerant spleen cells transferred; D - tolerant serum transferred; and E - ear challenge only, negative control.

GENERAL DISCUSSION - SESSION I

T CELL TOLERANCE

Richard T. Smith, Chairman

SCOTT: I would like to address a question to Henry Claman. Battisto and Bloom (Fed. Proc. 25:152, 1966) demonstrated eight years ago that TNP-coupled autologous spleen cells were excellent tolerogens in terms of contact sensitization to picryl (TNP) chloride. Since TNBS injected systemically will bind quite well to a variety of cells and serum proteins in vivo, it is possible that cells from tolerant donors contain TNP-coupled to a syngeneic super-carrier tolerogen and that this is responsible for the "suppressor cell" effect. TNP-coupled T cells might be especially good at transferring this effect due to their migratory characteristics. Have you tried to eliminate TNP-bearing cells with anti-TNP, and if so, what effect does this have on the transfer of this suppressor effect?

CLAMAN: No, we have not done this experiment.

PAUL: I also wish to address a question to Dr. Claman concerning the failure of specific proliferation of lymph node cells from mice which have received tolerant cells. If this form of tolerance is mediated by a population of specifically reactive lymphocytes, one might anticipate that these suppressive cells would themselves divide upon contact with antigen. Does the failure to observe such proliferation imply that suppressor cells fail to divide upon antigen contact?

CLAMAN: There is evidence that "suppressor T cells" may proliferate in vivo in response to tolerogen. First, it takes time to develop optimal suppression. Second, we showed years ago (but didn't understand very well) that actinomycin in vivo will inhibit the development of tolerance to BGG (Claman and Bronsky, J. Immunol. 95:718, 1965). One might expect that the antigen would stimulate LN cells from tolerant mice in vitro--but they don't. Maybe they are fully stimulated by in vivo tolerogen. Otherwise, I really don't know why they don't "turn" on with DNBSO$_3$.

NOSSAL: At first sight the discrepant results of tolerance mechanisms with heterologous serum globulins are puzzling. Chiller and Weigle find that human gamma globu-

lin (HGG) can cause B cell tolerance in mice. Basten
reports that fowl gamma globulin (FGG) and even HGG
fails to cause B cell tolerance but rather raises T
suppressor cells. I wonder whether the resolution of
this dilemma can be found in the capacity of stimulated
T cells to prevent B cell tolerogenesis. For example,
contaminating endotoxin or residual small aggregates
in some batches of globulin could cause T cell activation possibly being towards suppressor cells. We are
currently sorting out this possibility in double transfer experiments. However, one thing is clear, and that
is that we can get excellent tolerance to FGG and also
to DNP (using lightly-substituted DNP-HGG) in nude
mouse spleen cells, and even in anti-θ treated nude
mouse spleen cells. In other words, not all forms of B
cell tolerance are dependent on suppressor T cells. I
shall be presenting some data tomorrow that are more
consistent with a T-independent "clonal abortion".

FELDMANN: With regard to Gus Nossal's comment, I am personally not surprised that even with the one antigen, HGG
there are differences in experimental results as to
whether T suppressor cells are involved in different
laboratories. There are two other reasons which may
account for these differences: First, at a practical
level, it is possible that suppressive effects may be
very transient, and may be missed if looked for at only
one time point or at too widely spaced intervals. In
an in vitro assay for suppressor cell action on B cells,
R. Huchet and I only found suppressors at day 3-5 after
injection of 2.5mg HGG. Secondly, at a theoretical
level, it is possible, even likely, that the same end
result, which we call "tolerance" may be arrived at in
different ways. It is possible that T cell suppressor
effects may result in a B cell (or T cell) block or deletion. For teleological reasons, in view of the importance of self tolerance it may be an advantage to
have different pathways of tolerance mechanisms.

WAKSMAN: The focus of all these presentations has been the
spleen. Here Dr. Nossal's remark that B-cells can be
directly made tolerant without participation of T-cells
is very telling. However, we are ignoring the biological role of tolerance which serves the function of
protecting us against autoimmunization. The first lymphoid population in which self-antigens come in contact
are those of the thymus. We showed between 1964 and

130

1968, in a variety of experiments in both rats and mice, that tolerance can be induced within the thymus (Isakovic, TouÏlet). With tolerance to protein antigens and with transplantation tolerance, both induced at birth, later transfer of the thymus to neonatally thymectomized or thymectomized, irradiated, bone marrow-restored recipients transfers tolerance (Fig. 1).

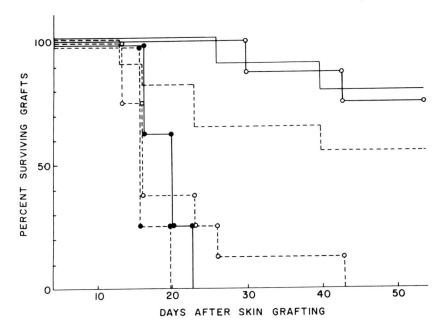

Figure 1. Rejection of skin allografts from CBA (————) and C57Bl/Ks (-----) donors by neonatally thymectomized A-strain mice, either untreated or after transfer to these mice of normal A thymocytes (●) or thymocytes from A mice with neonatally induced tolerance to CBA. Cell transfer and grafting were at 3 and 5 weeks, respectively. From TouÏlet, F.T. and Waksman, B.H. J. Immunol. 97: 686, 1966.

Injection of antigen in very small doses into the thymus of irradiated (Staples) or normal animals (Horiuchi) produced tolerance. Thymocytes from normal animals given a large dose of BGG 1-3 days earlier effectively transfer BGG-tolerance to normal syngeneic recipients (Fig. 2). Tolerance was antigen-specific in each case and controls in these experiments ruled out

the possibility that transfer of antigen could account
for the results. The ability of tolerant thymocytes to
transfer tolerance was not affected by mitomycin C or
actinomycin D, but was abolished by antimycin A and
cycloheximide (not shown). With these points in mind,
it seems to me that tolerance induced in cells outside
the thymus--and this applies to the findings with
B-cells-- must be regarded as a second line of defense.

EFFECT OF DRUGS ON ACTIVITY OF "SUPPRESSOR" THYMOCYTES

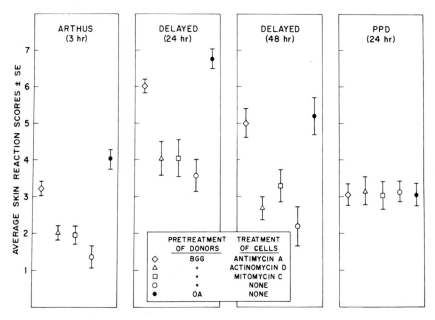

Figure 2. Suppression of skin reactions to BGG in normal
    Lewis rats given 10^9 thymocytes from syngeneic donors
    who had 2 days previously received 100 mg BGG i.v. The
    cells were treated in vitro with various drugs and trans-
    ferred after thorough washing. Recipients were challen-
    ged 1 day after transfer with BGG in adjuvant and skin
    tested 10 days later. The suppressor effect was abro-
    gated by antimycin A and cycloheximide (not shown) but
    not by mitomycin C or actinomycin D.

BENACERRAF: Since Dr. Waksman now interprets his earlier
    data on tolerance as resulting from the generation of
    specific suppressor T cells, I would like to ask the
    question to everyone whether there is any evidence at

present that "T cell deletion" or "T cell inactivation" types of tolerance exist in any system, and whether all T cell tolerance cannot be interpreted as resulting from the generation of suppressor T cells.

GERSHON: My recollection of the original Billingham, Brent and Medawar experiments is that they had a great deal of difficulty in breaking tolerance with normal cells; they usually used immune cells for the adoptive break-age of tolerance. These results are in line with Cla-man's point that his suppressor cells are ineffective when tested with immune target cells. We believe that one of the changes that occurs during the differentia-ation process that creates memory cells is the develop-ment of resistance (immunity?) to T cell-dependent sup-pressor factors. I will develop this point further in my talk on Tuesday.

FELDMANN: Baruj Benacerraf asked for the evidence for di-rect inactivation of T cells, apart from indirect ef-fects via "suppressor" T cells. Unfortunately, the ex-perimental techniques we have available do not as yet permit a resolution of this question, as with unprimed T cells, and the in vitro tolerance protocols (which are the most direct way of testing for tolerance in isolated cell populations). It is not possible to ex-clude the possibility that antigen first acts on sup-pressor cells which mediate or facilitate "tolerance" in T helper cell precursors,

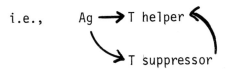

i.e.,   Ag ⟶ T helper
                      ⟍
                       ⟶ T suppressor

until we have a good reproducible way of separating the 2 populations. All our attempts in that direction so far have failed.

BENACERRAF: I realize that the demonstration of the exis-tence of "specifically tolerant T cells" or "deleted T cells" may be a technically difficult task. However, one cannot avoid having to resolve the issue whether these phenomena exist in T cell tolerance. An answer to this question may be provided by taking advantage of possible differences in the properties of suppressor and helper T cells such as their susceptibility to X-irradiation.

G. MÖLLER: You could equally well reverse the question raised by Dr. Benacerraf and ask what is the evidence for the existence of suppressor T cells as a distinct subpopulation. So far this hypothetical population has not been isolated or recognized by distinct markers. Its existence is postulated from a variety of phenomenological evidence such as X-ray sensitivity. Actually, we have no evidence for a separate population. If you have activated T cells in a number that cause optimal helper effect in culture in the absence of serum and in a parallel set of cultures add serum, the helper effect disappears and is replaced by suppressor activity. Here the same cell population was either helping or suppressing depending on culture conditions. In addition, all treatments that are supposed to act selectively on suppressor T cells in essence reduce cell number, e.g. irradiation. It seems most likely (to me) that the same T cell population can help and suppress depending on quantitative factors. Suppressor T cells would represent "super-help".

KATZ: I disagree. I think the type of data presented by Tony Basten today, data of our own in which suppressor activities appear to be more radiosensitive than helper functions and data of Tomio Tada's that will be presented later in this conference all argue against the phenomenology being explained purely on quantitative terms. Moreover, studies in Byron Waksman's laboratory separating cells with suppressor functions on glass wool columns and those of Shraga Segal in Hugh McDevitt's laboratory doing the same on histamine columns promise technical tools to determine whether these are the same or different populations.

E. MÖLLER: As long as nobody has been able to purify helper cells on the one hand, and suppressor cells on the other, and shown that equal numbers of each cell population have either effect, the problem whether the suppressive phenomenon is quantitatively or qualitatively different will not be solved. General findings such as differences in radiosensitivity or anti-θ sensitivity will not help.

BASTEN: Dr. Nossal suggests that T suppressor cells protect B cells from tolerogenesis. My point is that the kinetic studies of appearance of T cell suppressors indicates a time relationship between duration of suppressor cells and disappearance from spleen of specific antigen-binding (B) cells. In other words, it is tempting in the HGG tolerance system to suggest that tolerance induction in B cells may depend on the presence of a population of T cell suppressors.

The data presented for suppression of antibody production imply that it is an active process. Preliminary experiments support this in that the suppressor effect of spleen cells appears to be mitomycin C sensitive.

HUMPHREY: Part of the confusion about the existence and activity of suppressor T cells may arise because we do not know how they work. Clarification might come best from examining the product which causes suppression. In the system described by Claman, G. L. Asherson and M. Zembala can show that suppressor T cells release soluble material which suppresses the activity of actively sensitized T cells in transferring sensitization. If we knew whether this was hapten-antibody, hapten-cell surface component, hapten-T cell product--or free from hapten, we would know better what questions to ask.

LESKOWITZ: The question originally proposed by Benacerraf that precipitated this discussion poses a dilemma. Tolerance by a mechanism involving suppressor T cells is experimentally demonstrable as a positive phenomenon and can be measured and pursued by many techniques. But tolerance as a clonal deletion or "shut down" is not as amenable to experimental demonstration in a positive way if the "tolerant" T cells do not exist or are quiet. This puts us back to where we were 6 years ago. What kind of evidence would you need to accept clonal deletion as a mechanism of tolerance since I gather you do not accept the negative results (i.e. non-suppression) of mixing tolerant and normal cells by Chiller as compelling?

BENACERRAF: Another question worthy of discussion if indeed specific suppressor T cells exist, as the data presented this morning indicates, is: What is the mechanism by which a suppressor T cell exerts its effect specifically on a T cell or a B cell capable of reacting with the same antigen. This phenomenon implies an antigen-mediated interaction or, alternatively, the production by the suppressor T cell of a suppressive factor which contains antigen.

KATZ: It appears that we could be correct in assuming that some forms of T cell tolerance may well be of the "deletional type" whereas others reflect the consequences of active suppression mechanisms. Does anyone recall the details of differences in low dose versus high dose tolerance systems that would perhaps speak to this point?

TAYLOR: The evidence on this point is conflicting. Mitchison was able to break low-dose tolerance to BSA by adoptive transfer of normal lymphoid cells, but some others have not. I found that normal thymus cells would still provide help to bone marrow cells responding to BSA when mixed with tolerant thymus cells, but at a lower level. These results suggest, as you say, that T-cell tolerance need not depend entirely on active suppression-- although in some circumstances such suppression can exist. This seems to be exactly the situation we have been discussing for B-cells.

DRESSER: Intermediate effects such as those seen by Taylor using serum albumin antigens were not seen when bovine γG was used. This may well be because the latter persists longer in a monimmunogenic form and succeeds in turning off the normal cells.

The pitfalls of impurities and aggregates in different γglobulin preparations which Nossal emphasized certainly can be demonstrated experimentally. In addition to T/B differences and dependences in tolerance induction, we must be aware of differences within each main population, namely helper T and suppressor T cells on the one hand and different classes of B cells on the other.

The inducibility of idiotype-specific tolerance in B cells by relatively low doses of antigen may point to an evolutionary explanation of the phenomenon of the inducibility of tolerance to γglobulin antigen in adults. As the concentration of a particular idiotype rises during immunization, the tolerance mechanism allows the induction of tolerance before anti-idiotype-autoimmunity intervenes. It is implicit that the normal concentration is so low that neither tolerance nor immunity is induced unless the concentration is increased in some way. Xenogeneic gamma globulins may not be discriminated against at this level.

BURNET: I still consider that T cell tolerance may be very largely a matter of deletion of various types. I do not think that it has yet been demonstrated that T cell tolerance is not 80 or 90% a matter of deletion and the experimental results concern a minority which is available for experimental study.

G. MÖLLER: A final point on suppressor T cells. It is clear that we do not know whether this is a separate subset of T cells. But the phenomenology is further complicated by the fact that suppression by T cells obviously can be of at least two types: specific and non-specific. The latter phenomenon is seen after GVH reactions or Con A stimulation and is directly caused by T cells, as far as we can see today. The specific T cell suppressors cause an intellectual problem, well illustrated by allotype suppression. How can antibody against allotype activate a T cell so that this T cell only inactivates B cells having the allotype against which the injected antibody was directed. We cannot, for the moment, interpret this rationally. It is my guess that many specific suppressor T cell phenomena will actually turn out to be mediated by specific B cell produced antibody. Since the production of this antibody is T cell-dependent, this possibility is compatible with most findings.

BENACERRAF: We plan at a later session to present data on suppressor T cells in a genetic system under Ir gene control which will illustrate differences in the properties of suppressor T cells and helper T cells with respect to their sensitivity to X-irradiation. Suppressor T cells are sensitive whereas helper T cells are resistant to X-irradiation.

B CELL TOLERANCE

GÖRAN MÖLLER, CHAIRMAN

ACTIVATION OF AND TOLERANCE INDUCTION IN DNP-SPECIFIC B CELLS: ANALYSIS WITH THREE DISTINCT DNP-CARRIER CONJUGATES

William E. Paul, Michael Karpf and Donald E. Mosier

Laboratory of Immunology
National Institute of Allergy and Infectious Diseases
National Institutes of Health
Bethesda, Maryland 20014

INTRODUCTION

The mechanism by which precursors of antibody-secreting cells (B lymphocytes) are activated to proliferate and differentiate is still poorly understood despite the substantial progress which has been made in recent years. In the analysis of B lymphocyte activation and of tolerance induction in such cells, attention has been paid both to events dependent upon the participation of thymus dependent (T) lymphocytes and their products and to antigen-driven events which are independent of T lymphocytes.

Because T-independent responses are, at least superficially, less complicated to analyze than T-dependent responses, they have received considerable emphasis. There has been the implicit assumption that understanding critical aspects of the structure and biologic function of T-independent antigens would provide important clues to the delineation of how B cells are activated. In turn, there has been the expectation that most such T-independent antigens would have similar characteristics. For example, the finding that several T-independent antigens were mitogenic for B lymphocytes (1, 2) led to the expectation that all T-independent antigens would be B cell mitogens and that such mitogenic capacity would be critical for the immunogenic properties of these antigens.

Recently, we have described a T-independent antigen which either lacked mitogenic activity for B lymphocytes or was an exceedingly poor mitogen (3-5). The immunogenicity of this material, 2,4-dinitrophenyl lysyl-Ficoll (DNP-Ficoll) has lead us to reexamine both the B cell stimulatory and tolerance-inducing capacities of DNP conjugates of a series of substances. In this presentation we compare the effects on B cells of DNP-Ficoll, the DNP derivative of the copolymer of D-glutamic acid and D-lysine (DNP-D-GL), and the DNP conjugate of bovine serum albumin (DNP-BSA). Each of these agents appears capable of activating certain responses of B lymphocytes in the absence of detectable T lymphocytes but important distinctions in their behavior are evident.

DNP-Ficoll is a 2,4-dinitrophenyl-lysyl derivative of Ficoll. The latter is the Pharmacia trade name for a synthetic polymer of sucrose, cross-linked with epichlorhydrin. It has a mean molecular weight 4×10^5 Daltons. The DNP-lysyl groups are introduced into Ficoll by activation of the latter with cyanuric chloride (2,4,6-trichloro-s-triazine) in the cold and subsequent formation of covalent bonds with DNP-lysine at room temperature. The preparation used in the bulk of these studies contained 32 DNP-lysyl groups per 4×10^5 Daltons (6).

We have previously shown that DNP-Ficoll is a "T-independent" antigen in a variety of mouse strains. Among its interesting characteristics is the magnitude of the primary response ($\sim$100,000 cells/spleen forming anti-DNP antibody of the IgM class at 7 days after primary immunization), a large T-independent IgG response and the lack of detectable immunologic memory (4).

When evaluated in vitro using Mishell-Dutton type primary responses, DNP-Ficoll proves to be a powerful antigen (5). Four days after initiation of culture, one obtains 2000 to 8000 cells capable of forming hemolytic plaques on 2,4,6-trinitrophenylated sheep erythrocytes (TNP-SRBC). As shown in Table I, the optimal antigen dose is $\sim$10 ng/ml and at 1 µg or greater the response falls off sharply. The peak of the plaque-forming cell (pfc) response occurs at 4 days and requires cell division, as vinblastine added for the final 24 hours of a 96 hours culture prevents any increase in pfc between 72 and 96 hours. Similarly, radioautographic studies of uptake of 14C-thymidine show that a majority of the pfc derive from cells which have divided in the 24 hours prior to assay.

The stimulatory activity of DNP-Ficoll has been shown to be "independent" of T lymphocytes by three different methods. Thus, BALB/c spleen cells treated with anti-θ and complement respond to DNP-Ficoll to an extent comparable to untreated cells; cells from congenitally athymic (nu/nu) BALB/c mice are similar in responsiveness to cells of littermate nu/+ (or +/+) BALB/c mice and cells of neonatally thymectomized BALB/c mice are comparable in responsiveness to cells from sham-thymectomized controls. All three T cell deprivation procedures abolish or markedly inhibit the response to SRBC (5). Nonetheless, it cannot be definitively ruled out that small numbers of T cells are important in the regulation of the response. Hence, T-independence must be interpreted in an operational sense.

TABLE I

IN VITRO RESPONSE TO VARIOUS CONCENTRATIONS OF $DNP_{32}FICOLL$

Antigen Concentrations ($\mu g/ml$)	4 Day DNP-Specific PFC/Culture	
	IgM	IgG
0	290 $\pm$ 35	40 $\pm$ 10
10^{-4}	2,350 $\pm$ 210	410 $\pm$ 40
10^{-3}	2,765 $\pm$ 185	645 $\pm$ 35
10^{-2}	3,370 $\pm$ 200	720 $\pm$ 45
10^{-1}	3,330 $\pm$ 400	180 $\pm$ 20
10^{0}	690 $\pm$ 40	65 $\pm$ 15

Cell cultures done in the experiments described in this and the accompanying tables utilized conditions described by Mishell and Dutton (7) and modifications previously described (8). Ten million BALB/c spleen cells were cultured for four days in the presence or absence of antigen and plaque-forming cells per culture enumerated with TNP-SRBC. IgM pfc are direct pfc. IgG were detected by inhibiting IgM pfc with a goat anti-μ serum and developing IgG pfc with an anti-γ serum.

Not only is the stimulatory activity of DNP-Ficoll apparently independent of T cells, but it appears also to be independent of macrophages. Thus, removal of adherent cells by multiple plating on plastic culture dishes does not diminish the ability of the remaining cells to respond to DNP-Ficoll. Indeed, as shown in Table II, in the absence of macrophages, supraoptimal concentrations of DNP-Ficoll which would have led to a meager or absent response become quite stimulatory. This suggests that macrophage-associated DNP-

Ficoll not only is not required for activating B cells but may be inhibitory under certain conditions.

TABLE II

THE RESPONSE OF NORMAL AND MACROPHAGE-DEPLETED BALB/C SPLEEN CELLS TO DNP-FICOLL

Antigen Concentration (μg/ml)	4 Day IgM DNP-Specific PFC/Culture	
	Normal Spleen Cells	Non-Adherent Spleen Cells
0	350 $\pm$ 40	640 $\pm$ 80
10^{-4}	3,655 $\pm$ 340	5,040 $\pm$ 420
10^{-3}	2,875 $\pm$ 300	6,950 $\pm$ 580
10^{-2}	2,840 $\pm$ 250	5,905 $\pm$ 460
10^{-1}	1,960 $\pm$ 200	4,695 $\pm$ 380
10^{0}	1,230 $\pm$ 140	3,305 $\pm$ 350
10^{+1}	320 $\pm$ 20	2,795 $\pm$ 300

Culture conditions are described in legend to Table I. Non-adherent cells were prepared as previously described (9).

We have not as yet obtained evidence that DNP-Ficoll is tolerogenic in vitro. Thus, preincubation of spleen cells cultures for up to 24 hours with DNP-Ficoll at 100 μg/ml followed by extensive washing does not diminish the responsiveness of these cells to an optimally immunogenic concentration (10 ng/ml) of DNP-Ficoll (Table III). Under the very same conditions, as noted below, DNP-D-GL would have induced a profound degree of tolerance. We have not yet evaluated the capacity of DNP-Ficoll to induce tolerance to a subsequent challenge with a T-dependent antigen (e.g. TNP-SRBC) so that we cannot be certain as to whether this agent is non-tolero-genic. However, the finding that high concentrations of DNP-Ficoll do not diminish responsiveness to optimal concentra-tions of DNP-Ficoll suggest an important distinction between this agent and other DNP derivatives of T-independent anti-gens, such as type III pneumococcal polysaccharide (SIII) and levan.

TABLE III

HIGH DOSES OF DNP-FICOLL FAIL TO INHIBIT A SUBSEQUENT
IN VITRO RESPONSE TO AN OPTIMAL DOSE

24 hr. Preincubation with	Cells Washed, Cultured With	4 d. DNP-Specific IgM PFC/Culture
0	0	440 ± 55
	10^{-2} µg/ml DNP$_{32}$Ficoll	$2{,}545 \pm 260$
	10^{+2} µg/ml DNP$_{32}$Ficoll	510 ± 45
10^{-2} µg/ml DNP$_{32}$Ficoll	0	$1{,}540 \pm 120$
	10^{-2} µg/ml DNP$_{32}$Ficoll	$3{,}800 \pm 245$
	10^{+2} µg/ml DNP$_{32}$Ficoll	955 ± 85
10^{+2} µg/ml DNP$_{32}$Ficoll	0	810 ± 80
	10^{-2} µg/ml DNP$_{32}$Ficoll	$3{,}635 \pm 320$
	10^{+2} µg/ml DNP$_{32}$Ficoll	480 ± 60

Spleen cells were incubated at 10^7/ml with or without DNP-Ficoll for 24 hours. They were washed twice, recultured at 10^7/ml for 4 days and pfc measured.

A variety of mechanisms have been proposed to explain the activity of T-independent antigens and the requirements for B cell stimulation. Three of them have received considerable attention. They are:

1) T-independent antigens are "intrinsic" stimulants of B cells, and this stimulus is provided by the interaction of some region of the molecule other than the antigenic determinant with critical nonimmunoglobulin receptors on the cell surface. In this construction, the principal role of the immunoglobulin receptor on the specific B cell would be to form a high energy bond with the antigen. This, in turn, would create a high local concentration of the intrinsically stimulatory substance and lead to the selective activation of specific B lymphocytes. As the antigen is intrinsically stimulatory in this view, a sufficiently high general concentration would cause activation of cells without the requirement for binding to the specific immunoglobulin receptor. Thus, T-independent antigens would be viewed as general B cell stimulants or "polyclonal" activators (1, 2).

2) A second distinct proposal for the critical requirements for B cell activation is that two independent signals are required (10). One such signal would be delivered by the interaction of the antigen with the immunoglobulin receptor of the B lymphocyte, and the second signal might be delivered either by another portion of the same molecule or by an independent moiety. One suggestion in this regard is that activated C3 binding to the complement receptor of B lymphocytes might provide the second signal (11). In this theory all T-independent antigens should share the characteristic of activating C3, either by the direct or alternate pathways. Of course, a variety of other methods of generating a "second-signal" can be envisioned, including the cooperative activity of T lymphocytes. The predictions of this theory differ from those of the first principally in that they do not require that all B cells be directly stimulable by T-independent antigens; stimulation should be limited to those cells with receptors specific for the determinants of the antigen even when the antigen concentration becomes very high.

3) The third major proposal for B cell activation is that the critical feature is the presentation of antigenic determinants in an appropriate array or matrix. In this view the role of the "carrier" moiety is neither to deliver an independent signal or a second signal but rather to act as a passive carrier of antigenic determinants, albeit in a

critical spatial orientation. The latter leads to a type of cross-linking of surface receptors postulated to be required for activation.

Several characteristics of the response to DNP-Ficoll are of relevance in attempts to choose among these, and other, possible mechanisms of B cell activation. Firstly, in a large series of experiments we have found that DNP-Ficoll either fails to stimulate measurable uptake of ^{3}H-TdR by BALB/c spleen cells or causes very little stimulation ($\sim$2 fold over background). This is true over a wide dose range both in serum-containing and serum-free medium. Furthermore, DNP-Ficoll fails to cause any measurable increase in background pfc specific for sheep erythrocytes in Mishell-Dutton cultures. Both of these characteristics suggest that DNP-Ficoll is not a potent "polyclonal" activator and that the thesis that T-independent antigens are "intrinsic" B cell stimulants does not adequately explain its activity. Similarly, DNP-Ficoll fails to activate C3 by the direct or alternate pathways at concentrations up to 150 µg/ml, suggesting that a two-signal theory dependent on C3 activation is unlikely. One additional feature of the in vitro response to DNP-Ficoll which suggests the possibility that Ficoll is principally an "inert" carrier of appropriately spaced determinants is that addition of Ficoll in concentrations up to 10 mg/ml does not significantly effect the in vitro anti-DNP response to 10 ng/ml of DNP-Ficoll (Table IV).

Although our results to this time do not as yet allow a definitive conclusion as to the precise mechanism by which DNP-Ficoll activates DNP-specific B cells, the following points appear important:

1) Responses to DNP-Ficoll are T-independent;

2) Responses to DNP-Ficoll are macrophage-independent;

3) DNP-Ficoll does not induce tolerance to a T-independent antigen in vitro; and

4) DNP-Ficoll fails to stimulate generalized B cell DNA synthesis and appears not to be a "polyclonal" activator.

TABLE IV
FICOLL FAILS TO INHIBIT DNP-FICOLL RESPONSE IN VITRO

Ficoll concentration in culture (μg/ml)	DNP-Ficoll (μg/ml)	4 d. IgM DNP-specific PFC/culture + S.E.M.
0	0	960 $\pm$ 40
0	10^{-2}	6,160 $\pm$ 320
10^{+4}	"	4,870 $\pm$ 440
10^{+3}	"	4,840 $\pm$ 320
10^{+2}	"	4,680 $\pm$ 180
10^{+1}	"	4,470 $\pm$ 830
10^{0}	"	4,700 $\pm$ 200
10^{-1}	"	4,280 $\pm$ 240
10^{-2}	"	6,060 $\pm$ 400
10^{-3}	"	7,080 $\pm$ 620
10^{-4}	"	5,570 $\pm$ 510
10^{-5}	"	5,730 $\pm$ 340

Cells were cultured in the presence of various concentrations of Ficoll and 10^{-2} μg/ml of DNP-Ficoll.

Let us now turn to a consideration of a second type of DNP conjugate. The DNP derivative of the copolymer of D-glutamic acid and D-lysine was originally described as a powerful B cell tolerogen. This agent induces DNP specific tolerance in vivo in guinea pigs (12) and mice (13) at concentrations of 100 μg or above and leads to a profound diminution in the number of detectable cells capable of binding radioactive DNP-conjugates (12, 14). In vitro DNP-D-GL at concentrations of 1 μg/ml or above leads to tolerance induction as measured by capacity to give primary anti-DNP response to DNP-polymerized flagellin in vitro (15) or to DNP-protein upon transfer to irradiated syngeneic recipients (13).

Recently, we have explored the in vitro activity of DNP-D-GL (M.W. 109,000 Daltons; 75 DNP groups/mole) over a wider dose range than has previously been reported. We find that over a range of doses of from one picogram (10^{-6} mg) per ml to one nanogram (10^{-3} μg) per ml, DNP-D-GL leads to a substanial DNP-specific pfc response on the part of normal spleen cells. In the experiment illustrated in Table V. the peak response was ∿1200 pfc /culture. At concentrations over 1 ng/ml the response falls off and at 1 μg/ml, no DNP specific pfc are observed. Independent studies confirm that this concentration of DNP-D-GL if added for 1 hour, completely inhibits a subsequent response to DNP-Ficoll.

The response of mouse cells to DNP-D-GL appears to be independent of T cells (with the reservation expressed above) as shown by responsiveness of nu/nu spleen cells and of spleen cells depleted of T lymphocytes by anti-θ and C. Thus, DNP-D-GL is a T-independent antigen which differs from DNP-Ficoll in that it induces a profound state of tolerance at 1 μg/ml. One other critical and apparently related distinction between how these agents affect B cells is their differing requirement for macrophages. Incubating spleen cells depleted of macrophages with DNP-D-GL fails to lead to any measurable pfc response; moreover, preincubating non-adherent spleen cells with DNP-D-GL and adding back adherent cells after excess DNP-D-GL has been washed away does not allow a response of these cells, indicating that nutritional effects of macrophages are not the limiting feature in the response of B lymphocytes to DNP-D-GL. On the other hand, adding adherent cells which have been pulsed with DNP-D-GL (1 ng/ml to 10 μg/ml) to nonadherent cells which have not been preincubated with DNP-D-GL results in a substantial response (Table V).

This result strongly suggests that DNP-D-GL directly interacting with DNP specific B cells fails to stimulate these cells and, if the concentration is sufficiently high, renders them tolerant. On the other hand, macrophage-associated DNP-D-GL within an appropriate concentration range is a powerful B cell stimulant. Indeed, it seems likely that the inhibition seen when adherent cells pulsed with high DNP-D-GL concentrations are mixed with nonadherent cells is due to the release from macrophages of sufficient DNP-D-GL to render DNP-specific B cells tolerant by direct contact.

TABLE V

IN VITRO RESPONSE TO SOLUBLE OR CELL-BOUND DNP-D-GL

DNP-D-GL Concentration (μg/ml)	Normal Spleen Cells + Continuous DNP-D-GL	A Cells Pulsed With DNP-D-GL + Normal NA Cells	Normal NA Cells Continuous DNP-D-GL
0	200	420	190
10^{-6}	820	645	180
10^{-5}	880	770	200
10^{-4}	1,230	920	170
10^{-3}	1,440	1,760	180
10^{-2}	665	1,810	175
10^{-1}	325	1,800	160
10^{0}	180	1,365	145
10^{+1}	145	510	120
10^{+2}	95	440	90
10^{+1}	90	355	85

Spleen cells or non-adherent spleen cells from BALB/c mice were cultured in the continuous presence of DNP-D-GL and pfc measured after 4 days. Adherent spleen cells were exposed to DNP-D-GL for one hour, washed and then mixed with non-adherent cells. PFC in such cultures, not otherwise exposed to antigen, were measured after 4 days. A cells = adherent cells; NA cells = nonadherent cells.

150

Thus, DNP-D-GL is a T-independent antigen which differs from DNP-Ficoll in several critical ways:

1) It is a potent tolerogen and direct interaction of DNP-D-GL with DNP specific B cells inactivates them. On the other hand, direct interaction with soluble DNP-Ficoll can activate specific B cells.

2) Presentation of DNP-D-GL on macrophage surfaces (or associated with macrophages), at least within certain concentration ranges, leads to B cell activation. Macrophage-associated DNP-Ficoll is not superior to free DNP-Ficoll in B cell activation.

In closing this presentation, we wish to consider a third type of DNP conjugate which differs from the first two in several interesting ways and which provides important contrasts with them. DNP-BSA and DNP-keyhole limpet hemocyanin (DNP-KLH), which have been traditionally regarded as T-dependent antigens (16), appear to lead to certain T-independent responses on the part of specific B cells. Indeed, our initial studies on in vitro stimulation of spleen cells by these conjugates were of considerable surprise to us. Our goal was to develop an in vitro assay of mouse T cell responsiveness, using incorporation of tritiated thymidine (^{3}H-TdR) by cells from primed animals. We found that DNP-KLH (13 moles DNP/100,000 grams) did stimulate incorporation of ^{3}H-TdR by cells from primed animals; however, substantial stimulation of unprimed spleen cells also occurred. Table VI shows mean results from 4 experiments in which DNP-KLH caused an approximately 10-fold stimulation of ^{3}H-TdR incorporation on the part of unprimed cells and a 15-fold response by primed cells. Both phenomena have been described previously (17, 18), but the magnitude of the response of the unprimed cells observed here is striking. Furthermore, we found that treatment of primed cells with anti-θ and C did not diminish (and, indeed, enhanced) their response to DNP-KLH although it markedly inhibited the response to phytohemagglutinin (PHA) (Table VII). This indicated to us that "T-dependent" antigens, in fact, cause in vitro DNA synthesis by B cells, even in the absence of detectable numbers of T lymphocytes, and that this phenomenon might provide important insights into the mechanism of B cell activation.

Consequently, we examined the effect of DNP-BSA (4 moles DNP/mole), DNP-KLH and DNP-D-GL, all at 100 μg/ml, on spleen cells from unprimed nu/nu mice. The results showed

151

that these agents reproducibly stimulated DNA synthesis either in medium supplemented with serum or in serum-free medium. Table VIII shows a representive experiment using both serum-free and serum-supplemented media. In this particular experiment, DNP-BSA and DNP-KLH caused responses in excess of the lipopolysaccharide (LPS) response in serum-free medium. The magnitude of responses in serum-supplemented medium, although often smaller than those in serum-free medium, were more reproducible and mean results for from 2 to 4 experiments with each stimulant are shown in Table VIII.

TABLE VI

RESPONSE OF UNPRIMED AND PRIMED CELLS TO DNP-KLH

(n=4)

Stimulant	Unprimed	Primed
0	732 $+$ 209	234 $+$ 329
PHA	62,127 $+$ 10,633	77,147 $+$ 7,725
DNP-KLH	7,695 $+$ 1,968	18,107 $+$ 1,042

Spleen cells from control or DNP-KLH primed C57BL/10 mice were cultured in Microtiter wells 5 x 10^6/ml. ^{3}H-thymidine incorporation in response to no stimulation, phytohemagglutinin (1 µg/ml) or DNP-KLH (13 groups DNP/100,000 Daltons; 100 µg/ml) was determined at 72 hours. The results presented are mean $\pm$ standard error of 4 individual experiments.

One obvious explanation for the capacity of DNP-proteins to stimulate DNA synthesis by unprimed B lymphocytes is that such stimulation represented the effect of contamination of the antigen preparation with bacterial lipopolysaccharide. However, assays for LPS activity by the limulus hemolymph gelation assay (kindly performed by Dr. Ronald Elin) indicated that DNP-protein preparations which were highly stimulatory at 50 or 100 µg/ml contained the weight equivalent of less than 1 part LPS in 10^{+6}. Moreover, as shown in Table IX, responses of nu/nu cells to LPS are not significantly inhibited by the presence of purified anti-mouse κ antibody (100

TABLE VII

EFFECT OF ANTI-Θ AND C ON PROLIFERATIVE RESPONSES OF LYMPHOCYTES FROM PRIMED MICE

Stimulant	Serum-Supplemented		Serum-Free	
	BA anti-Θ (cpm)	Anti-Θ (cpm)	BA anti-Θ (cpm)	Anti-Θ (cpm)
0	3,349 ± 199	1,745 ± 407	1,744 ± 173	939 ± 92
PHA	183,547 ± 14,872	3,499 ± 591	72,308 ± 6,485	2,837 ± 116
LPS	16,537 ± 1,950	11,062 ± 1,341	14,792 ± 1,660	17,319 ± 488
DNP-KLH (100 μg/ml)	12,926 ± 1,632	23,518 ± 23	26,861 ± 766	34,454 ± 5,396

Spleen cells from DNP-KLH-primed C57BL/10 mice were exposed to anti-C3H-Θ serum or to brain-absorbed (BA) anti-Θ and complement. They were then cultured in serum-supplemented or serum-free medium and stimulated with nothing, PHA, lipopolysaccharide (LPS) or DNP-KLH.

153

μg/ml) in culture, while responses to both DNP-BSA and DNP-KLH are markedly inhibited. This result provides further evidence that the effect of DNP-KLH and DNP-BSA is not a function of LPS contamination. Moreover, it indicates that activation by DNP-BSA and DNP-KLH requires interactions with immunoglobulin, presumably as cell surface receptors. This strongly suggests that both DNP-BSA and DNP-KLH actually induce proliferation in B cells with some degree of specificity for DNP-BSA and DNP-KLH, even in the absence of T lymphocytes.

TABLE VIII

^{3}H-TdR INCORPORATION BY UNPRIMED NU/NU CELLS

	Experiment 1 (cpm)		Summated Data (E/C)
			n = 2 to 4
Stimulant	+ Serum	− Serum	+ Serum
0	1,986 + 213	1,338 + 281	1.0
PHA	2,008 + 245	3,184 + 373	1.25 + .16
LPS	13,221 + 2,738	20,127 + 6,372	10.35 + 2.60
DNP-BSA	8,290 + 1,443	39,776 + 4,899	6.59 + 2.00
DNP-D-GL	10,996 + 1,587	7,100 + 566	5.77 + .23

Spleen cells from unprimed congenitally athymic nu/nu outbred mice were incubated in serum-supplemented or serum-free media and stimulated with nothing, PHA, LPS or DNP-BSA (4 moles DNP/mole BSA; 100 μg/ml). Results presented are cpm incorporated for a single experiment and mean experimental to control ratios (E/C) for 2 to 4 experiments with standard errors.

This "T-independent" stimulation is particularly interesting in the case of DNP-BSA which is a classical T-dependent antigen (16). We have thus far been able to obtain primary in vitro anti-DNP responses to DNP-BSA nor does this antigen cause a non-specific increase in the number of pfc specific for sheep erythrocytes after a 4 day culture.

TABLE IX

INHIBITION BY ANTI-κ OF THE DNA SYNTHESIS RESPONSE

OF UNPRIMED NU/NU LYMPHOCYTES

Stimulant	Control	+ Anti-κ	% Response in Presence of Anti-κ
0	3,644 + 408	1,593 + 2,854	-----
LPS	33,275 + 1,201	24,100 + 5,126	91 + 24
DNP-BSA	27,334 + 3,197	1,480 + 269	19 + 8.9
DNP-KLH	35,674 + 2,854	3,890 + 581	6 + 3.0

Spleen cells from unprimed congenitally athymic nu/nu outbred mice were cultured in the presence or absence of rabbit anti-mouse κ antibody (100 μg/ml). Responses to nothing, LPS, DNP-BSA and DNP-KLH are presented for a single experiment. In addition, mean percent responsiveness in the presence of anti-κ + standard error for 5 experiments is presented.

Finally, analysis of stimulation of in vitro immunoglobulin (Ig) synthesis suggests that DNP-BSA causes relatively little Ig synthesis by nu/nu spleen cells in comparison to that obtained with either LPS or DNP-KLH, although DNP-BSA causes considerable DNA synthesis. Thus, a classical T-dependent antigen (DNP-BSA) has a profound, if unexpected, effect on B cells leading to cell proliferation with little or no Ig synthesis. Recent studies of in vivo responses of T-deprived mice to DNP-BSA indicate that B cell priming does ccur in such animals (19), providing an in vivo counterpart of these in vitro experiments.

Our results indicate at least three distinctive types of antigen-B cell interaction which occur in the absence of T cells (or in the presence of undetectable numbers of T cells). Specific activation including differentiation into antibody secretion without general B cell activation is mediated by direct B cell contact with DNP-Ficoll. Specific inactivation by direct antigen-B cell contact but activation by macrophage-associated antigen within an appropriate dose range occurs with DNP-D-GL. Stimulation of proliferation, with little or no antibody synthesis, is mediated by DNP-BSA.

Our data is clearly too fragmentary to yet draw definitive conclusions on the mode of activation of B cells by antigen. Nonetheless, our results indicate that "T-dependent" antigens may stimulate B cell proliferation with little differentiation to antibody synthesis, suggesting a critical role for T cells or their factors in such differentiation. In addition, the ability of DNP-Ficoll, a highly polymeric cross-linked molecule with little mitogenic capacity, to directly stimulate B cells supports a model of B cell activation in which form of presentation is critical. Finally, the immunogenicity of macrophage-associated DNP-D-GL and the tolerance-inducing capacity of free DNP-D-GL, which is of relatively low molecular weight, suggests that the view that tolerance induction requires more (and more highly ordered) interactions with a cell than does activation (20) is not generally correct. Indeed, one of the major puzzles in our experiments is the distinction between DNP-Ficoll and DNP-D-GL in their stimulatory capacity. If size and degradability are the sole critical factors in determining the activity of an antigen, one might anticipate that a higher molecular weight DNP-D-GL would be a very powerful antigen and lower molecular weight DNP-Ficoll would behave as a potent tolerogen.

The utilization of this series of antigens promises to provide important insights into the mechanisms by which B cell activation and tolerance induction are achieved. Such information may provide techniques to more precisely regulate tolerance induction and cell activation in clinically relevant situations.

ACKNOWLEDGMENTS

We thank Dr. Ronald Elin for assays of endotoxin activity and Dr. Michael M. Frank for testing the capacity of DNP-Ficoll to activate C3. The skillful technical assistance of Miss Lula Jackson and Mrs. Barbara Johnson is gratefully acknowledged.

REFERENCES

1. Coutinho, A. and Möller, G., Nat. New Biol. 245:12,1973.

2. Coutinho, H., Gronowicz, E., Bullock, W.W. and Möller, G., J. Exp. Med. 139:74, 1974.

3. Paul, W.E., Sharon, R., Davie, J.M. and McMaster,P.R.B., In Cellular Selection and Regulation in the Immune Response, edited by G.M. Edelman, Raven Press, N.Y. In press.

4. Paul, W.E., Sharon, R., Kask, A.M., Owens, J.D. and McMaster, P.R.B., Fed. Proc. 33:756, 1974.

5. Mosier, D.E., Johnson, B.M., Paul, W.E. and McMaster, P.R.B., J. Exp. Med. 139:1354,1974.

6. McMaster, P.R.B. Manuscript in preparation.

7. Mishell, R.I. and Dutton, R.W., J. Exp. Med. 126:423, 1967.

8. Mosier, D.E., J. Exp. Med. 129:351, 1969.

9. Mosier, D.E., Science (Wash., D.C.) 158:1575, 1967.

10. Bretscher, P. and Cohn, M., Science. 169:1042, 1970.

11. Dukor, P. and Hartmann, K., Cell Immunol. 7:349, 1973.

12. Katz, D.H., Davie, J.M., Paul, W.E. and Benacerraf, B., J. Exp. Med. 134:201, 1971.

13. Katz, D.H., Hamaoka, T. and Benacerraf, B., J. Exp. Med. 136:1404, 1972.

14. Breitner, J.C.S. and Paul, W.E., (unpublished observations).

15. Nossal, G.J.V., Pike, B.L. and Katz, D.H., J. Exp. Med. 138:312, 1973.

16. Gershon, R.K. and Paul, W.E., J. Immunol. 106:872, 1971.

17. Osborne, D.P., Jr. and Katz, D.H., J. Immunol. 111: 1164, 1973.

18. Phanuphank, P., Moorehead, J.W. and Claman, H.N., J. Immunol. 112:849, 1974.

19. Davie, J.M. and Paul, W.E. Manuscript in preparation.

20. Feldmann, M., J. Exp. Med. 136:532, 1972.

DISCUSSION FOLLOWING WILLIAM PAUL

DIENER: Your method of removing adherent cells may be quite insufficient. Dr. Lee in my laboratory has shown that removal of A cells with the conventional adherence technique abolishes the same response to SRC but not to POL. However, when using magnetic force, A cells bound to iron particles can be removed to such an extent that the POL response is now abolished. Control experiments show that this effect is not due to removal of immuno-competent cells.

PAUL: Although we have made serious efforts to remove mac-rophages from our culture system, we cannot exclude the possibility that very small numbers of these cells may play a role in the response to DNP-Ficoll. Nonetheless, our observation that depletion of adherent cells in-creases the response to DNP-Ficoll strongly suggests that macrophages are not critical for the in vitro response we have observed.

FELDMANN: Does DNP-BSA induce memory in purified B cells in vitro?

PAUL: Our attempts to demonstrate an expansion in "memory" in vitro have not led to definitive results.

GERSHON: In your studies of macrophage dependency have you looked at differences for the requirement of the physi-cal presence of macrophahes versus supernatants of macrophage cultures?

PAUL: We have not yet examined the effect of supernatants of macrophage cultures on in vitro responsiveness to DNP-D-GL or DNP-Ficoll.

HUMPHREY: You commented that you found no evidence of DNP memory elecited by DNP-Ficoll. Was there any evidence of exhaustion, i.e. failure of DNP response to subse-quent challenge with an unrelated antigen such as 1° response to DNP-KLH?

PAUL: In our initial studies with McMaster and Sharon, we had the impression that the high affinity response to DNP-KLH was ablated by prior challenge with DNP-Ficoll. However, we have not yet excluded a "treadmill" effect as an explanation for that observation.

UNANUE: Do the spleen cells from mice given DNP-D-GL which lack free anti-DNP receptors contain DNP-D-GL on their membranes?

PAUL: We have not examined these cells for the presence of DNP-D- GL on their membranes.

SMITH: Have you used varying concentrations of anti-kappa serum in showing a differential effect on LPS versus DNP-D-GL, or DNP-BSA? In our hands the concentration is critical in demonstrating depression of LPS mito-genicity in vitro.

PAUL: We have used a single, but relatively high, concen-tration of a specifically purified rabbit anti-mouse kappa serum. In all these studies, 100 µg of anti-kappa was used, which should be more than sufficient to saturate all membrane Ig sites.

BRITTON: B cell mitogenicity as measured by ability to increase number of background PFC in vitro should be measured at day 2 after addition of mitogen. The peak mitogenicity is then reached and thereafter rapidly falls. A determination at day 4, as you have done, is therefore not illustrative.

Have you tried to inhibit the B cell mitogenicity of DNP-BSA with homologous anti-DNP or anti-BSA anti-bodies instead of with heterologous anti-kappa anti-body?

PAUL: In response to your first question, Mosier has measured the response at day 2 as well as day 4 and has not observed a non-specific increase in the sheep erythrocyte specific PFC as a result of DNP-Ficoll ad-dition to spleen cell cultures. We have not yet exam-ined the effect of anti-DNP or anti-BSA antibody on the in vitro DNA synthetic response to DNP-BSA.

LESKOWITZ: The way you prepared your DNP-Ficoll leads to a lot of cross-linking and the possibility of a lattice type molecule with a lot of the DNP groups ending up in the interior of the molecule where they are perhaps inaccessible to lymphocyte receptors. Do you have another technique for preparation of DNP-Ficoll which gives a more linear product resembling the DNP-D-GL you reported on, and if so, how does it work?

PAUL: Although all the work we have reported here was carried out with DNP-Ficoll prepared by the cyanuric chloride technique, other preparative procedures are possible. John Inman has prepared an amino-Ficoll to which haptens may be added without the additional cross-linking which cyanuric chloride may cause. I should point out, however, that Ficoll itself is already highly cross-linked and thus DNP-Ficoll should be structurally quite different from DNP-D-GL even if prepared by more controllable techniques.

THREE CATEGORIES OF B CELL TOLERANCE INDUCED BY POLYSACCHARIDES: CHARACTERISTICS, INTERRELATIONSHIPS AND GENERAL IMPLICATIONS

James G. Howard

Department of Experimental Immunobiology
Wellcome Research Laboratories
Beckenham, Kent BR3 3BS

Polysaccharides have proved to be a useful group of natural antigens with which to analyze the mechanisms involved in T cell independent tolerance in B cells. Their attributes include: 1) a tendency to persist in vivo which facilitates the induction of high zone tolerance without recourse to repeated administration; 2) availability of information concerning their polymeric composition and, frequently, epitope size; 3) progressive depolymerization to a low molecular weight does not incur loss of specificity; and 4) hapten/polysaccharide conjugates with high epitope density are potent B cell tolerogens.

The pertinent structural features of the three principal polysaccharides we have used are summarized in Table I. All characteristically produce IgM responses in the mouse strains studied, which have been measured by direct PFC assays (using polysaccharide-sensitized sheep erythrocytes) (1, 2, 3) supplemented by passive hemagglutination titration of corresponding sera. An unexpected outcome of the work has been the predominant reversibility of B cell tolerance to SIII (4, 5) as compared with the "irreversible" nature of the levan counterpart (6), despite the similarly prolonged unresponsive states which both induce in the intact animal. One possibility arising from this distinction, that the extent of branching of a polymer might influence its tolerogenic activities, led us to extend the comparison to include highly branched dextran B1355, linear dextran B512 and a low molecular weight linear β2-6 levan. Investigations on the second and third of these are still insufficiently complete to be included in this report.

In spite of their superficial similarities as antigens, the three polymers in Table I have each shown dissimilar features with regard to B cell tolerance, which clearly can no longer be regarded as a single entity arrived at by a unique pathway. I hope that the following provisional classification encompasses all the categories of polysaccharide tolerance which I (and others) will discuss in this Symposium (Table II). The following is a summary of the main features of each in relation to our own experience, with the exception of category B2 which will be the subject of Dr. Baker's contribution.

TABLE I

STRUCTURE OF POLYSACCHARIDES STUDIED

	LEVAN	DEXTRAN B1344	S III
Av.Mol.Wt.	2×10^7	4×10^7	2×10^5
Chain Composition	Fructose, linked β2-6	Glucose, linked α1-6, α1-3 and α1-4 (few)	4β-glucurono-glucose, linked β1-3
Linkage and frequency of branch points	β1-2 (6-11%)	α1-3 (7%)	None
Epitope Specificity	β2-6 linkage	α1-3 linkage	4β-glucurono-glucose

TABLE II

CATEGORIES OF B LYMPHOCYTE TOLERANCE INDUCED BY POLYSACCHARIDES

A. Cell deletion

1. via direct inactivation
2. via exhaustive immunization
3. via suppression with cyclophosphamide

B. Reversible inactivation (tolerant cells)

1. surface blocking by excess antigen
2. mediated by "suppressor" T cells

A.1. B cell deletion by direct inactivation.
This category of tolerance clearly underlies classical
"high dose" tolerance to some, although not all, polymeric
antigens. The equivalent zone with others (e.g. SIII and
LPS) represents reversible blocking of B cells (Category B1).
Tolerance by direct inactivation is exemplified by the outcome of injecting 100 times or more the optimal immunizing
dose (10 µg) of levan (Curve A in Fig. 1). A state of complete, specific unresponsiveness develops in both intact and
T-deprived mice which will begin to break around 3 months
after 1 mg but still persists undiminished at 5 months in
recipients of 10 mg (6). The induction time necessary for
acquisition of this tolerance in vivo, as revealed by cell
transfer experiments, is very short indeed. Spleen cells
from donors injected only 6 or 24 hours previously with 1 mg
levan are found to be, respectively, partially and totally
tolerant on transfer into irradiated (900r) syngeneic mice
(6). The slow recovery of responsiveness (2-2 1/2 months) in
these recipients of tolerized cell populations implies that
it involves a process of cell replacement by recruitment.
The contention that tolerization by a single high dose of
levan is independent of immune triggering per se, and represents direct B cell inactivation is based on two main observations. First, the brief induction period is neither accompanied nor preceded by detectable immunity. Second, and more
compelling, is that when the average molecular weight of
levan is depolymerized below 10,000, it loses immunogenicity
while retaining virtually unimpaired the capacity to tolerize rapidly. For example, mice injected with 5 mg depolymerized levan (M.W. <10,000) become specifically unresponsive to subsequent challenge with 10 µg native levan and
their spleen cells will transfer this tolerant state (6).
Thus,a non-immunogenic polymer of around 50 fructose units
(which retains full PFC neutralizing activity) resembles the
fully immunogenic native macromolecule, which is 2000 x
larger, in the capacity to induce direct tolerance rapidly
in B cells.

By contrast, dextran B1355, the other branched polysaccharide studied, was found to be ineffective for inducing
tolerance in vivo in a similar way (Curve A in Fig. 2) (7).
This response curve shows a 2 $\log_{10}$ dose shift to the right
as compared with the corresponding levan curve (c.f. A in
Fig. 1), so that 1 mg rather than 10 µg evokes optimal immunization. The partial PFC suppression found after 10 mg
suggests that a fully tolerogenic dose would be at least
100 mg, in theory--in practice it is lethal. This high

threshold to direct tolerization by dextran B1355 does not appear to be a consequence of the high responsiveness of the BALB/c strain used, for comparable resistance to induction by 10 mg was found in lower responder mice (CBA and C57BL). The inefficiency of dextran B1355 as compared with levan for inducing high zone tolerance suggests some difference in handling in vivo (such as more rapid phagocytosis), for as will emerge in other respects, it resembles levan much more than SIII as a tolerogen. Although only 500 µg of the latter will induce total and specific suppression of the PFC response (Curve A in Fig. 3), which persists over one year, this predominantly represents reversible blocking of B cells (Category 2A) (4, 5). The weak α1-6 specific response to linear dextran B512 is also suppressed by antigen doses from 1 mg upwards, but whether or not this is reversible has not been ascertained at the time of writing.

Tolerance can also be induced by 2 hours incubation of spleen cells in vitro with either native or depolymerized levan in concentrations of 25 µg - 10 mg per ml (8). Lethally irradiated (900r) recipients of such cells develop PFC responses upon challenge which are only slightly above normal background levels, an unresponsive state which is both specific and stable. Perhaps more striking, by virtue of the greater amplitude of the response suppressed, is the result of similar experiments with dextran B1355 in BALB/c mice (Fig. 4) (7). Suppression was profound in recipients of spleen cells which had been incubated in 2 mg/ml dextran when they were challenged 6 days after transfer but much less so when the interval was only 1 day. This suggests that many B cells must have been initially triggered by their brief exposure to the polysaccharide and that the process of tolerization is here more one of exhaustion (Category A2) than of direct deletion. The very slow recovery of responsiveness to dextran in recipients of in vitro tolerized cells again suggests a process of cell replacement. By contrast, tolerance was never induced in vitro by SIII in many similar experiments (8).

A.2. B cell deletion by exhaustive immunization.
The concept that high zone tolerance results not from direct deletion but from exhaustive terminal differentiation of reactive lymphocytes was developed by Sterzl (9, 10). He proposed that excess antigen induces an abortive response involving their differentiation without proliferation into short-lived antibody-secreting cells. This hypothesis has failed to establish itself as a general model for tolerance

and, indeed, subsequent work has revealed that the antigens studied by Sterzl (sheep erythrocytes, LPS and SIII) induce reversible suppression rather than deletion of B cells (4, 5, 11, 12, 13). Nevertheless, we have recently obtained data which support a modified version of this proposal, namely that tolerance succeeds optimal immunization with levan or dextran B1355 (i.e. following the dose which evokes the greatest direct PFC response) (14). For example, mice which develop a maximal PFC response 5 days after 10 μg levan (Curve A, Fig. 1) exhibit,when challenged with the same amount on day 14,only the same background levels as are found in high zone tolerant animals, (Curve B, Fig. 1). Mice suboptimally immunized with 0.001 - 0.1 μg, however, show neither suppression nor memory responses on similar re-challenge with 10 μg but merely attain the same PFC level as do normal mice. Unresponsiveness following optimal im-munization with levan was complete, specific, persisted for upwards of 8 weeks and could be transferred adoptively from which recovery took 2 weeks.

This form of tolerance appears to develop through an exhaustive utilization of B cells in the absence of memory cell accumulation, for no evidence to implicate any active suppression mechanism (cell or antibody mediated) could be found (14). In particular:(a) spleen cells from unresponsive donors (2 weeks after immunization with 10 μg levan) did not inhibit normal cells in a transfer system (Table III). (In the experimentally less decisive alternative, partial recov-ery was accomplished by transfer of normal cells into unres-ponsive mice); and (b) humorally-mediated suppression was. excluded as follows. Mice were injected with 10 μg LE and 14 days later joined by coelomic parabiosis with normal partners. Following 2 days of union the exchange of lymph-oid cells between parabionts is minimal, whereas their anti-body titres equilibrate by exchange of peritoneal fluid (Table IV). Both partners with similar anti-LE titres were challenged at this time with 10 μg levan. The ensuing PFC counts demonstrate unequivocally the persistence of suppres-sed and normal responses by the corresponding mice.

Dextran B1355, although it fails to induce direct high zone tolerance, produces analogous exhaustion following im-munization 2 weeks previously with 1-10 mg (Curve B, Fig. 2) (7). The suppression is long lasting (full recovery does not emerge within 4 months), but it is also less complete (Fig. 5) as compared with the effect achieved with 10 μg levan. Again, no evidence of active suppression could be

obtained by similar approaches. The corresponding exhaustive capacity of SIII was found to be much weaker (c.f.
Curves A and B, Fig. 3). A similar conclusion emerged from
earlier experiments with SII, where repeated optimal immunization resulted in only a minimal reduction of protective
immunity (15).

TABLE III

FAILURE OF "LE-EXHAUSTED" CELLS TO INHIBIT
NORMAL CELLS IN 900R RECIPIENTS

Donor spleen cells i.v. (x10^{-6})		PFC/spleen (day 6)	
Normal	LE-treated*	10 µg LE (day 1)	No challenge
100	0	8090 (1.25)+	929 (1.24)
50	0	5045 (1.27)	647 (1.79)
0	50	569 (1.59)	820 (1.14)
50	50	5560 (1.15)	3770 (1.10)

*10 µg LE day - 14

+Geometric means with standard error factor in parentheses
(n = 5).

A.3. Specific B cell deletion mediated by cyclophosphamide.
The alkylating agent cyclophosphamide (Cy) is a potent
immunosuppressive agent which, in the mouse and chicken at
least, preferentially inhibits B cells (16, 17). We have
found that the peak PFC response 5 days after all the 3 polysaccharides under consideration is totally suppressed if
150 mg/Kg Cy is injected i.p. at the time of immunization
(7, 14). This potent inhibition is, however, relatively
transient and near-total recovery of responsiveness is found
if similar immunization is delayed until 2 weeks after the
same immunosuppressive dose. Cy is also highly effective
for securing drug-induced tolerance with normally immunizing
doses of T-dependent antigens (e.g. sheep erythrocytes and
chicken γglobulin), but paradoxically, this has been demonstrated to be located in T cells (18, 19, 20). Analogous
experiments with levan, dextran B1355 and SIII have, never-

theless, established decisively that simultaneous administration of Cy facilitates tolerance induction in B cells,
although to differing extents (Curves C, Figs. 1, 2, 3).
Injection of $\log_{10}$ graded immunizing doses of levan together
with Cy results in direct dose-related impairment of specific responsiveness, revealed by challenge with 10 μg levan
14 days later, at the time of non-specific recovery (14).
A comparison of the Curves A, B and C in Fig. 1 shows that
to attain equivalent levels of PFC suppression via direct
deletion or exhaustion requires,respectively,10,000-fold and
100-fold higher doses of levan. A quantitatively similar
conclusion also emerges from the corresponding experiments
with dextran B1355 (Curve C, Fig. 2) (7). Commencement of
spontaneous escape in situ from Cy-induced tolerance with
minimum doses of levan (0.1 μg) or dextran (100 μg) is first
detectable after 2 and 1 months, respectively. This process
is accelerated somewhat by cell transfer, but still requires
1 month for completion. These data are again characteristic
of B cell deletion states.

TABLE IV

FAILURE OF HUMORAL EQUILIBRATION FOLLOWING BRIEF PARABIOSIS
WITH LE-EXHAUSTED MOUSE TO INHIBIT LE RESPONSIVENESS

Pair No.	Log_2 anti-LE 2 days post ∞		PFC/spleen (day 5) after challenge 2 days post ∞ with 10 μg LE	
	Normal partner	LE partner*	Normal partner	LE partner
1	5	4	5160	160
2	8	7	29760	3480
3	6	7	25280	1760
4	6	6	113960	680
5	7	7	30320	1000
Means:	6.4	6.2	Geom means: 26720	923

*10 μg LE 2 weeks before coelomic parabiosis

Although Cy totally suppresses the response to SIII when they are given together, a supra-optimal dose of 50 µg is necessary for this to develop into tolerance during the recovery period (Curve C, Fig. 3) (14). As 250 µg SIII alone will produce equivalent PFC inhibition, Cy promotes in this instance a mere 5-fold reduction in the tolerogenic dose.

To which of the aforegoing B cell tolerance categories these examples mediated by Cy should be assigned depends on involvement of the following possible mechanisms: 1) Antigen-induced triggering may lead to cell death because differentiation is blocked or perhaps G and S_2 phase cells are selectively vulnerable ("Exhaustion"); and 2) The membrane is "frozen" following binding of much smaller quantities of antigen ("Direct deletion"). Two considerations lend some support to the second of these alternatives, which would be influenced by the avidity of an antigen for receptors: 1) the minimal promotion by Cy of tolerance to SIII; and 2) Cy reduces the minimum tolerogenic dose of non-immunogenic levan (mol. wt.<10,000) as effectively as it does the native polysaccharide (21).

B.1. Antigen-mediated reversible suppression of B cells.
Only the salient features of this category of tolerance induced by SIII, which have been published previously in detail (4, 5),will be reiterated here. Doses of 250 µg SIII upwards render a mouse profoundly unresponsive for over a year, during which PFC levels remain suppressed below background levels (1, 4). Unlike levan, however, induction is preceded by an immune phase which is weakly detectable by PFC levels on day 3 but not subsequently (1). This immunity clearly persists, although masked, for such animals possess raised numbers of antigen-binding B cells (22, 23), and these seem likely to be the antecedents of the large numbers of PFC which emerge within 24 hours of the transfer of tolerant spleen cell populations to irradiated recipients (4). The PFC suppression found in high zone tolerance to SIII would seem to represent blocking of triggered cells by the antigen which is detectable in plasma for months and which probably recirculates in and out of macrophage depots (24). SIII clearly does not possess much ability to achieve B cell deletion (directly, by exhaustion or by Cy-mediation); it is not tolerogenic in vitro and its tolerogenicity in vivo is lost if the molecule is depolymerized below the threshold molecular weight necessary for immunogenicity (25). These observations collectively suggest that binding of SIII to B

cell receptors is weak and unstable. The consequence of this would be continuous dissociation and reformation of surface complexes which, in the case of a non-degradable antigen, could be envisaged as a kind of "treadmill" state existing on the membrane.

Although high doses of Esch. coli lipopolysaccharide (LPS) induce tolerance of shorter duration than SIII (about 1 month or so), this is likewise characterized by raised numbers of antigen-binding cells (26) and rapid recovery on transfer or in vitro incubation of spleen cells (13). One dissimilarity from SIII, however, is its capacity to induce tolerance in vitro (27).

GENERAL CONSIDERATIONS

The induction of B cell tolerance and its characteristics are clearly influenced quite as much by the structure of a polysaccharide as by the dose of it used. The cases cited illustrate that conditions can be so selected as to obtain predominantly direct inactivation, deletion via exhaustion or reversible blocking. One corollary of this is self-evident--that other, intermediate conditions must involve combinations of these. The following are two examples: 1) Induction of partial high dose tolerance with levan presumably involves direct inactivation of some B cells at the outset (Curve A, Fig. 1) and will proceed to complete tolerance by exhaustion of the remainder (Curve B, Fig. 1); and 2) The prolonged tolerance following 500 μg SIII is almost immediately reversible following cell transfer at any time after induction. Yet the fact that this early recovery is never total (least in extent at day 25) implies that some concomitant deletion must be involved (4).

These considerations elaborate further the currently emerging multi-component concept of tolerance.

Influence of antigenic structure and its possible basis
The numerous differences between levan and SIII tolerance (summarized here and discussed in detail in Refs. 6, 8, 14, 28) indicate: 1) that SIII has a far weaker propensity than levan to produce B cell deletion irrespective of differences in molecular weight; and 2) that this distinction reflects the relative intensity of binding between polymer and receptors.

What could be the structural basis for the very different properties of these two polysaccharides? Binding sites for carbohydrate epitopes are generally considered to be, individually, of relatively low affinity, although overall intensity of surface binding will reflect the summated energy of multi-point attachments. Highly branched polymers might attach to more binding sites than those of linear composition perhaps by virtue of greater flexibility or epitope presentation. The tolerogenic activity of branched dextran B1355, although weaker according to dose than that of levan, still bears it greater qualitative resemblance than it does to SIII. Alternatively, epitopes themselves may vary greatly in binding capacity. My colleagues and I are currently exploring these possibilities by comparing our earlier findings with the B cell deletive capacities of unbranched β2-6 levan and α1-6 dextran, and also of DNP conjugated with branched and unbranched polysaccharides.

Reversible Inactivation.
Blockade of B lymphocyte receptors with SIII is viewed as the continuous dissociation and reforming of surface complexes. While this is unlikely to be a common event with regard to all antigen-reactive cells, it could be linked to the well-known resistance to deletion of lower affinity cells by protein and haptenic determinants. If the outcome with SIII is attributable to unstable binding, then a similar trend towards potential reversibility of tolerance to protein antigens should exist with receptors of progressively lower affinity.

Another comment concerns signal discrimination hypotheses--are there functionally distinct, blocking configurations involved in prolonged reversible inactivation with SIII and irreversible inactivation with levan? Alternatively, would "two signal" theories with an obligate role for accessory cells postulate the existence in these cells of discrimitory interactions with high doses of the two polysaccharides.

Tolerance via exhaustion.
"Optimal" doses of levan and dextran B1355 can lead to total or partial B cell deletion through exhaustive utilization, but the data presented do not suggest that the responses involve any impairment of proliferation. Rather, three attributes of these antigens seem likely to determine this uncommon sequel to immunization: 1) slow elimination from the body; 2) inability to induce accumulation of memory

cells, due perhaps to an inherent capacity to drive triggered cells into fully differentiated antibody-secreting cells; and 3) high efficiency of binding with B cell receptors. (Relatively lower binding by SIII could explain its weaker exhaustive propensity.) This pathway to tolerance would, therefore, seem a minor alternative if it is, indeed, restricted solely to IgM responses to certain T-independent antigens, and it is still uncertain to what extent it might involve IgG responses to T-dependent antigens. For example, adult mice (29) and rabbits (30) become unresponsive after repeated injections of large doses of BSA, but following an immune response which has been measured in terms of indirect PFC's (30). Whether this represents an obligate step towards tolerance or concomitant and conflicting immunization is a fine distinction according to which the final unresponsive state depends wholly or partially on an exhaustive process. One possibility in this type of system is that the anticipated prior induction of T cell tolerance may favor B cell exhaustion by removal of the normal amplification mechanism.

Direct inactivation.
This is the classical "high dose" phenomenon involving strong binding to receptors, which is favored by their possessing high affinity, or by structural features of the antigen, such as epitope density (31, 32) and possibly branching. While the minimum tolerogenic dose of levan in the mouse (1 mg) can be considered large, this is not invariably so. Taussig (33), for example, found that the corresponding value obtained with DNP-rabbit globulin is as low as 30 μg. Neither is the induction time necessarily slower than it is for T cells, as was suggested by the earliest relevant studies. Numerous polymers (see review 28) including levan and dextran B1355 will induce tolerance in vitro within a few hours. In vivo also, the induction time with levan is measurable in hours not days, while the T-independent conjugate DNP-D-GL studied by Dr. David H. Katz and his colleagues requires only 1 hour (34). The greater time and dose requirements reported initially for B cell tolerance are now seen as those pertaining to monomeric antigens (see 28).

Alternative theoretical mechanisms of direct inactivation will be discussed by others, but I wish to close by mentioning an, albeit unfashionable, yet simple possibility which has not so far been disproved.

According to one view, the first stage involves receptor immobilization by cross-linkage according to the Diener-

Feldmann lattice hypothesis (35). While the resultant second stage could involve signal discrimination, it may depend on the inability of the cell to shed or endocytose its antigen coat which would render it subject to physical elimination by phagocytosis. The alternative view denies the lattice hypothesis and substitutes a first stage identical with immune triggering but postulates a second stage dependent on failure of signal 2 generation (36). Even here cells will be rendered effete--are they not also candidates for elimination?

REFERENCES

1. Howard, J.G., Christie,G.H. and Courtenay, B.M., Proc. R. Soc. (London) (B.). 178:417, 1971.

2. Miranda, J.J., Immunology. 23:829, 1972.

3. Howard, J.G., Courtenay, B.M. and Desaymard, C., Eur. J. Immunol. In press.

4. Howard, J.G., Christie, G.H. and Courtenay, B.M. Proc. R. Soc. (London) (B.). 180:347, 1972.

5. Howard, J.G., Transplant. Rev. 8:50, 1972.

6. Miranda, J.J., Zola, H. and Howard, J.G., Immunology. 23:843, 1972.

7. Howard, J.G. and Courtenay, B.M. In preparation.

8. Kotlarski, I., Courtenay, B.M. and Howard, J.G., Eur. J. Immunol. 3:496, 1973.

9. Sterzl, J., Nature (London). 209:416, 1966.

10. Sterzl, J., Sima, P. ,Medlin, J., Tlaskalova, H., Mandel, L. and Nordin, A.A. In Developmental Aspects of Antibody Formation and Structure, edited by J. Sterzl and I. Riha, Academic Press, New York and London, 2:865, 1970

11. Gershon, R.K. and Kondo, K., Immunology. 21:903, 1971.

12. McCullagh, P.J., J. Exp. Med. 132:916, 1970.

13. Sjöberg, O., J. Exp. Med. 135:850, 1972.

14. Howard, J.G. and Courtenay, B.M., Eur. J. Immunol. In press.

15. Howard, J.G. and Siskind, G.W., Clin. Exp. Immunol. 4:29, 1969.

16. Turk, J.L. and Poulter, L.W., Clin. Exp. Immunol. 10: 285, 1972.

17. Lerman, S.P. and Weidanz, W.P., J. Immunol. 105:614, 1970.

18. Aisenberg, A.C. and Davis, C., J. Exp. Med. 128:35, 1968.

19. Many, A. and Schwartz, R.S., Proc. Soc. Exp. Biol. (New York). 133:754, 1970.

20. Basten, A. Personal communication.

21. Howard, J.G., Courtenay, B.M. and Moreno. Co. Unpublished data.

22. Howard, J.G., Elson, J., Christie, G.H. and Kinsky, R.G., Clin. Exp. Immunol. 4:41, 1969.

23. Howard, J.G., Christie, G.H., Courtenay, B.M., Leuchars, E. and Davies, A.J.S., Cell. Immunol. 2:614, 1971.

24. Howard, J.G., Christie, G.H., Jacob, M.J. and Elson, J., Clin. Exp. Immunol. 7:583, 1970.

25. Howard, J.G., Zola, H., Christie, G.H. and Courtenay, B.M., Immunology. 21:535, 1971.

26. Sjöberg, O., J. Exp. Med. 133:1015, 1971.

27. Britton, S., J. Exp. Med. 129:469, 1969.

28. Howard, J.G. and Mitchison, N.A., In Progress in Allergy. In press.

29. Mitchison, N.A., Proc. R. Soc. (London) (B.). 161:275, 1964.

30. Chiller, J.M., Romball, C.G. and Weigle, W.O., Cell. Immunol. 8:28, 1973.

31. Feldmann, M., J. Exp. Med. 135:735, 1972.

32. Desaymard, C. and Feldmann, M. In preparation.

33. Taussig, M.J., Nature. 245:34, 1973.

34. Katz, D.H., Hamaoka, T. and Benacerraf, B., J. Exp. Med. 136:1404, 1972.

35. Diener, E. and Feldmann, M., Transplant. Rev. 8:76, 1972.

36. Cohn, M., Ann. N.Y. Acad. Sci. 190:529, 1971.

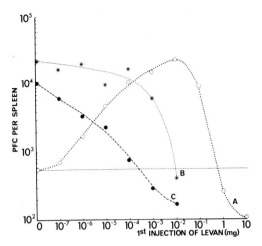

Fig. 1. Dose response curves in terms of PFC per spleen 5 days after: A. - One injection only of various doses of levan; B-C. - Challenge with 10 μg levan in mice given various first doses 14 days previous without (B) or with (C) 150 mg/Kg cyclophosphamide.
(Geometric means, n = 5)
(Normal background shown, n = 10).   CBA mice.
Note different tolerance thresholds -
            direct   1 mg (A)
            exhaustion 10 μg (B)
            Cy   0.1 μg (C)

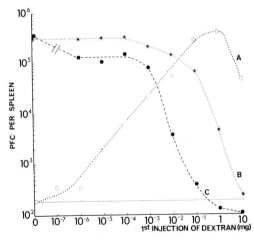

Fig. 2. As for Fig. 1, substituting dextran B1355 for levan and using a challenge dose on day 14 of 100 μg. BALB/c mice. Note only slight PFC suppression by 10 mg in direct response curve (A);
            tolerance by exhaustion with 10 mg (B);
            tolerance threshold with Cy - 100 μg (C).

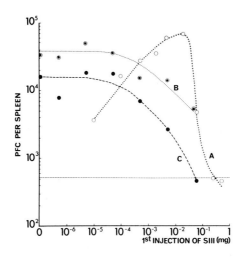

Fig. 3. As for Fig. 1, substituting SIII for levan and using a challenge dose on day 14 of 5 μg. CBA mice. Note PFC suppression by 250 μg in direct response curve (A); only slight exhaustion following optimal immunization (B) as compared with that in Figs. 1 and 2.

tolerance threshold with Cy - 50 μg (C).

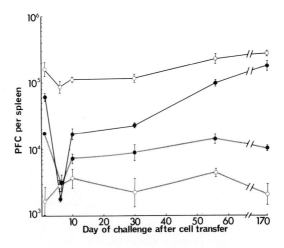

Fig. 4.

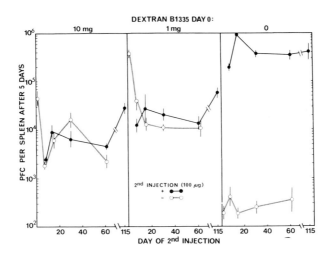

DEXTRAN B1335 DAY 0:

Fig. 5. Prolonged maintenance of raised PFC levels after single high doses of dextran B1355 (1 and 10 mg) with accompanying inability to respond to challenge with 100 µg. Note that pre-treated mice gave PFC counts which were only 1-10% of those in challenged normal controls (Box 0).

Fig. 4. Induction of tolerance _in vitro_ with dextran B1355. Spleen cells were incubated for 2 hours at 37⁰ with 2 mg per ml, washed 4 x and 8 x 10⁷ transferred to 800r - irradiated recipients. At intervals, PFC responses were taken 5 days after challenge with 100 µg B1355 (●——●) or in corresponding unchallenged mice (●ⁱⁱⁱⁱⁱⁱⁱⁱⁱⁱⁱ●). The results are compared with those in challenged (○——○) and unchallenged (○ⁱⁱⁱⁱⁱⁱⁱ○) recipients of normal cells. (Geometric means + S.E.).
    Note: 1) Complete PFC suppression 6 days after transfer of tolerized cells; and 2) slow recovery of responsiveness after early rise.

179

DISCUSSION FOLLOWING JAMES HOWARD

DRESSER: The different mechanisms of B cell "elimination" may act at different times during the course of immunocyte differentiation. For instance, exhaustion may eliminate more mature cells than direct elimination by antigen and one might expect a faster rate of recovery from a state of tolerance conferred by exhaustive immunization. Do different rates of recovery occur after the different tolerance induction protocols?

HOWARD: Recovery times in intact mice are directly related to the dose of levan and are asoociated with antigen retention. Results of cell transfer experiments, where antigen carry-over is minimal, however, support your proposal. Responsiveness returns rather more rapidly in recipients of cells tolerized by exhaustion (2 weeks) than in recipients of cells tolerized by direct deletion (2 months). If the latter involved elimination of a less mature cell, then it would appear to have a higher tolerance threshhold for levan than the mature B cell.

LESKOWITZ: The major difference between the polysaccharides you discussed is in their molecular weights, which differ by a factor of 10^2. Can you obtain S_{III} with a larger molecular weight or alternatively a levan with lower molecular weight and see if they shift categories of tolerance induction, i.e. S_{III} becomes non-reversible levan ,becomes reversible.

HOWARD: The widely differing capacities of native levan and S_{III} cannot be attributed to their respective molecular weights. Various depolymerized fractions of levan going down to below 10,000 daltons retain potent B cell deletive activities.

EFFECT OF TOLERANCE ON ANTIBODY-BINDING AFFINITY

Gregory W. Siskind

Division of Allergy and Immunology, Department of Medicine
Cornell University Medical College, New York, N.Y.   10021

It has been repeatedly shown by us (1-6) and by others (7-15) that the anti-hapten antibody formed by individual animal is generally heterogenous with respect to its affinity for the haptenic determinant, and that there is a progressive increase in antibody affinity with time after immunization. Furthermore, the rate of increase in affinity is faster after lower doses of antigen. These observations have generally been interpreted in terms of a selectional theory of antibody synthesis in which decreasing antigen concentration serves as the pressure to preferentially select high affinity B lymphocytes to proliferate and secrete antibody (16, 17). Thus, at least as far as B lymphocytes are concerned, the immune response behaves like a microevolutionary system.

Two factors appear to influence the affinity of serum antibody. First, as discussed above, the selective pressure of decreasing antigen concentration is a major factor. Second, the rate of cell proliferation appears to play an important role. For selection of high affinity antibody-forming cells to proceed efficiently, it is necessary to have a vigorous immune response. That is, a large population of dividing B lymphocytes is essential if decreasing antigen concentration is to operate effectively as a selective force. If the immune response is of low magnitude, efficient selection cannot occur and affinity will remain relatively low. That is, the rate of increase in affinity should be related not only to the antigen dose, but also, at least to some extent, to the magnitude of the immune response. For example, we have shown that non-specific augmentation of the immune response with adjuvants tends to increase the average affinity of the serum antibody, while non-specific depression of the immune response with cyto-toxic drugs tends to slightly lower antibody affinity (5). Non-specific depression of the immune response as a result of antigen competition will also depress antibody affinity but only when competition is very marked (18-19). It might be expected that antibody affinity and concentration would be correlated. Later after immunization no such correlation is observed. However, early after immunization at that time when antibody concentration and affinity are increasing most rapidly, we have found a highly significant correlation to exist between antibody concentration and affinity (20).

In general, specific modifications of the immune response (e.g. antigen dose, B cell tolerance, antibody-mediated immune suppression) tend to have a marked effect on antibody affinity relative to their effect on the magnitude of the response. On the other hand, it appears that non-specific modifications of the immune response have a comparatively small effect on affinity relative to their effect on the magnitude of the immune response.

With this in mind, two factors would appear potentially important in determining the effect of tolerance on antibody affinity: 1) the particular cell population rendered tolerant and 2) the depressed magnitude of the immune response. Since tolerance can result from different mechanisms and can result in varying degrees of depression of the immune response, it would not be surprising to observe different effects of tolerance on antibody affinity under different conditions.

Over the course of time we have examined the effect of tolerance on antibody affinity in several experimental models and obtained three different types of results: 1) a marked decrease in affinity; 2) a slight or no decrease in affinity; and 3) an increase in affinity.

Tolerance to 2, 4-dinitrophenylated-horse serum albumin (DNP-HrSA) induced by the injection of a large dose of antigen into neonatal rabbits resulted in a profound decrease in antibody affinity (21). In fact, the degree of depression in affinity seemed out of proportion to the degree of depression in the amount of antibody formed. A 47% depression in the magnitude of the antibody response was associated with a decrease in affinity from $\Delta F° = -8.67$ to $\Delta F° = -6.61$ kcal/mole. An experimental model of hapten specific B cell tolerance has been described by Davie et al. (22) which is also associated with a marked decrease in antibody affinity.

In several studies on tolerance induction in adult animals, we have found little or no effect on affinity. For example, adult rabbits made tolerant to bovine serum albumin (BSA) by a series of increasing, intravenous doses of soluble BSA showed no change in the avidity of the anti-BSA antibody synthesized after challenge with BSA in complete Freund's adjuvant (CFA) despite the fact that there was a 72% depression in the amount of antibody formed (23).

In another series of experiments (24), tolerance was induced in adult rabbits by a single intravenous injection of 0.5 mg DNP-bovine gamma globulin (DNP-BGG). Upon immunization with DNP-BGG in CFA the animals showed a 70% depression in the magnitude of their anti-DNP antibody response. The average affinity of the antibody produced by normal rabbits was $\Delta F° = -11.66 \pm 0.11$ (average $\pm$ standard error) as compared with -11.15 ± 0.07 kcal/mole for tolerant animals. This difference, while small, was statistically highly significant ($\underline{P} < 0.001$).

DNP-poly-L-lysine (DNP-PLL) genetic nonresponder guinea pigs synthesized large amounts of anti-DNP antibody when immunized with DNP-PLL coupled electrostatically to BSA (DNP-PLL-BSA) (25). However, when adult nonresponder animals were rendered tolerant to BSA by the repeated intravenous injection of soluble BSA, their anti-DNP response to DNP-PLL-BSA was decreased both with regard to amount and affinity (26). In this case tolerance induction could not possibly directly effect DNP-specific B lymphocytes. It is most likely that the effect of tolerance, in this system, was the result of decreased T lymphocyte helper function. It should be noted that in these experiments an 84% decrease in the amount of antibody formed was associated with a decrease in affinity from $\Delta F° = -8.20$ to $\Delta F° = -7.32$ kcal/mole. Thus, a rather marked depression in the amount of antibody synthesized was again associated with a relatively small change in affinity.

Finally, we have recently been studying a tolerant state induced in adult mice by a single intravenous injection of 0.5 mg DNP-BGG. This procedure results in an 80% reduction in the number of indirect plaque-forming cells associated with an increase in antibody affinity.

Thus, tolerance induced by different experimental procedures can have very different effects on the affinity of the residual antibody formed. Undoubtedly, this is due to the complexity of the factors controlling antibody affinity (cell selection by antigen and cell proliferation) and to the fact that a number of different mechanisms can lead to a state of specific immunological tolerance.

Specific tolerance in the B cell population results in a marked depression in antibody affinity. This is presumably due to the fact that high affinity B lymphocytes preferentially capture antigen and are, thus, preferentially rendered tolerant.

Specific tolerance of T lymphocytes might be expected to have a less dramatic effect on antibody affinity than does B cell tolerance. However, it has been shown that depletion of helper T lymphocytes tends to depress antibody affinity (27). Similarly, it has been shown that elimination of suppressor T cells activity results in a increase in both the amount and affinity of serum antibody (28). Since the mechanism of T cell helper of suppressor activity is not known, the precise explanation for the effects of T lymphocytes on antibody affinity cannot be stated with certainty. However, one possible explanation is that the increased cell proliferation associated with an increase in the magnitude of the immune response results, peri pasu, in more efficient selection of high affinity antibody-forming cells. Thus, it would be predicted that pure T cell tolerance, of moderate degree, would result in no change or in a slight decrease in antibody affinity. Very marked depression of the immune response, as a result of T cell tolerance, would be expected to prevent efficient selection for high affinity antibody synthesis and consequently, block the increase in affinity normally seen with time after immunization. A pattern of this sort has been observed with non-specific depression of the immune response due to antigenic competition. A moderate degree of competition has little or no effect on affinity while marked competition greatly reduces antibody affinity (18,19,29). This pattern is in marked contrast to B cell tolerance where slight depression in the magnitude of the response appears to be associated with a marked decrease in affinity.

We have shown that specific suppression by passive antibody preferentially effects low affinity antibody synthesis (2, 23). A tolerance model which we have been studying recently appears to be mediated by the production of a small amount of high affinity antibody which suppresses further antibody synthesis. This model will be discussed in greater detail later in this meeting. In this type of tolerance we have observed the presence of a subpopulation of high affinity antibody-forming cells earlier after immunization in the tolerant than in the normal animals.

In conclusion, a variety of different observations have been made regarding the effect of tolerance on antibody affinity. Depending on the type of tolerance, one can see either a marked depression of affinity, slight or no depression in affinity, that T cell tolerance leads to no change or a modest depression in affinity and that antibody-mediated tolerance results in an increase in affinity.

ACKNOWLEDGMENTS

This work was supported in part by a research grant from the U.S.P.H.S., N.I.H. number AM-13701 and by a contract from the Office of Naval Research, number N00014-70-A-0412-0002. Dr. Gregory W. Siskind is a Career Scientist of the Health Research Council of the City of New York under Investigatorship I-593.

REFERENCES

1. Eisen, H.N. and Siskind, G.W., Biochemistry. 3:996, 1964.

2. Siskind, G.W., Dunn, P. and Walker, J.G., J. Exp. Med. 127:55, 1968.

3. Goidl, E.A., Paul, W.E., Siskind, G.W. and Benacerraf, B., J. Immunol. 100:371, 1968.

4. Werblin, T.P., Kim, Y.T., Quagliata, F. and Siskind, G.W., Immunology. 24:477, 1973.

5. Mond, J., Kim, Y.T. and Siskind, G.W., J. Immunol. In press.

6. Kim, Y.T. and Siskind, G.W., Clin. Exp. Immunol. In press.

7. Nisonoff, A. and Pressman, D., J. Immunol. 80:417, 1958.

8. Karush, F., Advan. Immunol. 2:1, 1962.

9. Klinman, N.R., Rockey, J.H., Frauenberger, G. and Karush, F., J. Immunol. 96:587, 1966.

10. Parker, C.W., Godt, S.M. and Johnson, M.C., Biochemistry. 6:3417, 1967.

11. Andersson, B., J. Exp. Med. 132:77, 1970.

12. Davie, J.M. and Paul, W.E., J. Exp. Med. 135:660, 1972.

13. Miller, G.W. and Segre, D., J. Immunol. 109:74, 1972.

14. Moller, E., Bullock, W.W. and Makela, O., Eur. J. Immunol. 3:172, 1973.

15. Huchet, R. and Feldmann, M., Eur. J. Immunol. 3:49, 1973.

16. Siskind, G.W. and Benacerraf, B., Advanc. Immunol. 10: 1, 1969.

17. Werblin, T.P. and Siskind, G.W., Transplant. Rev. 8: 104, 1972.

18. Brody, N.I. and Siskind, G.W., J. Exp. Med. 130:821, 1969.

19. Kim, Y.T., Merrifield, N., Zarchy, T., Brody, N.I. and Siskind, G.W., Immunology. In press.

20. Werblin, T.P., Kim, Y.T., Mage, R., Benacerraf, B. and Siskind, G.W., Immunology. 25:17, 1973.

21. Theis, G.A. and Siskind, G.W., J. Immunol. 100:138, 1968.

22. Davie, J.M., Paul, W.E., Katz, D.H. and Benacerraf, B., J. Exp. Med. 136:426, 1972.

23. Heller, K.S. and Siskind, G.W., Cell. Immunol. 6:59, 1973.

24. Weksler, M.E., Merrits, L.L., Werblin, T.P. and Siskind, G.W., J. Immunol. 110:897, 1973.

25. Green, I., Paul, W.E. and Benacerraf, B., J. Exp. Med. 123:859, 1966.

26. Theis, G.A., Green, I., Benacerraf, B. and Siskind, G.W., J. Immunol. 102:513, 1969.

27. Gershon, R.K. and Paul, W.E., J. Immunol. 106:872 1971.

28. Taniguchi, M. and Tada, T., J. Exp. Med. 139:108, 1974.

29. Harel, S., Ben-Efraim, S. and Liacopoulos, P., Immunology. 19:319, 1970.

HAPTEN-SPECIFIC TOLERANCE INDUCED BY THE DNP DERIVATIVE OF D-GLUTAMIC ACID AND D-LYSINE (D-GL) COPOLYMER

David H. Katz

Department of Pathology
Harvard Medical School
Boston, Massachusetts 02115

INTRODUCTION

Nearly four years ago, in studies designed to delineate the possibility that the "allogeneic effect" in guinea pigs (1) was mediated through a direct interaction of transferred allogeneic T cells with primed DNP-specific B lymphocytes of the host recipient, Bill Paul, Baruj Benacerraf and I fortuitously discovered a molecule with unique and potentially applicable properties--the synthetic random copolymer of D-glutamic acid and D-lysine (D-GL). Our choice of this molecule was based on the following reasoning. In order to demonstrate that the allogeneic effect resulted from direct stimulation of host B cells, it followed that we should utilize the fact that strain 13 guinea pigs, which lack the PLL gene, are genetic non-responders to L-GL and its DNP-derivative and, moreover, manifest this genetic deficiency by an absence of T cell helper functions as well as other parameters of cell-mediated immunity (2). Thus, if one demonstrated that an allogeneic effect induced by transfer of strain 2 guinea pig lymphoid cells into strain 13 recipients permitted the latter to respond to a challenge with DNP-GL, then a forceful argument could be made for the foregoing hypothesis. However, at that time we had not yet obtained definitive evidence which ruled out the remote possibility that cells in the unprimed donor inoculum might be contributing to the antibody response by themselves responding to the eliciting DNP-carrier conjugate. Since strain 2 guinea pigs are genetic responders to DNP-L-GL, we elected to circumvent this potential objection by using a carrier molecule which was truly "non-immunogenic" in both strains of guinea pigs - hence, our choice of the D-rotatory isomer of the copolymer of GL.

Preliminary experiments were performed to determine whether or not DNP-D-GL was immunogenic in both strains of guinea pigs and it was in the course of these studies that we first realized the potent tolerogenic properties of this molecule. Then, in collaboration with Joe Davie we carried

out a series of experiments in the guinea pig model to characterize the nature of the tolerance induced by DNP-D-GL (3,
4). Subsequently, this tolerance model was studied in the
mouse both in vivo and in vitro in collaboration with
T. Hamaoka (5-8) and in vitro with Nossal and Pike (9). Most
recently, experiments with Ault and Unanue have been directed
to delineation of the mechanism by which tolerance is induced
by this molecule using cytological analyses (10). In this
short presentation, I will direct attention primarily to the
basic phenomenology of this tolerance model with some mention
of its potential therapeutic applicability for certain allergic and possibly autoimmune disorders. In the following session (this volume, Katz and Benacerraf), I will discuss at
greater length the possible mechanisms involved in B cell
tolerance induced by the haptenic derivative of D-GL as compared to other mechanisms of B cell tolerance induced by more
conventional antigens.

The basic phenomenology of DNP-D-GL-induced B cell tolerance can be summarized as follows: 1) Tolerance can be
induced in both unprimed animals or in animals previously
primed to DNP and producing anti-DNP antibodies at the time
of initial treatment; 2) The tolerance is highly specific--
only DNP-specific B cell precursors and/or antibody-secreting
cells are affected by treatment with DNP-D-GL; 3) The tolerant state is relatively long-lasting; 4) The tolerant state
is accompanied by a significant diminution of DNP-specific
antigen-binding B cells and results in a preferential depression of the high affinity anti-DNP antibody response;
5) Tolerance can be induced by exposure of cells to DNP-D-GL
in vitro as well as in vivo, and in the latter case either
in intact animals or in an adoptive transfer recipient;
6) DNP-specific B cells of the IgE as well as IgG and IgM
antibody classes can be rendered tolerant by DNP-D-GL; and
7) Suppressor T cells are not involved.

TOLERANCE INDUCTION IN INTACT ANIMALS

The capacity to render unprimed BALB/c mice tolerant to
immunization with a highly immunogenic DNP-carrier conjugate,
in this case DNP-KLH (keyhole limpet hemocyanin), by pre-
treatment with DNP-D-GL is illustrated in Fig. 1 (5).
Figure 2 depicts tolerance induction in strain 13 guinea
pigs that had been primed with DNP-OVA (ovalbumin) two weeks
earlier and were, therefore, in the process of developing
antibody responses, by administering an intervening treatment with DNP-D-GL or DNP-L-GL (3). The capacity to induce

tolerance so effectively with the L-rotatory copolymer in
this case is dependent upon the fact that these animals are
genetic non-responders to GL. I will address this point in
greater detail in the following session when we present data
on tolerance induction in mice with DNP-L-GL. Figure 2 also
presents data illustrating the DNP specificity of the tolerant state, since administration of either DNP-D-GL or DNP-
L-GL, which completely abolished anti-DNP responses (left
panel), had no significant effect on antibody responses to
the OVA carrier (right panel). Comparable results have been
obtained in mice.

The tolerant state induced by DNP-D-GL is relatively
long-lasting, a feature reflecting, in part, the fact that
administration of this compound results in a substantial
diminution in both DNP-specific precursor B cells and antibody-secreting cells (3, 4) and, in part, the fact that
being non-metabolizable it is likely to remain for long
periods of time in intact animals. Figure 3 illustrates the
diminution in DNP-specific antigen-binding cells in peripheral blood of DNP-D-GL-treated guinea pigs. Studies in which
avidity subgroups of DNP-specific plaque-forming cells (PFC)
and binding affinities of serum anti-DNP antibodies of control and DNP-D-GL-induced tolerant guinea pigs were compared
demonstrated a clear preferential depression of high affinity antibody-producing cells in the tolerant animals (4).

TOLERANCE INDUCTION IN ADOPTIVE TRANSFER SYSTEMS

A) Exposure of Cells to DNP-D-GL In Vivo.
The somewhat unique feature of the DNP-D-GL tolerance model is the relative ease with which tolerance can be
established in previously immunized animals (3-5). We took
advantage of this feature to develop an adoptive transfer
tolerance-induction system which offers potential capacity
for manipulation of tolerant cells in a variety of ways for
subsequent analysis of the cellular events involved in the
phenomenon.

The data in Table I illustrate two modes of tolerance
induction that can be used in adoptive transfer systems in
which the cells employed are exposed to DNP-D-GL in vivo (5).
In the first case, DNP-KLH-primed spleen cells were transferred to syngeneic irradiated recipients which were then
treated with either saline (group A) or DNP-D-GL (group B)
3 days prior to secondary challenge with DNP-KLH. In the
second case, DNP-D-GL was administered to the donors of DNP-

KLH-primed spleen cells 7 days prior to cell transfer (group C and D). Note that profound suppression of the secondary anti-DNP antibody response occurred in both cases. The fact that one dose of DNP-D-GL induced marked suppression when administered to DNP-KLH-primed donors prior to cell transfer illustrates the potent tolerogenic properties of this compound since these donors were immunized with DNP-KLH in complete adjuvant. Moreover, it is of considerable importance that the tolerant state was still expressed after adoptive transfer (group C) since this is not the case in some models of tolerance in which this has been studied (11-14); this point will be approached in greater detail in the next session (see this volume, Katz and Benacerraf). Although not shown in this experiment, tolerance can be induced by administering DNP-D-GL to the adoptive recipient in doses as low as 10 µg per mouse. Moreover, DNP-D-GL will induce tolerance in adoptive <u>primary</u> anti-DNP antibody responses in suitably treated irradiated recipients of unprimed syngeneic spleen cells (Fig. 4).

B) <u>Exposure of Cells to DNP-D-GL In Vitro</u>.
Two systems have been employed for rendering DNP-primed spleen cells tolerant by <u>in vitro</u> exposure to DNP-D-GL (5). In the first (Fig. 5), primed cells are incubated under standard Mishell-Dutton conditions (15) either with saline or DNP-D-GL for varying periods of time, washed thoroughly and then transferred to irradiated syngeneic recipients. As shown in Fig. 5, these conditions of DNP-D-GL exposure result in suppression of secondary anti-DNP responses at all times tested but most optimally after 48 hours. The second method (Fig. 6) involves incubation of primed spleen cells in stationary tubes for shorter periods of time at $37^{\circ}C$ in a standard 5% CO_2-air atmosphere. Cells incubated with DNP-D-GL under such conditions are essentially maximally tolerized within 1-4 hours (Fig. 6).

In a series of collaborative studies performed with Nossal and Pike in Melbourne (9), it was demonstrated that exposure of cells to DNP-D-GL in appropriate dose ranges prior to initiation of <u>in vitro</u> antibody responses prevented the development of anti-DNP antibody responses to both T-dependent and T-independent DNP-carrier conjugates. More importantly, Nossal et al demonstrated the capacity of DNP-D-GL to effectively tolerize spleen cells from athymic nude mice, thus arguing against any substantial role of, or necessity for, T cell participation in the tolerance-inducing sequence in this model (9).

TABLE I

INDUCTION OF DNP-SPECIFIC TOLERANCE IN ADOPTIVELY TRANSFERRED DNP-KLH-PRIMED
A STRAIN SPLEEN CELLS BY THE ADMINISTRATION OF DNP-D-GL

Group	PROTOCOL* Treatment of donors of DNP-KLH-primed cells	Treatment of recipients of DNP-KLH-primed cells	No. of Recipients	ANTI-DNP ANTIBODY (μg/ml)[+] Day 7 after 2° challenge
A	None	None	10	424.8 (1.21)
B	None	500 μg DNP-D-GL	10	0.02 (1.50)
C	1.0 mg DNP-D-GL i.p. 7 days before sacrifice	None	10	28.2 (1.34)
D	1.0 mg DNP-D-GL i.p. 7 days before sacrifice	500 μg DNP-D-GL	10	0.01 (1.0)

*Irradiated (500 R) A/J mice were injected intravenously with spleen cells (50 x 10⁶/recipient) from syngeneic donor mice which had been primed with 100 μg of DNP-KLH in CFA 46 days earlier (groups A and B). Recipient mice in groups C and D were injected with spleen cells from donors which had been identically primed with DNP-KLH but also treated with 1.0 mg of aqueous DNP-D-GL intraperitoneally 7 days prior to sacrifice. Immediately after cell transfer recipients were either treated with 500 μg of aqueous DNP-D-GL i.p. (groups B and D) or not treated (groups A and C). Three days later all mice were secondarily challenged with 100 μg of DNP-KLH i.p. in saline.

+The data are expressed as geometric means of serum anti-DNP antibody levels 7 days after secondary challenge. Numbers in parentheses represent standard errors. A comparison of geometric mean antibody levels gave the following results: Comparison of group A with group B and group C with group D yielded P values of 0.001 > P in both cases. Comparison of group A with group C yielded a P value of 0.001 > P (taken from Ref. 5).

193

INDUCTION OF DNP-SPECIFIC TOLERANCE IN BOTH
IgE AND IgG ANTIBODY CLASSES BY DNP-D-GL

In a recent study we investigated the capacity of DNP-D-GL to induce tolerance in DNP-specific B cells of the IgE antibody class (6). The reason for interest in this particular antibody class concerns the potential clinical applicability of such a tolerance model to a wide variety of allergic disorders. Thus, by taking advantage of parameters established recently in our laboratory for the successful adoptive transfer of DNP-specific IgE antibody responses (16) and the aforementioned conditions for tolerance induction by DNP-D-GL in adoptive transfer systems (5), the experiment depicted in Fig. 7 was undertaken (6). Donor mice were primed under conditions designed to induce both IgE and IgG DNP-specific B lymphocytes and then treated with either saline or DNP-D-GL 7 days prior to a secondary challenge. The top right panel of Fig. 7 illustrates the absence of detectable anti-DNP antibodies of either IgE or IgG classes 7 days after challenge. When spleen cells from these donor mice were adoptively transferred to syngeneic irradiated recipients, the cells from tolerant donors were markedly suppressed as compared to controls in the development of either IgE or IgG responses following subsequent challenge (bottom right panel, Fig. 7). Other experiments also demonstrated that unprimed DNP-specific IgE B lymphocytes could be effectively tolerized by pretreatment of mice with DNP-D-GL prior to primary immunization (6).

Thus, although it is not known whether the mechanism of specific cell inactivation by DNP-D-GL is the same or different for IgG and IgE B cell precursors, certain features such as the capacity to induce tolerance in previously primed lymphocytes and maintenance of unresponsiveness after adoptive transfer clearly apply to both antibody classes. Furthermore, even if there are slight mechanistic differences between the two classes, these observations represent the first demonstration of restricted B cell tolerance of the IgE antibody class and provide, therefore, a starting point for many areas of experimentation ultimately destined to solve many therapeutic problems concerning clinically allergic patients.

In the following session many of the phenomenological observations described here will be applied to more intensive analyses of the critical cellular events underlying the mechanism(s) of tolerance induction by this unique molecule, (this volume, Katz and Benacerraf).

ACKNOWLEDGMENTS

I am deeply indebted to all of our colleagues who participated in the studies described herein, in particular, Drs. Toshiyuki Hamaoka and Baruj Benacerraf, without whom many of these observations would not have been possible. I am also grateful to Ms. Candace Maher for excellent secretarial assistance in preparation of the manuscript. We also thank the publishers of the Journal of Experimental Medicine for permission to reproduce certain Figures presented herein.

This work was supported in part by Grants AI-10630 and AI-09920 from the National Institutes of Health, U.S. Public Health Service.

REFERENCES

1. Katz, D.H., Paul, W.E., Goidl, E.A. and Benacerraf, B., J. Exp. Med. 133:169, 1971.

2. Benacerraf, B., Green, I. and Paul, W.E., Cold Spring Harbor Symp. Quant. Biol. 32:569, 1967.

3. Katz, D.H., Davie, J.M., Paul, W.E. and Benacerraf, B., J. Exp. Med. 134:201, 1971.

4. Davie, J.M., Paul, W.E., Katz, D.H. and Benacerraf, B., J. Exp. Med. 136:426, 1972.

5. Katz, D.H., Hamaoka, T. and Benacerraf, B., J. Exp. Med. 136:1404, 1972.

6. Katz, D.H., Hamaoka, T. and Benacerraf, B., Proc. Nat. Acad. Sci. 70:2776, 1973.

7. Hamaoka, T. and Katz, D.H., J. Exp. Med. 139:000, 1974.

8. Katz, D.H., Hamaoka, T. and Benacerraf, B., J. Exp. Med. 139:000, 1974.

9. Nossal, G.J.V., Pike, B.L. and Katz, D.H., J. Exp. Med. 138:312, 1973.

10. Ault, K.A., Unanue, E.R., Katz, D.H. and Benacerraf, B., Proc. Nat. Acad. Sci. 1974, in press.

11. Byers, V.S. and Sercarz, E.E., J. Exp. Med. 132:845, 1970.

12. Howard, J.G., Transplant. Rev. 8:50, 1972.

13. Sjöberg, O., J. Exp. Med. 135:850, 1972.

14. Möller, E. and Sjöberg, O., Transplant. Rev. 8:26, 1972.

15. Mishell, R.J. and Dutton, R.W., J. Exp. Med. 123:423, 1967.

16. Hamaoka, T., Katz, D.H., Bloch, K.J. and Benacerraf, B., J. Exp. Med. 138:306, 1973.

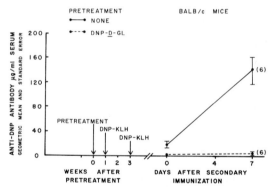

Fig. 1. Specific suppression of anti-DNP antibody production in BALB/c mice as a result of administration of DNP-D-GL prior to primary immunization. Normal BALB/c mice received a series of injections of 200 μg of aqueous DNP-D-GL intraperitoneally (i.p.) daily for 3 successive days. Control mice received saline injections during this period. One week later all mice were primarily immunized with DNP-KLH (500 μg i.p. in saline daily for 3 successive days). This was followed 14 days thereafter (day 0) by secondary immunization with 500 μg of aqeous DNP-KLH i.p. Serum anti-DNP antibody concentrations just before secondary challenge and on day 7 are illustrated. Numbers in parentheses refer to the number of animals in the given groups. Statistical comparison of the responses of untreated and DNP-D-GL treated animals yielded a P value of 0.001 >P (taken from Ref. 5).

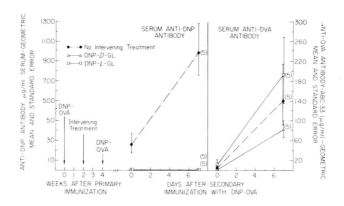

Fig. 2. DNP-specific tolerance induced in DNP-OVA-primed guinea pigs as a result of an intervening treatment with DNP-D-GL or DNP-L-GL. Strain 13 guinea pigs received a primary immunization with 3.0 mg of DNP-OVA administered intraperitoneally in saline at week 0. Two weeks later an intervening treatment with 3.0 mg of either DNP-D-GL or DNP-L-GL in saline or saline alone was carried out. Four weeks after primary immunization, the animals were challenged with 0.1 mg of DNP-OVA in saline. Serum anti-DNP and anti-OVA antibody concentrations just prior to challenge and on day 7 are illustrated. The numbers in parentheses refer to the number of animals in the given groups (taken from Ref. 3).

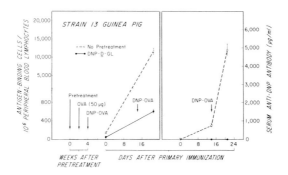

Fig. 3. Diminution of DNP-specific antigen-binding cells in strain 13 guinea pigs rendered tolerant by pretreatment with DNP-D-GL. Strain 13 guinea pigs were either pretreated with 3.0 mg of DNP-D-GL intraperitoneally (1.0 mg per day for 3 successive days) or not pretreated at week 0. Two weeks later both groups (6 animals per group) were pre-immunized with 50 μg of OVA in CFA followed 2 weeks thereafter by primary immunization with 3.0 mg of DNP-OVA in saline intraperitoneally. Fourteen days later all animals were challenged with 1.0 mg of DNP-OVA in saline. The numbers of DNP-specific antigen-binding lymphocytes in the peripheral blood (left panel) and levels of serum anti-DNP antibodies (right panel) at the time of primary immunization with DNP-OVA and 7 days after secondary challenge are illustrated. The differences between tolerant and control groups for both antigen-binding cells and serum antibodies were $0.001 > P$ (taken from Ref. 3).

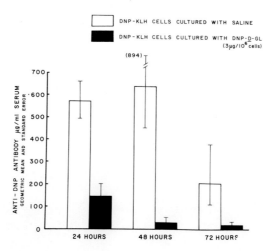

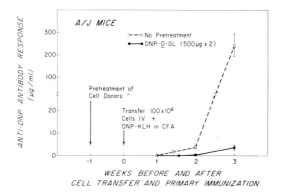

Fig. 4. Induction of DNP-specific tolerance in adoptive primary anti-DNP antibody responses by pretreatment of un-primed cell donors with DNP-D-GL. Normal A/J mice were either not treated or pretreated with 500 µg of DNP-D-GL intraperitoneally on 2 successive days. One week later cells from pretreated and control donor mice were transferred intravenously to syngeneic, irradiated (500 R) recipients (100 x 10⁶ cells per mouse). Recipients were then primarily immunized with 100 µg of DNP-KLH in CFA i.p. The serum anti-DNP antibody responses of the two groups (10 mice per group) on days 7, 10, 14 and 21 after primary immunization are illustrated. The difference at day 21 was 0.001 > P.

Fig. 5. Induction of DNP-specific tolerance in vitro by incubation of DNP-KLH-primed cells with DNP-D-GL in Mishell-Dutton cultures prior to adoptive transfer. Spleen cells from A/J mice, primed 2 months earlier with 100 µg of DNP-KLH in CFA, were cultured in slightly modified Mishell-Dutton conditions (cell density 30 x 10⁶/ml) with either saline or DNP-D-GL (3 µg per 10⁶ cells). At intervals of 24, 48 and 72 hours, cells were harvested from the dishes and washed three times with MEM. Equal numbers of viable saline-control cells and cells incubated with DNP-D-GL were transferred intraperitoneally to respective groups (5 mice per group) of irradiated (450 R), syngeneic recipient mice. The numbers of viable cells of each type transferred to individual recipients were 42 x 10⁶ at 24 hours, 38.5 x 10⁶ at 48 hours and 20 x 10⁶ at 72 hours. All mice were secondarily challenged with 100 µg of DNP-KLH in saline i.p. immediately after cell transfer. Serum anti-DNP antibody levels on day 7 after secondary challenge are illustrated. Statistical comparisons of the responses of recipients of saline-control cells and cells exposed to DNP-D-GL yielded P values of 0.005 >P >0.001 in all cases (taken from Ref. 5).

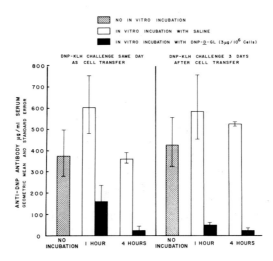

Fig. 6. Induction of DNP-specific tolerance in vitro by incubation of DNP-KLH-primed cells with DNP-D-GL in stationary cultures prior to adoptive transfer. Spleen cells from A/J mice, primed 30 days earlier with 100 µg of DNP-KLH in CFA, were incubated in stationary tubes with or without DNP-D-GL (3 µg per 10^6 cells) for 1 or 4 hours in a 5% CO_2-air environment. At the end of the incubation cells were washed three times and then injected intraperitoneally (66 x 10^6 cells per recipient) into irradiated (450 R), syngeneic recipients. Additional control mice received DNP-KLH-primed cells which had not been incubated at all in vitro. Certain groups of recipients were challenged with 100 µg of DNP-KLH in saline i.p. immediately after cell transfer (left panel) whereas other groups did not receive secondary challenge until 3 days after cell transfer (right panel). Mean serum anti-DNP antibody levels of groups of 5 mice on day 7 after secondary challenge are illustrated. Statistical comparisons of the responses of recipients of saline-control cells and cells exposed to DNP-D-GL yielded the following results: a) left panel: 1 hour - 0.05 > P > 0.025; 4 hours - 0.01 > P > 0.005. b) right panel: 1 hour - 0.005 > P > 0.001; 4 hours - 0.005 > P > 0.001 (taken from Ref. 5).

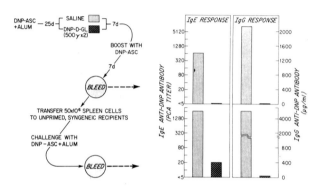

Fig. 7. Protocol depicted on left of figure. The serum IgE and IgG anti-DNP antibody responses of the DNP-ASC (Ascaris extract)-primed donors of spleen cells (top right panel) and recipients of those cells (bottom right panel) on day 7 after challenge are illustrated. Each group consisted of 5 mice. Statistical comparisons of the IgG responses of donors and recipients of control cells vs. DNP-D-GL-treated cells yielded P values of 0.001 > P in all cases (taken from Ref. 6).

TOLERANCE IN ISOLATED B-CELL POPULATIONS IDENTIFIED BY AN ALLOTYPE-MARKER: ROLE OF T-CELLS IN INDUCTION

R.B. Taylor and C.J. Elson

M.R.C. Immunobiology Group, Department of Pathology, University of Bristol, Britain

Recent literature contains much evidence that states of partial, or reversible tolerance may exist (review in 1). There is also evidence that T cells may in some circumstances exert suppressive effects on the responsiveness to antigen of other T cells and of B cells (2,3). If such suppressive effects occur, then particular care must be taken before making the unequivocal statement that B cells can be made tolerant. We have begun studies by which we intend to test rigorously the tolerance of B cells in various situations. With the use of an allotype marker we can study the response of a transferred population of putatively tolerant B cells in the presence of other cells which are responding, and thus test for the presence of suppressive influences.

Another question which we have approached with the use of this allotype marker is that of the possible role of T cells in the induction of B cell tolerance. There is already evidence that thymectomy may interfere with the induction of tolerance (4,5). However, in view of the many examples of partial or reversible tolerance (e.g. 6), it needs to be ascertained whether T cells help to induce irreversible tolerance in B cells or merely hold them in a state of temporary suppression.

MATERIALS AND METHODS

The mice were CBA/H and a congenic line bearing the Ig^b allele (CBA/H/Ig^b or "Ig^b"). The antigens will be more fully described elsewhere. They include TNP_{14} sheep serum globulin (TNP-SG); TNP_{34} bovine serum albumin (TNP-BSA); human IgG (HIgG) and TNP-sheep red cells (TNP-SRBC). Antibody was estimated by an adaptation of a radioimmunoassay (7), in which purified ^{125}I-labelled preparations of either polyvalent anti-mouse Ig or anti-Ig^b were used to assay total or allotype-bearing (Ig^b) antibodies respectively (3). Hapten-specific tolerance was tested by challenge with the hapten on a new

carrier protein not used in tolerance induction, and this
was given an alum-precipitate with B. pertussis as adjuvant
(indicated by "AP", e.g. TNP-SG (AP)). T cells were killed
(where indicated) by incubation with either anti-theta or
anti-brain sera and complement. These treatments left B
cells functionally intact (3).

EXPERIMENTS AND RESULTS

Hapten-specific tolerance.
We tried to induce tolerance to trinitrophenyl (TNP)
with procedures described by Fidler and Golub (8). However,
the tolerance induced either by the simple injection of 5 mg
TNP-sulphonate (TNPS) or by this with the additional injection of TNP-sheep red cells given one hour later and was
barely detectable after the challenge with adjuvant. It was
only when the injection of TNPS was followed by a more
powerful immunogenic stimulus (TNP-BSA (AP)) that a depressed
response was obtained, and then only in the response to secondary challenge (Fig. 1). Eventually, a satisfactory level
of tolerance was obtained by giving five injections of 5 mg
TNPS and following the last with TNP-BSA (AP). This procedure was used in all subsequent experiments.

When lymph node cells from TNP-tolerant Ig^b donors were
transferred to irradiated CBA recipients and challenged with
TNP-SG, they retained a high degree of tolerance (Fig. 2).
This was specific in that the response to HIgG was given by
an additional inoculum of non-tolerant CBA cells; nor did
these non-tolerant cells "break" the tolerance of the Ig^b
population.

Tolerance in lymph node cells persisted for at least
15 weeks without evidence of recovery, although during this
time the competence of the irradiated host had recovered
almost to normal. On the other hand, spleen cells from tolerant donors showed no tolerance--in fact, they responded
slightly better than those from normal donors (see results
with HIgG tolerance in Fig. 3. Similar results were obtained
with TNP tolerance.) This led us to consider the possibility
that unresponsiveness of lymph node cells might be due to
emigration of TNP-specific cells--perhaps to the spleen.
However, splenectomy did not prevent induction of tolerance
(Fig. 2).

Tolerance was also undiminished in Ig^b lymph node cells
treated so as to remove suppressor T cells (3), although the

B cells remained intact, as shown by their response to HIgG in the presence of CBA T cells (9).

Effect of T cell depletion on induction of B cell tolerance to HIgG.

Thymectomized or non-operated control Ig^b mice were irradiated and repopulated with bone marrow cells. These "ATxBM" mice were injected with 2.5 mg deaggregated HIgG as tolerogen, and tolerance was tested in their lymph node or spleen cells after transfer to irradiated CBA recipients. In addition, all recipients received an injection of CBA spleen cells as a source of non-tolerant T cells. These cells would not contribute to the Ig^b titres but would indicate by the total titres whether a state of general suppression existed in the response to HIgG. As in the case of TNP-tolerance, the lymph node cells of non-operated mice were highly tolerant, but by contrast no tolerance was detected in the lymph node cells of ATxBM mice (Fig. 3). There was no evidence of "infectious tolerance", in that CBA spleen cells responded normally in the presence of tolerant Ig^b lymph node cells. More recently we have been able to restore the tolerizability of the ATxBM mice by injecting them with normal lymph node cells but not with tolerant lymph node cells (9).

DISCUSSION

In these experiments tolerance not only occurred in lymph node cells at the level of hapten recognition and resisted transfer to irradiated recipients but also survived attempts to circumvent putative suppressor mechanisms. It is hard to escape the conclusion the permanent tolerance, in the sense of clonal elimination, can exist in B cells.

The absence of tolerance in spleen cells may only reflect the fact that the spleen (but not lymph node) contains haemopoietic stem cells. These would divide in the irradiated host and might regenerate a sufficient population of new B cells to produce as mush antibody as the non-tolerant cells. There is evidence (10) that bone marrow from HIgG-tolerant mice also showed no tolerance after transfer - and that the cell population responsible could be separated by density-gradient centrifugation from a B cell population which remained tolerant. Nevertheless, we should be prepared to find subclasses of B cells with differing susceptibilities to tolerance.

Of the different means of inducing tolerance to TNP, it was remarkable that the most immunogenic was (if given after TNPSO the most efficient. This suggested the involvement of tolerance, rather than the simple interaction of antigen with cellular receptors which is often envisaged. This idea was re-inforced by the finding that B cell tolerance could not be induced in ATxBM mice. These latter results confirm using a different antigen, the original work of Gershon and Kondo with sheep red cells (4). On the other hand, using nude mice rather than thymectomized, B cell tolerance has been induced to sheep red cells (11). Possibly, nude mice possess the particular type of cell which helps in tolerance induction. On the other hand, ATxBM mice may posses a few helper cells which in the absence of suppressors prevent tolerance induction in B cells.

If T cells are finally shown to play a necessary specific role in induction of B cell tolerance, it would suggest that the task of self-notself discrimination belongs to them, with B cells playing a subservient role.

ACKNOWLEDGEMENTS

We are grateful to Rodney Oldroyd and Hadyn Downs for technical help, and we thank Dr. A.J. S. Davies and Dr. H.S. Micklem for generous gifts of mice and Dr. Jean Dolby for the gift of B.pertussis vaccine. This work was supported by a grant from the Medical Research Council.

REFERENCES

1. Simpson, E., In Immunological Aspects of Transplantation Surgery, edited by R.Y. Calne, Med. and Tech. Publ. Co., Lancaster England, 1974.

2. Playfair, J.H.L., Clin. Exp. Immunol. In press, 1974.

3. Elson, D.J. and Taylor, R.B., submitted to Eur. J. Immunol.

4. Gershon, R.K. and Kondo, K., Immunol. 18:723, 1970.

5. Phillips-Quagliata, J.M., Bensinger, D.O. and Quagliata, F., J. Immunol. 3(6):1712, 1973.

6. McCullagh, P.J., J. Exp. Med. 132:916, 1970.

7. Klinman, N.R. and Taylor, R.B., Clin. Exp. Immunol.

8. Fidler, J.M. and Golub, E.S., J. Exp. Med. 137:42, 1973.

9. Elson, C.J. and Taylor, R.B., to be published.

10. Kaplan, A.M. and Cinader, B., Cell. Immunol. 6:442, 1973.

11. Mitchell, G.F., Lafleur, I. and Andersson, K., Scand. J. Immunol. 3:39, 1974.

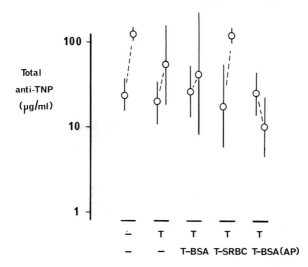

Fig. 1. Effect of different treatments designed to induce TNP-specific tolerance. Ig^b mice were injected with a single dose of 5 mg TNPS i.p. ("T") or left as controls. Other groups were given a further pretreatment one hour after the injection of TNPS: 1 mg TNP-BSA in solution (T-BSA); 2x 10^8 TNP-SRBC (T-SRBC) or 1 mg TNP-BSA(AP) all given i.p. They were challenged at 10 days with 250 mg TNP-SG(AP) (1st symbol of each pair), and again at 31 days (2nd symbol) after pretreatment. They were bled at 21 days after each challenge.

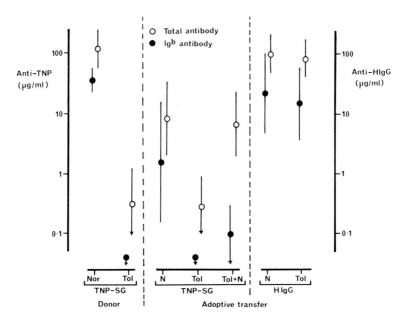

<u>Fig.</u>   2.   TNP-specific tolerance.   Some splenectomized
mice were given 5 injections of TNPS and one of TNP-BSA(AP)
("TOL"), and others left as non-tolerant controls ("N").
Ten days later some were killed and 2.5 x 10^7 of their lymph
node cells transferred to irradiated CBA recipients.   One
group also received 2.5 x 10^7 normal CBA spleen cells as a
source of T cells which had not had contact with the
tolerance procedure ("Tol + N").   One day after transfer,
some recipients were challenged with HIgG(AP) as a control
for specificity of tolerance; while the rest, and the
surviving donors, were challenged with TNP-SG(AP).   All
were bled 21 days after challenge.   The figure shows a high
degree of specific tolerance for the Ig^b antibody; slightly
less for total antibody - presumably because of contribution
by the irradiated host.

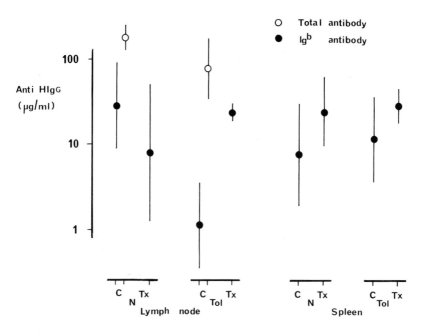

Fig. 3. Effect of T cell depletion on induction of B cell tolerance to HIgG. Some Ig^b mice were thymectomized at 2 months of age, and others left as controls. Six weeks later they were all irradiated (850 r) and repopulated with 5×10^6 anti-theta-treated Ig^b bone marrow cells. After a further 6 weeks half of them were each injected with 2.5 mg deaggregated HIgG. Fourteen days after this they were killed and their cells (2.5×10^7 spleen or 10^7 lymph node) transferred to irradiated (500 r) CBA recipients. Each recipient was also given 10^7 CBA spleen cells as a source of non-tolerant T cells. All recipients were challenged a few hours after transfer with 250 mg HIgG(AP). The figure shows tolerance induced in lymph node B cells of the <u>non operated, but not of the thymectomized donors</u>. No tolerance is evident in the splenic B cells. In addition, the figure shows that the tolerant lymph node cells did not affect the ability of CBA spleen cells to respond to HIgG.

B CELL TOLERANCE INDUCED BY NON-METABOLIZED
OR TOXIC ANTIGENS

John H. Humphrey

National Institute for Medical Research
The Ridgeway, Mill Hill
London NW7 1AA

My colleagues and I have been examining the stimulation and inactivation (tolerization) of B cells in mice by hapten-conjugated T cell independent carriers in the hope of learning more about the way in which epitopes on the antigen interact with specific receptors on the B cells, so as either to stimulate these into antibody secretion or to inactivate or eliminate them. Most of our experiments have involved stimulation of B cells in vivo, and they complement (and to some extent complicate) the elegant in vitro experiments done by Feldmann and his colleagues using hapten-conjugated T independent antigens. Although we hoped with our systems to eliminate the need to consider the role of T cell cooperation (which means that for many, though not all, biologically relevant antigens our analysis may not apply), we are aware that consideration of the role of macrophages in capturing, holding and releasing the antigens and any special anatomical considerations is also omitted. Nevertheless, it is possible to reach some tentative generalizations about the mode of action of T-independent antigens whose conclusions are relevant to and broadly in agreement with the conclusions of others presented at this meeting.

Early experiments (1) using DNP-lys-S3 showed that small amounts of DNP-lys-S3 added either in vivo or in vitro could specifically inactivate DNP-primed B cells so that no or a negligible IgG anti-DNP response resulted on stimulation with DNP on the original carrier. This was attributed to interaction of the DNP-lys-S3 with B$^\gamma$ memory cells with anti-DNP receptors, coupled with failure to recruit carrier specific T cells. Without an additional stimulus from T cells, the B cells would be inactivated and perhaps eliminated, rather than activated to proliferate and secrete Ig. The question was left open whether persistence of DNP-lys-S3 in the circulation and failure to be degraded at the cell surface was a contributory factor.

We have now examined the behavior in C3H or (CBA x C57) Fl hybrid mice of several more hapten conjugates of carriers which are T-independent immunogens (or not even immunogenic) in respect of their capacities to induce primary anti-hapten and/or anti-carrier responses; of their capacity to induce primary unresponsiveness; of their ability to inhibit secondary anti-hapten IgG responses and the effect of mild graft versus host reactions (allogeneic effect) upon such inhibition. The conjugates used were $DNP_{0.6}$-lys-S3, $DNP_{2.5}$-lys-S3, $DNP_{4.6}$-lys-S3, $DNP_{1.9}$-lys-levan (LE) and $DNP_{2.9}$-lys-hyaluronic acid (HA). The carriers are all large molecules made up of simple multiply repeated units and are slowly metabolized (even hyaluronic acid had a half life of 5 days in the mouse). They not only have multiply repeated epitopes of their own, but the attached hapten is also multiply repeated.

Immunogenicity:

Anti-hapten responses. All conjugates induce a markedly dose dependent IgM response with little or no IgG anti-hapten antibody. The response is transient, despite the fact that all the hapten carrier complexes persist in the body (and in small amounts in the tissue fluids) for weeks or months (2).

Anti-carrier responses. S3 and LE elicited dose dependent IgM responses very similar to the anti-hapten responses, as already described by Howard and his colleagues. Hyaluronic acid, being widely present in connective tissues, is not immunogenic, and antibody responses against it have not been detected despite many attempts to elicit them (3).

Primary tolerogenicity:

At higher doses (e.g. 1 mg) DNP-lys-S3, DNP-lys-LE, S3 or LE induce complete unresponsiveness both to hapten and carrier or to the relevant carrier. When the mice were challenged 14 days later, neither IgM nor IgG responses were elicited (measured as PFC). However, tolerance to LE in no way diminished the anti-DNP response to an immunogenic dose of DNP-lys-LE (Table I) nor did tolerance to DNP (induced by DNP-lys-S3) affect the anti-LE IgM response (Table II). The presence or absence of T cells had no effect on the response to DNP-lys-LE. S3 and LE are also thymus independent immunogens (J.G. Howard, this volume).

It is clear, therefore, that both positive IgM antibody responses and/or tolerance to DNP, to LE and to S3 must be elicited by interaction of the hapten carrier complex with separate populations of B^{μ} cells which recognize repeated

212

suitably spaced carrier epitopes or repeated DNP groups suitably spaced on a large carrier molecule and that there is no evidence for B cell-B cell cooperation. Furthermore, in agreement with this, the carrier need not itself be immunogenic. The effects appear to be due to direct interaction of immunogen with B^μ cells (possibly with the intervention of macrophages and other factors such as C3 activation) and to be comparable to the findings of Feldmann and his colleagues with T independent antigens in in vitro systems. The notably brief duration of the IgM response may well be attributable to conversion of the stimulatory antigen array to an inhibitory lattice by antibody (4).

TABLE I

FAILURE OF PARALYSIS TO LEVAN TO AFFECT
THE ANTI-HAPTEN RESPONSE TO DNP-LYS-LEVAN

	Immunization		PFC/spleen (x 10^{-3})[a]	
Group	Day 0	Day 10	Anti-DNP	Anti-LE
1	LE (1.0 mg)	DNP-Lys-LE (50 µg)	85.0 $\pm$ 14.6	0.34 $\pm$ 0.15
2	0	DNP-Lys-LE (50 µg)	60.8 $\pm$ 10.9	8.2 $\pm$ 1.9
3	LE (1.0 mg)	LE (50 µg)	ND	0.33 $\pm$ 0.09
4	0	LE (50 µg)	ND	17.2 $\pm$ 5.8

ND - not done

a - assays performed on Day 14; data presented as arithmetic means $\pm$ standard errors of groups of 4 mice.

Student's t test: anti-DNP PFC - GP 1 vs. GP 2, p=0.25; anti-LE PFC - GP 1 vs. GP 2, p=0.005; GP 3 vs. GP 4, p=0.01.

Tolerization of B^Y cells. Pretreatment with DNP-lys-S3 in vivo or in vitro of primed anti-DNP IgG precursor cells very readily rendered them unable to make an IgG anti-DNP response (1). It was proposed that hapten-reactive B^Y cells, which reacted with hapten on a carrier which failed to stimulate T cells, would be inactivated if no additional signal for proliferation were forthcoming. This explanation has been reinforced by observations in other experimental systems (5, 6). DNP-primed B^Y cells transferred to irradiated recipients with as little as 1 µg $DNP_{2.5}$-lys-S3 became tolerized so that on boosting with the original antigen no IgG anti-DNP is formed (see Fig. 1). They can also be tolerized by $DNP_{2.9}$-lys-HA in a similar system, but 2000 µg is required to produce a comparable effect. Since DNP-lys-HA is degradable _in vivo_ relatively rapidly (and is susceptible to hyaluronidase), this suggests that the great effectiveness of non-degradable conjugates as tolerogens may be due to their persistence after binding at the cell surface. Unprimed B^Y as well as B^μ cells can also be tolerized by DNP-lys-S3, so that they will not respond to a potent immunogen such as DNP-KLH, but the concentration required is substantially higher (Fig. 2). This suggests that binding of the DNP-lys-S3 by unprimed B cells (or their precursors) is less firm or less liable to form an inhibitory lattice.

TABLE II

FAILURE OF HAPTEN-SPECIFIC TOLERANCE TO AFFECT THE ANTI-CARRIER RESPONSE TO HAPTEN POLYSACCHARIDE CONJUGATES

Group	Immunization Day 0	Day 10	PFC/Spleen $(\times 10^{-3})$[a] Anti-DNP	Anti-SIII	Anti-LE
1	DNP-Lys-LE (1.0 mg)	DNP-Lys-LE (50 µg)	0.33 + 0.1	ND	0
2	DNP-Lys-SIII (1.0 mg)	DNP-Lys-LE (50 µg)	1.31 + 0.52	ND	7.9 + 1.9
3	0	DNP-Lys-LE (50 µg)	46.2 + 6.5	ND	9.1 + 1.3
4	DNP-Lys-SIII (1.0 mg)	DNP-Lys-SIII (50 µg)	0.48 + 0.13	2.6 + 0.5	ND
5	0	DNP-Lys-SIII (50 µg)	1.14 + 0.21	6.3 + 1.7	ND

ND - not done
a - PFC assays performed on Day 14 on groups of 5 mice; data given as arithmetic means + standard errors.
Student's t test: anti-DNP PFC - GP 2 vs. GP 3, p<0.001; GP 4 vs. GP 5, p<0.05; GP 1 vs. GP 3, p<0.001.
anti-carrier PFC - GP 2 vs. GP 3, not significant; GP 4 vs. GP 5, p<0.1.

Effect of epitope density. Tolerization of DNP-primed B cells by $DNP_{0.6}$-lys-S3 and $DNP_{2.5}$-lys-S3 was compared in an adoptive transfer system. Washed spleen cells (30×10^6) from (CBA x C57)F1 mice primed with $DNP_{11}OVA$ 3 months previously were injected i.v. into 650r irradiated syngeneic recipients, followed by 1, 10 or 50 μg of each preparation or 50 μg unconjugated S3. One day later they were challenged with 20 μg aqueous DNP OVA and splenic anti-DNP IPFC measured 9 days after transfer. $DNP_{2.5}$-lys-S3 completely suppressed the IgG response at all dose levels; $DNP_{0.6}$-lys-S3 caused almost complete suppression, but a small number of IPFC (1000-3000 per spleen) were detected which may represent relatively low affinity B^Y cells which escaped inhibition (Fig. 1). Unconjugated S3 had no effect on the anti-DNP response.

The effects on a primary response were compared as follows: C3H mice were given 2 or 4 mg $DNP_{0.6}$-lys-S3 or 0.5 or 1 mg $DNP_{2.5}$-lys-S3 one week before challenge with 200 μg alum precipitated DNP-KLH plus 2×10^9 B. pertussis. Spleen direct and indirect anti-DNP PFC were measured 8 days later. Compared with control mice, pretreatment with both doses of $DNP_{2.5}$-lys-S3 caused substantial inhibition of the IgM and almost complete inhibition of the IgG response; neither dose of $DNP_{0.6}$-lys-S3, however, diminished (and may even have increased) the IgM or IgG responses (Fig. 2). The observation that lightly substituted DNP-lys-S3 was not tolerogenic in a primary response in vivo accords with the in vitro findings of Desaymard and Feldmann (8) in respect of primary IgM responses to DNP-lys-S3 or DNP-lys-LE. The very potent tolerogenic effect on primed B^Y cells of even lightly substituted DNP-lys-S3 would not have been observed in their in vitro system. It appears that in the case of B^Y cells with high affinity receptors, so long as the hapten binds by multipoint attachment via a persistent polymeric carrier; the end result will be irreversible inactivation unless a second stimulus from T cells is provided in time.

Effect of concomitant T cell stimulation (allogeneic effect). Although anti-DNP B^Y cells were not stimulated by DNP-lys-S3, DNP-lys-LE or DNP-lys-HA--and, indeed, appeared to be inactivated by them--it seemed possible that interaction of T cells with the potentially responsive B^Y cells, in a graft versus host reaction, might overcome the inhibition (as described in other situations by Katz and colleagues (9, 10)). (CBA/H x C57BL/6)F1 mice which received CBA/H spleen cells (50×10^6 was an optimal dose) at the

same time as the immunogens (in normally immunogenic doses)
showed not only a markedly (up to 20 fold) increased IgM response, both to hapten and carrier, but also developed res-
pectable IgG anti-DNP responses, measured as indirect PFC.
The tolerance threshold was also raised, though at high doses
(e.g. 500 µg DNP-lys-LE), the IgM and especially the IgM
responses both began to diminish (Fig. 3). The allogeneic
effect did not prolong the response to either hapten or carrier moiety, and whatever mechanism cuts the response off
was still operative (11).

Although the T cell help provided by the allogeneic
effect clearly enabled primary stimulation of anti-DNP BY
cells, there was no detectable stimulation of IgG PFC in
response to the carrier moieties S3 or LE. Although this
might be due to technical failure to demonstrate IPFC, an
alternative explanation is that polysaccharide specific BY
cells either do not exist (which is unlikely) or that they
do exist but are inactivated by binding with the polysaccharides as presented with their very high epitope density despite any T cell-derived signal.

For comparison with the DNP on T-independent carriers,
Klaus and McMichael (11) also tested DNP attached to various
T-dependent protein carriers KLH, OVA and BGG. When given in
fluid form without adjuvants, 250-500 µg elicited minimal
splenic IgM and IgG anti-DNP PFC responses at 4 and 6 days;
but when allogeneic cells were also given,the IgM responses
were increased up to 8 fold and the IgG up to 30 fold. These
findings suggest that in certain circumstances non-specific
(allogeneic) T cell activity can also enhance specific
(isologous) T cell help.

The influence of epitope density on induction of B cell
tolerance by hapten protein conjugates. Klaus and Cross
(12, 13) have studied the immunogenic and tolerogenic properties in mice of DNP-BSA at hapten conjugation ratios varying from 5 to 50 DNP groups per mol. Heavily conjugated
$DNP_{50}BSA$ behaved in many ways like the T-independent conjugates discussed above, i.e. it induced a dose dependent primary IgM anti-DNP response, with relatively little IgG and
little or no immunological memory. No antibody response was
detected against serologically detectable native BSA or to
any neodeterminants resulting from dinitrophenylation.
Nevertheless, the response to DNP was highly T-dependent
(presumably due to recognition by T cells of determinants
not recognized by B cells). This indicates that a high

216

density of repeating epitope alone is not sufficient to make an immunogen T-independent, and that for this the carrier must have other characteristics such as size, shape and flexibility. $DNP_{50}BSA$ was, however, quite an effective hapten specific B cell tolerogen. Adult (CBA x C57)F1 mice were given multiple injections (5 mg 3 x per week for 2-8 weeks) of $DNP_{50}BSA$, and tolerance to DNP was assayed by challenge with DNP-KLH. Anti-DNP responses were completely suppressed by $DNP_{50}BSA$. A similar course of DNP_5BSA was a much less effective one. However, when DNP-BSA was administered during an intensive 2 week course, such that the amount of DNP hapten given as DNP_5BSA equalled that given as $DNP_{50}BSA$, they were equally able to suppress the anti-hapten response. This implies that B cell tolerance can be induced in vivo by conjugates with a low epitope density, provided that a critical concentration of epitope is maintained for long enough.

A point of considerable interest in relation to the relative ease with which B^μ and B^γ cells can be tolerized arose in studying the recovery of anti-DNP DPFC and IPFC responsiveness to stimulation with DNP-KLH after partial tolerization with $DNP_{50}BSA$ (6 x 3 mg for 2 weeks). The IgM response was less completely suppressed than the IgG and recovered more rapidly (75% compared with 15% at 6 weeks, Fig. 4). This is another indication that B^γ cells are more readily tolerized than are B^μ cells.

Recovery of B cells from tolerance or elimination. In a completely different set of experiments, we have been studying the inactivation of hapten-specific B cells by incubation with DNP attached to carrier protein or polypeptide made highly radioactive with ^{125}I (c.f.14). In this system, which has been termed "radioactive suicide", B cells are preferentially inactivated. Inactivation of all B cells reactive with the hapten is usually not achieved, and recovery of the capacity to make anti-DNP occurs within 3-4 weeks. However, by treating spleen cells from unprimed mice or mice primed with DNP-OVA with very highly radioactive DNP-^{125}I p-TGL, followed by transfer of 25 x 10^6 cells to lethally irradiated syngeneic mice, we could in some conditions achieve complete "suicide" of those DNP-specific B cells able to interact significantly with DNP-OVA. In some of the recipient mice, although carrier (OVA)-sensitized cells were present, and the antibody response to OVA was unimpaired compared with that of control cells treated with nonradioactive antigen, responsiveness to DNP (even measured by the sensitive phage inactivation test) did not begin to recover for at least 5 and up to 8 or more weeks (15). This seems to represent the time taken to generate or regenerate B cells with receptors able to respond to DNP from the stem cells present in the 25 x 10^6 million cells transferred. It is interesting that a similar time period seems to be needed for recovery of B^γ cells from tolerance induced by soluble proteins (16). Since "radioactive suicide" is presumably the result of cell death, this implies that tolerant B^γ cells are actually killed or eliminated rather than held in check by residual antigen.

CONCLUSIONS

Although most of the experiments discussed above have involved atypical immunogens, they suggest some differences between susceptibility to and perhaps mechanisms of tolerization of B^μ and B^γ cells.

B^μ cells, with IgM's receptors of variable but never very high affinity for an epitope, can bind large flexible polymeric molecules which present the epitopes in a suitable array to cause stimulation and IgM antibody secretion. Accessory factors such as "mitogenicity" (17) or C3 activation (18) and presentation via macrophages are probably not essential but may potentiate such interaction (discussed in 19) as may an allogeneic reaction. At higher concentrations (or when the antigen is not readily degradable),the cells binding antigen are tolerized. This may involve reversible or irreversible blocking or their elimination (J.G. Howard in this symposium and 2).

Receptors on B^γ cells, especially from primed animals, behave as though they have a high affinity for the epitope. Mitchell (20) among other interesting suggestions proposes that B^γ cells derived from B^μ cells, as a result of antigenic stimulation, are bound to have a high affinity for the antigenic determinant which caused such a switch to occur. Binding of polymeric antigen molecules inhibits instead of stimulating such cells unless a second stimulatory signal is provided. In the absence of a second signal inhibition becomes irreversible and/or the cell may be physically eliminated. T cell help resulting from a graft versus host reaction is an effective second signal; the B cell mitogenic stimulus provided by lipid A in bacterial lipopolysaccharides may be another (21).

15. Willcox, H.N.A., Humphrey, J.H. and Cross, A.M., in preparation.

16. Chiller, J.M. and Weigle, W.O., J. Immunol. 110:1051, 1973.

17. Coutinho, A. and Möller, G., Nature New Biol. 245:12, 1973.

18. Dukor, P. and Hartmann, K.U., Cell. Immunol. 7:349, 1973.

19. Greaves, M., Janossy, J., Feldmann, M. and Doenhoff, M., In Genes, Receptors and Signals, edited by A. Williamson and E. Sercarz, Academic Press, 1974.

20. Mitchell, G.F., In The Lymphocyte: Structure and Function, edited by J.J. Marchialous, Marcel Dekker Inc., New York, 1974.

21. Louis, J.A., Chiller, J.M. and Weigle, W.O., J. Exp.Med. 138, 1481, 1973.

ABBREVIATIONS

DNP-lys   - dinitrophenyl lysine (The ratio of DNP-lys to carrier is expressed as moles/50,000 daltons molecular weight.)

DPFC   - direct plaque-forming cells

IPFC   - indirect plaque-forming cells

S3   - high molecular weight capsular polysaccharide from diplococcus pneumoniae Type III

LE   - branched chain levan from Aerobacter aerogence

HA   - hyaluronic acid purified from human umbilical cords

OVA   - hen ovalbumin

BGG   - bovine gamma globulin

One mystery which particularly needs solving is why T-independent antigens apparently do not themselves react with T cells. Are there no T cells with receptors capable of interacting with the epitopes involved (which seems unlikely)? Or, if they exist, are they inevitably tolerized by the antigen and unable to cooperate with B cells? We are currently trying to answer these questions.

REFERENCES

1. Mitchell, G.F., Humphrey, J.H. and Williamson, A.R., Eur. J. Immunol. 2:460, 1972.

2. Klaus, G.G.B. and Humphrey, J.H., accepted for publication in Eur. J. Immunol.

3. Humphrey, J.H., (unpublished).

4. Diener, E. and Feldmann, M., J. Exp. Med. 132:31, 1970.

5. Katz, D.H., Hamaoka, T. and Benacerraf, B., J. Exp. Med. 136:1404, 1972.

6. Mitchell, G.F., LaFleur, L. and Andersson, K., Scand. J. Immunol. 3:39, 1974.

7. Klaus, G.G.B., (unpublished data).

8. Desaymard, C. and Feldmann, M., in preparation.

9. Katz, D.H., Paul, W.E., Goidl, E.A. and Benacerraf, B., J. Exp. Med. 133:169, 1971.

10. Katz, D.H., Transplantation Reviews. 12:141, 1972.

11. Klaus, G.G.B. and McMichael, A.J., accepted for publication in Eur. J. Immunol., 1974.

12. Klaus, G.G.B. and Cross, A.M., accepted for publication in Cellular Immunology, 1974.

13. Klaus, G.G.B. and Cross, A.M., submitted to Journal of Experimental Medicine.

14. Golan, D.T. and Borel, Y., J. Exp. Med. 134:1046, 1971.

KLH   - keyhole limpet haemocyanin

B^{μ} cell - B cell precursor of IgM antibody-secreting
                    cell

B^{γ} cell - B cell precursor of IgG antibody-secreting
                    cell

IgM's   - subunit of IgM with 2H and 2L chains

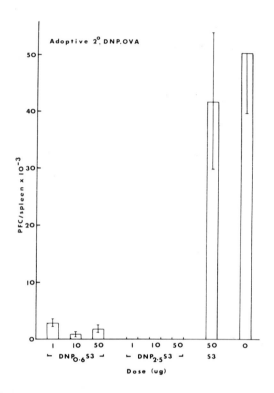

Fig. 1.   Effect of DNP-lys-S3 with different epitope densities on an adoptive 2⁰ response to DNP.
    Donors: (CBA x C57)F1 mice primed with 200 µg alum precipitated DNP_{11} OVA + 2 x 10^9 B. pertussis 3 months previously.
    Recipients: 650r irradiated F1 mice.   Each received 30 x 10^6 thrice washed spleen cells i.v., followed by 1, 10 or 50 µg $DNP_{0.6}$ lys-S3 or $DNP_{2.5}$-lys-S3 or 50 µg S3 or nothing.   The mice were challenged with 20 µg aqueous DNP-OVA the next day, and splenic indirect anti-DNP PFC measured 9 days after transfer.

222

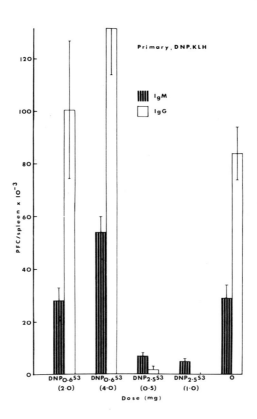

Fig. 2. Effect of DNP-lys-S3 with different epitope densities on 1° response to DNP.

C3H mice were injected i.p. with $DNP_{0.6}$-lys-S3 (2 or 4 mg); $DNP_{2.5}$-lys-S3 (0.5 or 1 mg), or not injected. One week later they were challenged with 200 µg DNP_{100} KLH + 2 x 10^9 B. pertussis. Direct and indirect anti-DNP PFC were measured in the spleen 8 days after challenge.

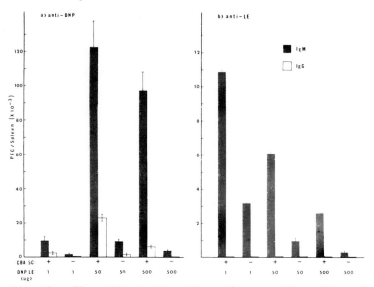

Fig. 3. The effect of antigen dose on the allogenic effect in response to DNP-lys-LE.
 (CBA x C57)F1 mice were given varying doses of $DNP_{2.5}$-lys-LE with or without 50×10^6 parental spleen cells (± CBA SC). Anti-DNP (a) and anti-LE (b) direct PFC were assayed on day 4 and indirect PFC on day 6.

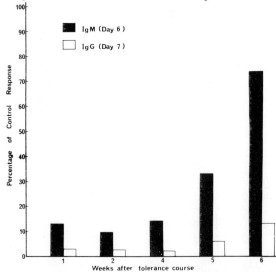

Fig. 4. Recovery of IgM and IgG anti-hapten responses after induction of partial tolerance by DNP_{50} BSA.
 Groups of CBA mice received 3×3 mg DNP_{50} BSA/week for 2 weeks. Groups of tolerized or non injected mice were then challenged with 100 µg alum-precipitated DNP-KLH + 2×10^7 B. pertussis at various time intervals after the last injection of tolerogen. IgM and IgG anti-DNP PFC were assayed in the spleen 5 and 6 days after challenge.

EFFECT OF EPITOPE DENSITY ON
THE INDUCTION OF TOLERANCE IN VITRO

Catherine Desaymard
Marc Feldmann
Paul Maurer

Department of Experimental Immunobiology, Wellcome Research
Laboratories, Beckenham, Kent, England;
I.C.R.F. Tumour Immunology Unit, Department of Zoology,
University College, London, England;
Department of Biochemistry, Jefferson Medical College,
Philadelphia, Pennsylvania

INTRODUCTION

Relatively little is yet known about the mechanisms by
which antigens induce responses in lymphocytes. Certain
antigens can induce responses in purified populations of
B cells in vitro, i.e. macrophage and T cell depleted spleen
(1). Such antigens, which have been termed "thymus
independent" (TI) directly trigger B cells, thus offering a
simple experimental model for the study of the immunogenic
or tolerogenic interactions of antigen molecules with the
surface of B cells.

It has previously been reported that the physical
structure of antigen molecules determine their capacity to
directly trigger B cells. For example, the polymerized form
of flagellin (POL), a long linear polymer, or its haptenic
conjugates, readily triggers B cells, whereas the monomeric
form does not, requiring the cooperation of both T cells
and macrophages (2,3) under the experimental conditions
studied. Thus, direct triggering of B cells depended on a
"polymeric" structure. While studying dinitrophenylated
derivatives of POL, it was found that highly conjugated DNP
POL was not immunogenic but was tolerogenic. Lower conjugates were immunogenic but never tolerogenic (4). Thus, the
number of haptenic groups conjugated per POL molecule or
"epitope density" markedly influences its capacity to
"signal" to B cells to induce immunity or tolerance.

Since this conclusion was based on studies with a
single polymeric carrier, POL, which was a protein and may
have been "denatured" by the conjugation, it was felt
essential to verify this conclusion with different carriers,

e.g. polysaccharides or synthetic antigens. This report indicates that high epitope density is required for B cell tolerance induction with DNP pneumococcal type III polysaccharide (DNP-SIII), DNP-levan (DNPLE) and DNP conjugated to a copolymer of D amino acids, glutamic acid and lysine (DNP-D-GL).

METHODS

Culture techniques for the induction of antibody responses and for tolerance induction were essentially as reported previously. The preparation of DNP-SIII, DNP-LE was as detailed elsewhere (Desaymard and Feldmann, manuscript in preparation).

DNP-D-GL of varying substitutions were prepared by using either DNP sulphonic acid or dinitrofluorobenzene under alkaline conditions (4,5). For comparison with flagellin, all substitutions of polymers, which are of polydisperse molecular weights, are expressed as no.groups/ 40,000 daltons; the 40,000 being the molecular weight of monomeric flagellin.

RESULTS

DNP-POL. Only highly conjugated DNp-POL induces tolerance. Figure 1 indicates that a substantial degree of tolerance requires about 3 DNP groups/40,000 daltons of the polymer. No tolerance was found with less than 2 groups/ 40,000 using up to 100µg/ml to induce tolerance for up to 6 hours at 37°.

DNP-SIII. SIII, obtained from J.G.Howard of Wellcome Research labs, was conjugated with various numbers of DNP groups. The results shown in Table I indicate that highly conjugated DNP-SIII induced tolerance within 4 hours in vitro, provided it had at least 1.7 DNP groups/40,000 MW of SIII. No tolerance was induced with 1 DNP/40,000. DNP-SIII induced tolerance at somewhat lower concentrations (< 1µg/ ml) than DNP-POL (4).

DNP-LEVAN. Various batches of DNP-Levan were tested for their capacity to induce DNP specific tolerance in mouse spleen cell suspensions. The results in Table II indicate that tolerance to DNP-LE also depended on the conjugation ratio;for example DNP$_{1.1}$LE did not induce tolerance even with up to 100µg/ml, whereas DNP$_{1.5}$LE and DNP$_{2.5}$LE did at concentrations of 5µg/ml or greater and 3µg/ml, respectively.

TABLE I

INDUCTION OF TOLERANCE WITH DNP-SIII IN VITRO

INDUCTION	CHALLENGE	IgM anti-DNP response (%)
NIL	DNP-LE	100
1 µg/ml $DNP_{1.1}SIII$	"	103
" $DNP_{1.7}SIII$	"	39
" DNP_2SIII	"	21
" DNP_8SIII	"	9

4 hour preincubation of normal CBA mouse spleen with DNP-SIII at 37^0 prior to challenge with 0.5 µg/ml $DNP_{1.7}LE$.

TABLE II

INDUCTION OF TOLERANCE WITH DNP-LE IN VITRO

INDUCTION	CHALLENGE	IgM anti-DNP response (%)
NIL	DNP-LE	100
20 µg/ml LE	"	98
20 $DNP_{1.1}LE$	"	99
20 $DNP_{1.7}LE$	"	9.5
3 µg $DNP_{2.5}LE$	"	36

4 hour preincubation of normal CBA mouse spleen with LE or DNP-LE at 37^0 prior to challenge with 0.5 µg/ml $DNP_{1.7}LE$.

DNP-D-GL. DNP-D-GL has been reported by Katz et al (6) to be a uniquely powerful tolerogen, both in vivo and in vitro perhaps because it is nonimmunogenic and not easily degraded. It was thus of interest to know whether the epitope density effect was also true for DNP-D-GL. Thus, a wide range of DNP-D-GL batches were prepared and tested. Low conjugates were found to be nontolerogenic (Table III) and were, in fact, strong thymus-independent antigens (unpublished data).

TABLE III

INDUCTION OF TOLERANCE WITH DNP-D-GL IN VITRO

INDUCTION		CHALLENGE	IgM anti-DNP Response (AFC/culture)
NIL		NIL	113
NIL		DNP-LE	705
10 µg DNP-D-GL	(3/1)	"	593
10 "	(3/3)	"	563
10 "	(3/10)	"	630
10 "	(3/30)	"	580
10 "	(3/100)	"	350
1 "	"	"	613
1 "	(high)	"	127
10^{-1} "	"	"	250
10^{-2} "	"	"	533

Normal spleen cells were incubated for 4 hours at 37° with DNP-D-GL before being washed and challenged with 0.5 µg of $DNP_{1.7}LE$. Figures in brackets represent ratio DGL to DNP sulphonic acid in reaction mixture during preparation. "High" refers to a preparation made with dinitroflurobenzene. Approximate coupling ratios (based on spectophotometry) 3/1-1.2 DNP/4 x 10^4; 3/3-0.5 DNP/4 x 10^4; 3/10-1 DNP/4 x 10^4; 3/30-2 DNP/4 x 10^4; 3/100-4 DNP/4 x 10^4; "high"-14 DNP/4 x 10^4.

TNP-coated beads. The "antigen presentation" concept of thymus independence suggests that a thymus-dependent (TD) antigen bound to a surface will become thymus independent. This prediction was verified with TNP conjugated to keyhole limpet haemocyanin (TNP-KLH) covalently coupled to sepharose (7). With this antigen as well, immunogenicity depended on the amount of TNP-KLH conjugated per bead. Too highly conjugated beads were nonimmunogenic, as shown in Fig. 2. However, it is difficult to do tolerance experiments with beads, as a diminution of the response of spleen cells incubated with beads could be due to physical removal of the cells (immunoadsorption) rather than tolerance. At the moment it is not certain whether these highly conjugated beads are tolerogenic.

DISCUSSION

The importance of a high epitope density for the induction of high zone tolerance in B cells in vitro, reported initially with DNP-POL (4), is now confirmed with several, quite different polymeric carriers. Results were reported with two polysaccharides, linear SIII (Table I) and the highly branched levan (Table II) with a linear synthetic polypeptide of D amino acids, D-GL (Table III)and also with hapten coupled into the surface of beads (7). Thus,the validity of the principle of high epitope density for the induction of B cell tolerance with thymus independent polymeric antigens in vitro seems established. In fact, it has been possible to induce transferable tolerance in vitro with DNP-SIII, whereas SIII by itself does not (8), indicating that the incapacity of SIII to tolerize was not due to its physical structure but rather due to its chemical nature. There are other forms of tolerance induction in vitro, where the importance of epitope density is not yet clear. Antibody-mediated tolerance induced by complexes of antigen and antibody (9) can be envisaged as having the same mechanism, i.e. initiated by the presentation of a crowded matrix of determinants (10). Such a concept is currently being tested using lightly coupled hapten-protein conjugates. Similarly, specific T cell suppression in vitro (11), which is thought to be caused by the direct interaction of IgT-antigen complexes with the surface of lymphoid cells, is envisaged as having a similar mechanism. Again, the role of epitope density has not been tested.

There is increasing evidence that high epitope density is of importance for the induction of B cell tolerance in vivo. Highly conjugated DNP-D-GL is a potent tolerogen (6). DNP-SIII, DNP-LE and DNP dextrans of varying conjugations are being tested in vivo; the preliminary results confirming the ones obtained in vitro (Desaymard, unpublished data).

Despite the importance and generality of the epitope density effect in vitro and in vivo, there is little knowledge as to how tolerance is induced.

The epitope density phenomenon was found to be immunologically specific, i.e. high conjugation with DNP did not facilitate tolerance to small numbers of dansyl groups. This specificity rules out trivial explanations of the phenomenon, involving grossly altered properties of the carrier such as "denaturation".

Very basic questions remain unanswered. The first is the fate, on the surface of antigen binding cells, of tolerogens compared with immunogens. Diener and Paetku (12) obtained results with tritiated POL at high concentrations which were compatible with the notion that the receptors are "fixed". Whether this is also true for other tolerogens needs to be elucidated. It is also not clear how long a tolerogenic stimulus must remain at the surface to induce tolerance. Does this vary with different carriers or different concentrations of antigen? All these questions must be answered before in vitro tolerance in B cells begins to be understood.

SUMMARY

Evidence for the importance of high hapten density for the rapid induction of tolerance in unprimed B cells was presented by using DNP conjugates of a protein polymer, polymeric flagellin, or polysaccharide polymers, SIII and Levan and of a synthetic polymer of D amino acids. Nevertheless, the exact mechanism of this high epitope density effect remains unclear.

REFERENCES

1. Feldmann, M., Contemp. Topics Molecular Immunology. Volume 3, 1974. In press.

2. Feldmann, M. and Basten, A., J. Exp. Med. 134:103, 1971.

3. Feldmann, M., J. Exp. Med. 135:1049, 1972.

4. Feldmann, M., J. Exp. Med. 135:735, 1972.

5. Katz, D.H., Paul, W.E., Goidl, E.A. and Benacerraf, B., J. Exp. Med. 133:169, 1971.

6. Katz, D.H., Hamaoka, T. and Benacerraf, B., J. Exp. Med. 136:1404, 1972.

7. Feldmann, M., Greaves, M.F., Parker, D.C. and Rittenberg, M.D., Eur. J. Immunol. In press.

8. Kotlarski, I., Courtenay, B.M. and Howard, J.G., Eur. J. Immunol. 3:506, 1973.

9. Feldmann, M. and Diener, E., J. Exp. Med. 131:247, 1970.

10. Diener, E. and Feldmann, M., Transplant. Rev. 8:76, 1972.

11. Feldmann, M., Nature New Biol. 242:82, 1973.

12. Diener, E. and Paetku, V., Proc. Nat. Acad. Sci. (USA). 69:2364, 1972.

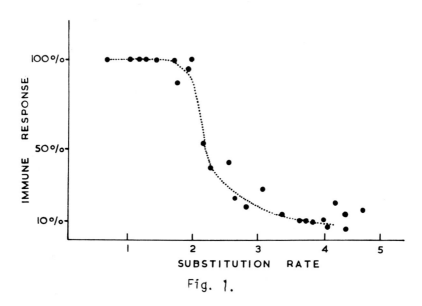

Fig. 1.

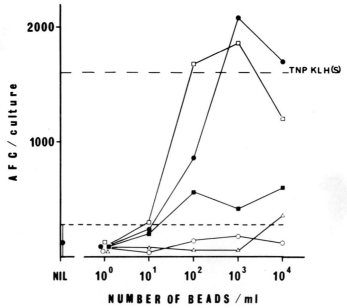

Fig. 2.

GENERAL DISCUSSION - SESSION II

B CELL TOLERANCE

G. Möller, Chairman

G. MÖLLER: I want to outline various possible mechanisms of
B cell tolerance in order to structure the discussion.
I will base the analysis on one postulate; namely, that
activation of B cells is caused by one nonspecific
triggering signal which is not delivered to the cell by
the Ig receptor. The relevant signal is either intrinsic to the antigen in the case of thymus-independent
(TI) antigens, which are all polyclonal B cell activators (PBA) or brought to the B cell by various helper
cells (T cells or macrophages) in the case of thymus-
dependent (TD) antigens. The role of the Ig receptor is
only to focus the antigen to the surface. The B cell
will be activated when a sufficient number of PBA signals have been generated at the surface. Since the Ig
receptors specifically concentrate the antigen, only
specific cells will be activated at immunogenic antigen
concentrations. The specific B cells will be turned
off (paralyzed) by superoptimal concentrations of the
inducer, as has been shown experimentally.

With this model as a background, I will analyze
possible mechanisms of paralysis. The available experimental evidence suggests the existence of several forms
of paralysis. The phenomena are complicated by the
facts that paralysis can be induced separately in T and
B cells and that the kinetics of induction and the persistence of paralysis are different between these cells.
Although this discussion deals specifically with activation and paralysis of B cells, it is necessary for the
sake of completeness to deal also with T cells. However, it is not necessary for an understanding of the
general principles to outline in detail my views on the
mechanism of activation and paralysis of T cells, except
for the general statement that we consider it likely
that T cells are activated by antigens binding to
specific receptors (whether or not these are immunoglobulins) and, therefore, that TD antigens are by themselves capable of activating T cells, in contrast to the
situation in B cells. I will not discuss various
phenomena that superficially resemble paralysis, such as
impairment of the expression of cell-mediated immunity,

233

since this may be caused by a variety of mechanisms not
necessarily related to the signal discrimination between
activation and paralysis. In order to discuss various
possibilities of inducing immunological paralysis, we
want to separate two main phenomena - induction of
paralysis to TI and TD.

Paralysis to TI Antigens

As pointed out previously, TI antigens are competent to activate B cells because they are PBA. It has
also been shown that superoptimal stimulation of B cells
by TI antigens results in paralysis. Antigen-specific
B cells reach the paralytic threshold of TI antigen concentrations that are much lower than those needed for
nonspecific B cells (because of the focusing function of
the Ig receptors), and therefore this type of paralysis
will appear as antigen-specific, even though the
mechanism is nonspecific. All the evidence suggests
that both activation and paralysis are due to the same
PBA signal delivered to the B cells in different quantities. Therefore, antigen-specific paralysis to TI
antigens is identical to the nonresponsiveness observed
in nonspecific cells exposed to superoptimal concentrations of PBA. Consequently, there can be only one zone
of paralysis (high) to TI antigens; this is also supported by experimental evidence. Therefore, it is
reasonable to conclude that the Ig receptors do not
deliver any signal (triggering or a paralytic) to B
cells. Thus, paralysis of B cells to TI antigens is
PBA-induced.

This type of paralysis is not dependent on T cells,
is usually specific (but can be nonspecific at high
doses of TI antigen), and occurs only at high antigen
concentrations (low-zone paralysis does not exist). It
may or may not be reversible (the evidence is not strong
for either possibility), but paralysis can never be
broken by activation by PBA (in contrast to many other
forms of paralysis to be discussed below).

Paralysis to TD Antigens

For the sake of simplicity I have deliberately
avoided discussing the activation mechanism of T cells.
However, for the present discussion I will assume (without giving the supporting evidence) that the triggering

event as well as the triggering receptors are different from those of B cells. As mentioned above, I will accept the concept that antigen interacting with the T cell receptors can directly activate or paralyze T cells, depending on the quantity of antigen reacting (in analogy with PBA-induced paralysis of B cells caused by TI antigens). Paralysis is easily demonstrable with TD antigens. On the basis of the available evidence I have differentiated between three types of paralysis to TD antigens.

1. TRUE B CELL PARALYSIS (inability of B cells to triggered by PBA). This phenomenon cannot be directly induced by TD antigens, since they are not PBA and therefore require the participation of T cells or other accessory cells. It is conceivable that an excessive T cell (or other types of accessory cells) activation results in the release of superoptimal concentrations of T-cell factors, which are PBA and therefore capable of paralyzing B cells at superoptimal concentrations. This type of paralysis is thus identical to that against TI antigens (caused by superoptimal PBA, the PBA being T-cell factor or other analogous factors produced by accessory cells). Examples of this type of paralysis are found in the suppressive effect of graft-versus-host reactions and in other cases of excessive T-cell activation (such as that induced by T-cell mitogens), whether specific or nonspecific. Quite often (although unsupported by direct, experimental evidence) this type of paralysis has been ascribed to the existence of a special type of suppressor T cells. Except for self-tolerance against histocompatability antigens (see below), this type of paralysis may be rare and most easily demonstrable in experimental systems that are specifically designed to detect it. When it operates naturally and is specific (as opposed to the suppressive effect of graft-versus-host reaction), it probably appears specific for the same reasons as B cells can be specifically activated by T-cell factors--namely, by a bridging mechanism between specific antigen-binding T and B cells. This is not a likely event after injection of a soluble foreign TD antigen, although it could occur in special situations because it requires that T cells are activated by antigen and, as a consequence, para - lyze B cells. Thus, true B-cell paralysis can occur only in high zone, is an indirect effect mediated by PBA secreted by accessory cells (T cells, macrophages),

is due to superoptimal activation, and, therefore, cannot be broken by PBA.

2. BLOCKED B CELLS. If the Ig receptors of specific B cells become occupied by TD antigens, the B cell cannot be activated by TD antigens, since the TD antigens lack PBA properties and since the blocked Ig receptors prevent linking between T and B cells. The term blocked B cells does not necessarily imply that the Ig receptors are permanently blocked by antigens. Conceptually, it is important that the interaction between TD antigens and the Ig receptors does not give rise to a paralytic signal. However, the cells that have interacted with antigen may be e.g. removed by phagocytosis, complement-mediated lysis or other mechanisms. Thus, they may not physically persist as blocked B cells. Thus, even if the T cell became activated by the TD antigen, little or no response is expected to occur. It is plausible that antigen-antibody complexes can block the Ig receptors more efficiently than free antigen, because of multiple binding (but this is not a necessary prerequisite for the existence of the phenomenon). Such B cells blocked by TD antigen can be activated by PBA. The experimental proof for the existence of this type of tolerance is that paralyzed B cells can be activated by PBA to produce their specific antibodies and that removal of the blocking antigen from the receptor by, for example, incubating the cells in vitro, trypsinizing them, or passing them through secondary hosts abolishes paralysis. However, the failure to demonstrate this does not exclude the concept (see above). This type of paralysis is specific, restricted to TD antigens, can be reversible, mostly but not always short-lasting, and may occur at antigen doses that activate T cells (it is at present impossible to predict precisely antigen dose and B-cell blocking versus T cell activation-paralysis because of lack of knowledge of the concentration gradients in the intact animal, the avidity of interaction between T and B cells and antigen, and so forth).

3. TRUE T CELL TOLERANCE. True T-cell tolerance is probably an important mechansim for establishment of paralysis to TD antigens. Because of the special properties of T-cell recognition of antigen (specificity of recognition and activation) a specific interaction

between antigen and T-cell receptors can either result in activation or paralysis, depending on the number of interacting antigen molecules (a quantitative concept). Thus, high doses of TD antigens can specifically paralyze T cells. If the T-cells are paralyzed, no response to TD antigens can be expected, even if immunocompetent specific B cells still persisted in the organism. (The mechanism of high- and low-zone paralysis- if they exist- is also outside the scope of this discussion. Receptor affinity for antigen on T and B cells is obviously of importance in this context and will be mentioned below. This type of paralysis can also be overcome by activating the B cells with PBA or by introducing cross-reacting TD antigens, as has been demonstrated by several investigators.

SELF-NON-SELF DISCRIMINATION has been considered to be an important function of the immune system. It seems most likely that functional self-reacting T cells do not exist, because their efficient killing action would endanger the existence of the individual. Self-reactive B cells may exist, although the risks for immune complex diseases and the possibility for antigen-antigbody complex-induced B-cell cytoxicity suggest that also the presence of anti-self B cells is dangerous. Such cells could be triggered by PBA or activated T cells and thus cause humoral autoimmunity.

B-cell activation can be achieved only by PBA, whereas failure of B-cell activation could be achieved in many ways, as outlined above. Even so, any scheme of activation-paralysis postulating that activation precedes paralysis invites the danger of anti-self reactivity. This dilemma can be overcome by the postulate that the first-appearing immunocompetent (T or B) cells during differentiation are susceptible only to paralysis (not to activation) by confrontation with an otherwise inductive stimulus. In other words, their threshold for triggering is so low that an interaction between ligand and the immunocompetent cells results in paralysis rather than induction. I will in turn consider the consequences of this model for self-paralysis in B and T cells.

A. B CELLS. True B-cell paralysis against self antigens could occur in two situations. (1) The self antigens are Tl antigens. As mentioned above, any

Tl antigen can cause paralysis by superoptimal stimulation. The dose necessary to establish paralysis will be higher than that needed to maintain paralysis, because in the former case already mature B cells must be paralyzed, and they require a higher PBA concentration, whereas maintenance requires lower doses because the immature B cells are more susceptible to paralysis induction. The self antigens are TD antigens and are membrane components of T cells. In such a case anti-self B cells bind to the T cells and thereby become physically linked to PBA-secreting cells. This requires that also nonactivated T cells secrete PBA. Such B cells would, therefore, be confronted with supraoptimal PBA concentrations and become paralyzed.

    B. T CELLS. True T-cell paralysis against self antigens also has to be explained by superoptimal antigen activation. However, anti-self reactivity may occur by such a mechanism, because antigen concentrations that are capable of paralyzing high-affinity cells will activate low-affinity cells. In natural paralysis to self antigens this need not be of major concern, because the first-appearing competent T cells would immediately be paralyzed by any recognition of self antigens. Any low-affinity T cells escaping paralysis could not be activated after they have matured because the threshold of triggering has been increased during differentiation. In experimentally induced paralysis, however, it is likely that both paralysis and activation will result after introduction of foreign antigen because of differences in affinities for the antigen in different cells. If it is assumed that the affinity of interaction needed for activation is lower than that needed for a detectable effector function of the activated T cells, the problem becomes less difficult. In this case T cells of low affinity for the antigen could be activated, but they could not express any function such as helper effect or cytotoxicity because these functions would require a higher degree of affinity for the antigen. Such cells would be nonsense cells without any biological significance. Possibly the recent demonstrations of anti-self reacting killer cells in F_1 hybrid and allophenic mice can be due to such a phenomenon: the in vitro systems used for the detection of killer cells may be capable of showing low-affinity cells not having any biological significance in vivo because of the extreme sensitivity of the in vitro detection system used. Analogous situations with B cells may be found where a high epitope density allows the detection of PBA induced anti-hapten-producing cells, which could not be immunologically induced by the same hapten.

GERSHON: I don't understand the deletion and exhaustion explanations, particularly the latter. What mechanism prevents new cells from differentiating into proper B cells? Residual antigen cannot be responsible since this occurs even when the total antigen dose used to produce tolerance is not tolerogenic and thus cannot be responsible for inducing tolerance. Further, the tolerance can be transferred even though Howard showed that not enough antigen is transferred to induce tolerance in other cells.

HUMPHREY: Point 1. The very short duration of the response to polymeric T-independent antigen is at least partly due to antibody feed back-despite persistence of the antigen (which is mostly not circulating).

Point 2. Radioactive suicide of DNP responsive "B" cells by DNP-p-TGL can be so complete that apparently all B cells able to interact significantly with DNP receptors are eliminated. When 25×10^6 suicided spleen cells are transferred to lethally irradiated mice, which are challenged at various time intervals, it takes 5-8 weeks before DNP-reactive B cells are detectable. This appears to be the time taken for new responsive cells to be generated from the stem cells in the cell population transferred.

PAUL: Göran, your thesis that all T-independent antigens are "PBA's" and that tolerance simply represents an excess of the stimulatory activities of the PBA would predict a 1:1 relationship between the immunogenic and tolerogenic capacities of molecules. James Howard's finding that levan of <10,000 daltons in size is tolerogenic and not immunogenic constitutes a serious problem for your thesis.

Moreover, one would anticipate that the most powerful T-independent antigens would have the most powerful "PBA" activity. Our results with DNP-Ficoll suggest that such a relationship does not obtain.

G. MÖLLER: Neither point is relevant to the idea. If a substance has been degraded to such an extent that it is not immunogenic, it is obviously not a thymus-independent antigen any longer. Since such a substance lost the PBA property, but posesses antigenic determinants it cannot activate B cells, but is fully competent to block these cells, in accordance with the hypothesis.

Your second point is not necessarily correct for several reasons, two of which I will comment upon. 1. The Ig receptors have a much higher affinity for the antigenic determinants than the PBA receptors have for the PBA determinants. The PBA receptors probably vary in their capacity to bind different PBA's. Therefore, a certain substance can be a TI antigen without obviously being a PBA, simply because the Ig receptors bind it much more efficiently than the PBA receptors. In essence, the ultimate test for PBA activity is thymus- dependence. 2. Different PBA's act on different subpopulations of B cells. Thus, dextran-sulphate acts on primitive B cells. Depending on what you study (antibody synthesis or DNA synthesis) the different PBA's will appear differentially "strong". Moreover, they are all PBA's, but active on different B subpopulations.

BENACERRAF: Göran, I think that you would be ill-advised to consider that all cases of tolerance to thymus-dependent antigens represent instances where there is an excess of mitogenic stimulus. There will be circumstances where the susceptibility of the antigen to be metabolized may be a very important factor.

G. MÖLLER: Baruj, I agree, but I do not think that is the case. Actually, I think it is very rare that tolerance to TD antigens is caused by excess mitogenic stimulus. It can occur in rare instances (GVH reactions) but is unlikely to be a normal phenomenon.

UNANUE: The concept of antigen blockade with metabolizable antigen is not substantiated by experimental evidence. All antigens that are metabolizable can be rapidly eliminated by the lymphocyte in the absence of T helper activity.

G. MÖLLER: The term blockade does not necessarily imply that the cells persist in a blocked form. Cells that have reacted with antigen may actually be removed by a

240

variety of mechanisms (e.g. phagocytosis). Therefore, it is irrelevant whether the antigen is metabolizable or not. However, it is relevant that a TD antigen (whether metabolizable or not) cannot give a relevant signal (activating or paralytogenic) to any B cell.

WEIGLE: I would like to support Emil Unanue's contention that the rapid turnover of receptors would not permit a prolonged blockade of B cells as a mechanism of B cell tolerance and offer another possibility. With HGG the amount of tolerogen in mice remaining at a time before B cell tolerance is terminated is between 5 and 10 μg of tolerogen. Since this tolerogen is super-processed, it is probably present in an amount sufficient to maintain tolerance in newly arriving B cells. Thus, blockade seems unnecessary and the absence of B cells with specific receptor would suggest the absence of potential competent B cells.

G. MÖLLER: I agree with the second part, which restates my notion that newly differentiated B cells are very susceptible to tolerance induction. I also restate that blocking must not be taken literally. It implies an absence of a signal to the B cell, but not any of a large number of possible (but non-basic) secondary consequences of the interaction between Ig receptors and the antigen.

FELDMANN: Göran, the scheme you have put up is interesting, but, as we have discussed before, I do not think that it fits many of the facts about tolerance induction or immunity. Firstly, the basic premise of B cell triggering by polyclonal B cell activation sites is, I think, greatly in doubt, and so must the converse, that B cell tolerance of a long lasting type is due to excess of a PBA signal. This model of tolerance induction does not explain, (1) tolerance induction by antigens shown not to have PBA activity, such as DNP-D-GL, (2) does not explain the epitope density phenomena in the induction of B cell tolerance which, as described above, is true for several substances, (3) does not explain antibody mediated tolerance, (4) does not explain the deletion type of tolerance reported by Howard by the nonimmunogenic hydrolyzed levan of low MW (10,000), which is still as tolerogenic as the high MW (2 x 10^7) strongly immunogenic native levan.

This low MW material, since it is nonimmunogenic, has no PBA activitiy, so clearly tolerance cannot be due to excess PBA. This is a very strong argument against the overactive model of B cell "deletion" type tolerance.

G. MÖLLER: I have tried to emphasize that there exist several forms of tolerance. Paralysis to TI antigens is caused by excess of triggering signals. Obviously paralysis to TD antigens cannot be caused by the same mechanism, since TD antigens lack PBA properties. Therefore your questions are wrongly posed, but I will answer them anyhow. (1) Tolerance to TD antigens are not caused by PBA signals, but by other mechanisms which I outlined before. (2) The importance of epitope density is obvious in my model for TI antigens, since the focusing function of the Ig receptors will depend on the epitope density. However, it is not possible--as you have done--to conclude from this that the epitope density as such is responsible for tolerance or triggering. (3) Antibody mediated tolerance is easily explained in our model if the antigen is a PBA. If the antigen is TD, other mechanisms listed above must be used. I do not see that you have explained this type of tolerance in a meaningful way. (4) I have already answered your last point. Obviously, if the substance that cannot be recognized by T cells is not immunogenic it can induce tolerance by blocking or consequences of blocking, such as removal of blocked cells.

I would like to point out that our model is testable and has predictive value. Your cross-linking ideas cannot lead to elucidating experiments, because you have so far failed to tell us the exact conditions leading to activation and tolerance. The vague nature of the cross-linking concept by itself makes the idea less attractive. I think you owe us an explanation for the dramatic differences between substitutions of 1 and 1.7 in your hapten experiments.

DRESSER: The B cell may not see the difference between 1 and 1.7 substitutions; these are averages and there is presumably a fairly wide variation around these mean values. Perhaps there is a threshold value for the number of molecules bound with substitutions much higher than 1.7, say 4 or 5. At an average of 1 substitution this threshold is simply not reached.

PAUL: Marc, one would anticipate that in DNP_1-D-GL a substantial fraction of all the D-GL molecules which bear any DNP groups bear 2 or more such groups. Consequently, it is somewhat surprising that you observe such a marked difference in the tolerogenic capacity of DNP_1-D-GL and $DNP_{1.7}$-D-GL. If the tolerogenic moiety is D-GL bearing 2 or 3 DNP molecules as I believe you might postulate, a sufficient concentration of DNP_1- D-GL should lead to tolerance induction in view of its content of such molecules.

CLAMAN: I am addressing this to Marc Feldmann. In view of the facts that a) the DNP substitutions on POL are average, and probably have a Poisson distribution, as Bill Paul just said, and b) many people think that "tolerance is dominant", then couldn't you get tolerance merely by increasing the dose of lightly-conjugated DNP-POL (eg., DNP_1-POL)? This would raise the number of "$DNP_{1.7}$-POL" which are in DNP_1POL and thus prevent turning on the cells.

LESKOWITZ: Marc, would you consider the possibility of another type of change with increasing DNP substitution? Namely, that not only is epitope density increasing but so is the hydrophobicity of the molecule and this might affect ability to induce tolerance by stickiness to cell surface.

DIENER: I object to the notion made in this discussion that a small increase in hapten substitution should have a minimal effect on the degree of receptor cross-linking. The optimal epitope density is the one which most accurately reflects the receptor spacing. Thus the relationship between epitope density and the degree of receptor cross-linking by the conjugate cannot be a linear one. Furthermore, no one here who works with hapten-carrier conjugates has provided any data which concern the effect of hapten substitution on the configuration of the carrier. Extrapolation, therefore, from the degree of hapten substitution to that of receptor cross-linking may not be meaningful. This criticism applies more to peptide carriers than to polysaccharides which have a much more rigid structure.

KATZ: I think the issues Marc Feldmann has raised are quite important and, in a very central way, the issue of what subpopulations of B cells are responding to thymus-independent vs. thymus-dependent antigens, to which he referred in his talk, is directly related. Could he please tell us what the data is that demonstrates this point?

FELDMANN: In response to David's question, we are being cautious not to over-interpret the existing data on the role of epitope density on tolerance induction. At the moment this data is available for B cells from spleen, producing a primary IgM response in vitro to thymus-dependent antigens. At the moment we are looking at IgG responses and 2° responses, and Catherine Desaymard and James Howard are looking to see if epitope density is of importance in the induction of B cells in vivo.

One important question which has been raised by work of Reg Gorczynski and myself is whether B cells responding to T-independent and T-dependent antigens are the same. It was found that spleen cells separated by size were heterogeneous in their response to T-independent and T-dependent antigens--some only respond to T-independent antigens. Thus it must be checked whether the role of epitope density is the same for both subpopulations of B cells. But David Katz's in vivo results with DNP-D-GL of high epitope density, would suggest that it would be the same.

G. MÖLLER: In response to both David Katz and Marc Feldmann I wish to point out that it has been quite clearly demonstrated by Eva Gronowicz that different TI antigens and consequently PBA act on subpopulations of B cells. The experiments makes it likely that these cells are in different stages of differentiation, but belong to the same cell line. The most mature cells appears to be those responding to PPD and PVP and most probably to T cell factors. However, the triggering event is the same in all of these cells. It is, therefore, illogical to conclude that the existence of subsets of B cells reflect different triggering mechanisms; a conclusion which has been made quite often.

NOSSAL: I am not as unsympathetic to the idea that a hapten-focussed excess of PBA or Signal 2 activity is a tolerogenic mechanism as were my colleagues Feldmann and Diener. For this reason, I want to set the record straight on three points. First, Schrader finds that allogeneic factors do not have PBA or signal 2 activity;

rather, they amplify clonal expansion, once a B cell has been triggered. Secondly, there is a T-independent tolerogenesis by antigen-antibody complexes, yet antibody does not have signal 2 activity. If this is purely blockade, it should not be irreversible, yet Diener and Feldmann claim it is. Thirdly, I do not believe in absolute distinctions between T-dependent and T-independent carriers. For example, $DNP_{20}HGG$ can give anti-DNP responses in nude mice. Perhaps Dr. Möller can comment on these three specific points.

G. MÖLLER: T cell factors have been found by several investigators to have PBA activity and to induce polyclonal antibody synthesis. However, they are rather weak PBA and need not necessarily be detected if the tissue culture conditions are such that strong PBA is already present, by eg., "good" sera. Furthermore, the T cell factors act on a very differentiated B cell population and it is likely that the effect is nore easily detected in primed cells, exactly as Schrader found. That he could not find that it had signal 2 activity probably depends on the fact that there are no signal 2. The synergy between PBA and antigen which is Schrader's test system has never been found to work with truly TD protein antigens such as gamma globulins. There are several explanations for this which we have outlined in Scan. J. Immunology. My main point now is to state the synergy is mostly due to trivial events when it occurs, that it is due to helper cells such as macrophages and does not represent a direct interaction at the B cell level between antigen and PBA.

If the experiments claiming that antigen-antibody complexes induce tolerance are correct they must be explained by blocking or selective removal of cells that have interacted with complexes. There is no reason and actually no data to show that a complex gives a signal to the B cell.

Finally, there is no sharp distinction between TI and TD antigens in many cases. Truly TI antigens are pure polysaccharides and truly TD antigens are pure Ig. Other antigens have both properties. Thus, KLH is a PBA but at the same time a TD antigen. Actually, LPS can be shown to be TD if it is present on bacteria with intact proteins. It is rather easy to see why this is so. If an antigen can be recognized by T cells it will receive T cell help even if it is a PBA. This help acts primarily on differentiated cells giving rise to IgG antibodies, whereas in the absence of T help the PBA property would have stimulated B cells by itself, but a different subpopulation giving rise to mainly IgM antibodies with most PBA. However, others (PVP) would also give rise to IgG even in the absence of T help, because the target B cell population for PVP is a differentiated cell.

GERSHON: We must distinguish between thymus-dependent antigens and thymus-dependent antibodies or B cells. The concept of thymus-dependent antigens is historical and misleading. All antigens are thymus-independent in that they can elicit an antibody response in nude mice, albeit poorly in some cases. Thus, the key question is, it seems to me, what difference is there in T-dependent and independent B cells in terms of triggering requirements. Some antigens trigger T-independent B cells well and some don't. A subset of the above also trigger T cells while another doesn't. A third group of antigens triggers T cells but not thymus-independent B cells. None of these antigens trigger thymus-dependent B cells without some form of T cell help. By framing the questions we ask in different forms, we may serve to identify problems requiring different explanations.

G. MÖLLER: I disagree with the interpretation, but not the facts. Subpopulations exist which are triggered by different antigens selectively, but this does not mean that the triggering event is different. Actually the work by Gronowicz and Coutinho strongly indicates that the triggering mechanism is identical.

MECHANISMS OF B CELL TOLERANCE

HUGH McDEVITT, CHAIRMAN

REVERSIBLE AND IRREVERSIBLE B CELL TOLERANCE: DISTINGUISHING PROPERTIES AND MECHANISMS

David H. Katz and Baruj Benacerraf

Department of Pathology
Harvard Medical School
Boston, Massachusetts 02115

INTRODUCTION

In the preceding session we briefly described the basic phenomenological features of DNP-specific B cell tolerance induced by exposure of cells either in vivo or in vitro to the DNP derivative of the copolymer D-glutamic acid, D-lysine (DNP-D-GL) (this volume, Katz, D.H.). The present session is broadly entitled "Mechanisms of B Cell Tolerance", a rather bold title inasmuch as we are still at a stage of relative guesswork concerning precise mechanisms involved in inactivation processes at the cellular and subcellular level. However, it is my optimistic belief that Immunologists working in this area have developed at the very least a more sophisticated capability in our guesswork that has permitted us to focus on the most pressing questions that need to be answered and, moreover, to recognize certain of the better technical approaches to follow or to develop to answer such questions.

In this presentation I will attempt to demonstrate two readily discernible forms of B cell inactivation with possibly distinct tolerogenic mechanisms which provide usable investigative models to: 1) further our understanding of tolerance mechanisms, and 2) develop clinically applicable methods for specifically abolishing deleterious antibody responses. Since it is not yet clear whether or not similar inactivation processes may occur in T lymphocytes, no deliberate analogy is either intended or warranted from the available data.

The two readily discernible forms of B cell inactivation to which I am referring are: 1) rapidly irreversible B cell tolerance of which the paradigm example is the DNP-specific inactivation induced by DNP-D-GL and perhaps comparable molecules, and 2) reversible B cell inactivation, probably best termed B cell refractoriness, which can be induced by appropriate exposure of cells either to:
a) metabolizable, conventional or autologous antigens in

which little or no helper T cell function exists and/or in which the activity of suppressor T cells may be involved, or b) a certain class of T-independent antigens, namely, pneumococcal polysaccharide (SIII) and lipopolysaccharide, which may or may not inactivate cells by comparable cellular events as the aforementioned substances.

RAPIDLY IRREVERSIBLE B CELL TOLERANCE INDUCED BY DNP-D-GL

There are three findings that collectively support the conclusion that DNP-D-GL rapidly induces a state of irreversible B cell tolerance: 1) The tolerant state of a cell population is not altered or reversed either by passive incubation of tolerant cells in vitro or by serial adoptive transfer in vivo (1-4); 2) The tolerant state of a cell population is not, once induced, altered or reversed by providing a very potent non-specific T cell stimulus such as that provided by the allogeneic effect (2, 5)--on the other hand, an allogeneic effect of appropriate magnitude induced at an appropriate time prior to administration of DNP-D-GL will prevent tolerance induction and, indeed, result in immune induction following encounter of the DNP-specific cells with the normally tolerogenic moiety (5-9); and 3) The tolerant state induced by DNP-D-GL is not readily reversed by enzymatic treatment of cells with trypsin at times and under conditions in which B cell refractoriness induced in other ways will be reversed by such treatment (1, 2). These observations are reviewed in detail in the following sections.

Failure to reverse tolerance by serial transfers and lack of suppressor cell activity in DNP-D-GL-induced tolerance.

The observations by several independent investigators that removal and transfer of lymphocytes from tolerant animals to nontolerant, syngeneic irradiated recipients results in rapid loss of the tolerant state (10-12), raise serious questions about the nature and mechanisms of central immunologic tolerance. When dealing with tolerance models involving both T and B lymphocytes, the matter of interpretative construction of results must of necessity be extremely complex. However, when the tolerant state being studied is shown to be an isolated B cell-specific tolerance, the issue becomes rather clear cut: In such instances tolerance either reflects a central (i.e. intra-cellular) inhibitory state or a surface (i.e. receptor-blocking) event. If the former is true, one would expect tolerance not to be easily reversible and not to depend (once fully induced) on the constant presence of tolerogen; the converse reasoning applies to the latter alternative. In the mouse adoptive transfer experiments described above in the preceding session we observed that DNP-keyhole limpet hemocyanin (KLH)-primed cells obtained from donors which had been treated with DNP-D-GL 7 days before adoptive transfer maintained a significant degree of tolerance in the untreated irradiated recipients. This result suggests a true central tolerizing event in this model. We performed the following series of experiments to approach this question more completely.

The protocol and results of the first experiment are summarized in Fig. 1. As shown in the earlier experiments, the secondary anti-DNP response in the first adoptive transfer was abolished by DNP-D-GL treatment of either the recipient immediately after cell transfer (groups II and IV) or of the DNP-KLH cell donors 7 days prior to transfer (group III). When these first transfer recipients were then used as donors for the second adoptive cell transfer, the results very clearly show that such manipulation does not result in a loss of the tolerant state. Thus, group I recipients of cells which had never been exposed to the tolerogen developed very good anti-DNP antibody responses. In contrast, recipients of cells which had been exposed to DNP-D-GL in the first transfer, but not subsequently (group III), manifested profound DNP-specific tolerance. Even more striking, however, is the fact that a highly significant degree of tolerance was evident in group V recipients whose cells had not been exposed to DNP-D-GL since the original donors were so treated 24 days earlier. It follows, therefore, that recipients in group VII should be tolerant, as indeed, they are. As expected, essentially no secondary response was obtained in recipient mice treated with DNP-D-GL after the second transfer (groups II, IV, VI and VIII).

These results immediately raised two questions in our minds as to the possible explanations of the data. The first possibility was that we were not only serially transferring tolerant cells but small tolerogenic doses of DNP-D-GL as well. The second possibility was that treatment with DNP-D-GL had induced a population of DNP-specific suppressor cells. We approached these questions by repeating and modifying the preceding experiment in part. Thus, groups I and II of the first adoptive transfer were set up as shown in Fig. 1. On day 7 after DNP-KLH challenge, the animals were bled (yielding comparable results as those shown in Fig. 1), and their spleen cells adoptively transferred intravenously to new recipients (50 x 10^6 cells/recipient). Certain groups of recipients of cells rendered tolerant by DNP-D-GL in the first adoptive transfer were also injected on the same day with varying numbers of spleen cells from DNP-KLH-primed donor mice. Comparable groups of mice which received only the respective numbers of these "fresh" DNP-primed cells were established as controls. Three days later all mice were secondarily challenged with 100 µg of DNP-KLH and then bled 7 days thereafter.

The data from the second transfer of this experiment is depicted graphically in Fig. 2. The left panel of this figure reiterates the observation made in the preceding experiment, namely, that the DNP-specific tolerant state is maintained in cells transferred to a second recipient (solid bar). However, when these tolerant cells are transferred simultaneously with freshly obtained DNP-KLH-primed cells, they do not exert a suppressive effect on the adoptive secondary anti-DNP response (open bars of right panel, Fig. 7). This was true even when relatively low numbers (12.5 x 10^6) of fresh DNP-primed cells were employed. It is not immediately clear why the combination of tolerant cells and fresh DNP cells gave somewhat better responses than fresh cells alone, although the differences are not statistically significant.

This experiment, therefore, argues strongly against the possibility that either: 1) Tolerogenic amounts of DNP-D-GL have been serially transferred or 2) DNP-D-GL treatment has generated suppressor cell activity in quantities sufficient to maintain the tolerant state in these cells and suggests rather the existence of a central, intracellular mechanism of specific paralysis.

Capacity of the Allogeneic Effect to Alter or Reverse Tolerance Induced by DNP-D-GL.

The allogeneic effect has been shown to be a potent T cell stimulus capable of influencing antigen-induced activation of B lymphocytes (8, 9, 13). Indeed, as pointed out in the preceding session, our fortuitous discovery of the tolerogenic properties of DNP-D-GL came about in our search for a suitable non-immunogenic molecule with which to test the hypothesis that allogeneic T cells were reacting directly with DNP-specific B lymphocytes. The positive results obtained in this type of experiment performed initially in guinea pigs (Fig. 3) constituted, in fact, the strongest early evidence that such cell interactions were taking place (5). As shown in Fig. 3, strain 13 guinea pigs primed to DNP-ovalbumin (OVA) three weeks earlier were injected with appropriate numbers of allogeneic (strain 2) lymphoid cells six days prior to secondary challenge. Under these conditions administration of DNP-D-GL resulted in elicitation of a clear secondary anti-DNP antibody response not statistically lower than that elicited by the immunogenic conjugate, DNP-bovine gamma globulin (BGG). Although not shown here, analysis of splenic DNP-specific plaque-forming cells in these animals demonstrated that equivalent numbers, and of the IgG class, were elicited by both DNP-D-GL and DNP-BGG in this experiment (5).

Precisely the same results have been obtained in secondary responses in mice undergoing an allogeneic effect (6, 9). Moreover, as shown in Fig. 4, an appropriately timed allogeneic effect in mice--namely, one induced prior to administration of antigen--can provide the necessary helper influence for generating primary antibody responses of the IgG class to DNP-D-GL (7). The reasons for failing to obtain augmented primary responses to conventional antigens in this system are discussed at length elsewhere (7). In addition, very recent observations in our laboratories have shown that a biologically active substance produced by T cells and released into supernatants of cultures of allogeneic cell mixtures can provide the necessary additional stimulus to permit DNP-primed B cells to respond to DNP-D-GL in vitro (14). Finally, it has recently been shown that DNP-D-GL can itself elicit primary in vitro anti-DNP responses, restricted to the IgM class, provided the molecule is either first attached to macrophage cell surface membranes or added to cultures in very low concentrations (15) or that the substitution ratio of DNP determinants is restricted to the low epitope density range (this volume, Desaymard et al).

The point of the preceding discussion has been to emphasize the critically important fact that the predominantly tolerogenic molecule DNP-D-GL can and does provide a specific immunogenic signal in the proper milieu or in a narrow concentration range. Thus, such observations provide a starting point to question certain parameters of B cell inactivation by DNP-D-GL. The most important of these concerns the degree of reversibility of such a tolerant state inasmuch as this feature offers an indirect view into possible mechanisms involved. The following series of experiments were designed to probe the capacity of the allogeneic

effect, a source of strong T cell action to alter the responsiveness of B cells subjected to various tolerance-
inducing regimens.

a) Induction of the allogeneic effect one day after
administration of DNP-D-GL in vivo.
     In a representative experiment in guinea pigs (Fig. 5),
strain 2 and strain 13 guinea pigs were treated with DNP-D-
GL one day prior to transfer of allogeneic lymphoid cells
(5). Such subsequent allogeneic cell transfer did not,
however, alter the tolerogenic effects of DNP-D-GL since pre-
treated animals were unable to develop augmented primary
anti-DNP antibody responses to a later immunization with
DNP-OVA in contrast to allogeneic cell recipient controls
not pretreated with DNP-D-GL. Figure 5 also reiterates the
DNP-specific nature of the tolerance induced by DNP-D-GL,
since anti-OVA antibody responses were clearly not affected
in treated guinea pigs.

b) When DNP-specific tolerance is induced by exposure
of DNP-KLH-primed cells to DNP-D-GL in vivo in adoptive
recipients.
     The protocol of this experiment is schematically de-
picted in the left panel of Fig. 6. As shown in the right
panel of Fig. 6, very good anti-DNP responses were elicited
in the second adoptive recipients of primed cells exposed
only to saline in the initial recipients, and these responses were not significantly affected by allogeneic cell transfer. In contrast, cells exposed to DNP-D-GL in the first
recipients developed markedly diminished responses, lower by
more than 90% of controls, irrespective of whether or not
allogeneic cells were included in the second transfer (2).

c) When DNP-specific tolerance is induced by incubation
of DNP-KLH-primed mouse cells in vitro with DNP-D-GL before
adoptive transfer.
     The far left panel of Fig. 7 summarizes schematically
the protocol for two experiments in which DNP-KLH-primed
cells were incubated with DNP-D-GL in vitro at different
temperatures (2). The left and right data panels depict the
results obtained with cells incubated at 4°C and 37°C,
respectively. Essentially no substantial differences attributable to temperature of incubation were observed. In both
experiments when no additional allogeneic cells were transferred, very good adoptive secondary anti-DNP antibody responses were obtained with control cells incubated with
saline provided secondary challenge with DNP-KLH was carried

out. Cells incubated with DNP-D-GL manifested poor responses to DNP-KLH challenge that were diminished by more than
95% irrespective of the temperature of incubation. When
additional allogeneic cells were transferred, the secondary
response of control saline-treated cells was enhanced in one
experiment (right panel, 37°C incubation) but not in the
other (left panel, 4°C). The responses to DNP-KLH obtained
with cells incubated with DNP-D-GL were increased as a result of allogeneic cell transfer in both experiments.
Whereas these increases are clearly statistically significant
when compared to responses of cells exposed in vitro to DNP-
D-GL and transferred without allogeneic cells, it should be
noted that the secondary responses in the presence of allogeneic cells were still diminished by more than 92% as compared to the responses of respective saline control cells in
the presence of allogeneic cells. Nevertheless, the fact
that a significant increase in response could be obtained as
a result of allogeneic cell transfer indicates the presence
of a sub-population of DNP-specific B cells capable of being
triggered by a sufficient T cell stimulus even after exposure to the tolerogenic signal.

Taken collectively, therefore, our best evidence leans
heavily towards the conclusion that a very potent T cell
activation mechanism, such as the allogeneic effect, which
is capable of providing sufficient helper function to permit
non-tolerant B cells to respond to DNP-D-GL in conditions of
appropriate timing, fails to reverse the tolerant state once
apparently the tolerogenic signal has been translated to the
DNP-specific B lymphocytes.

Capacity of enzymatic treatment of cells with trypsin
to alter or reverse DNP-specific tolerance induced by DNP-
D-GL.
In our initial studies with this system in mice (1), we
had been able to render DNP-KLH-primed spleen cells relatively unresponsive by exposing them for appropriate lengths
of time in vitro to either DNP-D-GL or a DNP conjugate of an
unrelated carrier protein such as OVA. Thus, as shown in
Table I, cells exposed to these reagents developed markedly
diminished adoptive secondary anti-DNP antibody responses
when transferred to irradiated recipients and challenged
with DNP-KLH. However, a difference in the unresponsive
states caused by DNP-D-GL as opposed to DNP-OVA was shown in
that gentle enzymatic treatment of such cells with trypsin
completely reversed the unresponsiveness in the case of cells
exposed to DNP-OVA, but not in the case of cells exposed to

TABLE I

FAILURE TO REVERSE TOLERANCE INDUCED IN VITRO WITH DNP-D-GL BY
TRYPSINIZATION OF CELLS PRIOR TO ADOPTIVE TRANSFER TO IRRADIATED RECIPIENTS

Cells Incubated in vitro with	PROTOCOL * No Trypsin			PROTOCOL * Trypsin-Treated		
	Group	Number of cells Transferred	Anti-DNP µg/ml **	Group	Number of cells Transferred	Anti-DNP µg/ml **
Saline	A	20×10^6	2471.3	B	10×10^6	1621.0
DNP-D-GL	C	20×10^6	107.4	D	13×10^6	55.8
DNP-OVA	E	20×10^6	172.4	F	10×10^6	1212.1
DNP-KLH	G	20×10^6	1384.7	H	7×10^6	447.3

*Spleen cells from BALB/c mice, primed and boosted 30 and 15 days, respectively, with 100 µg of DNP-KLH in CFA were incubated for 48 hours in vitro with saline, DNP-D-GL, DNP-OVA or DNP-KLH (the latter 3 at a dose of 3 µg/10^6 cells). At the end of the culture period, cells were thoroughly washed and then divided into 2 aliquots. One aliquot of each type was then incubated (20 minutes, 37°C) with trypsin (5 µg/10^6 cells) and then washed. The second aliquot of cells was left untreated. Groups of irradiated (500 R) syngeneic recipeints were injected i.v. with untreated or trypsinized cells of the type and in numbers as indicated above. Immediately after cell transfer, all mice were challenged with 100 µg of DNP-KLH i.p. in saline.

**The data are expressed as geometric means of serum anti-DNP antibody levels of groups of 5 mice 7 days after secondary challenge. A comparison of geometric mean antibody levels gave the following results: Comparison of group A or group B with groups C, D and E yielded P values of 0.001 > P in all cases. Comparison of group F with group E also yielded a P value of 0.001 > P. Comparison of group A with group G yielded a P value of 0.30 > P > 0.20.

DNP-D-GL (Table I). This observation formed a strong basis
for our contention that tolerance induction by DNP-D-GL involves complex, irrevocable intra- or subcellular events
following a tolerogenic signal probably generated at the
surface membranes of such cells consequent to specific binding of the molecule (1).

Our initial concept of how trypsin might have worked in
reversing DNP-OVA-induced unresponsiveness was by stripping
the cell membrane of its specific receptors and any DNP-OVA
attached to them. This, in turn, would result in resynthesis of surface receptors and the intact capability of such
cells to respond. The failure of trypsinization to reverse
the tolerant state induced by DNP-D-GL was explained in the
context of an irreversible intracellular inactivation process not subject to manipulations at the cell surface.
Another possible,explanation with altogether different implications for mechanisms of tolerance in this system, is
that being a non-metabolizable molecule, DNP-D-GL is not
itself subject to enzymatic degradation and may, thereby,
prevent accessibility of other surface membrane sites to the
enzyme. If this were the case, then the index of irreversibility by trypsin as a reflection of intracellular mechanisms of inactivation may be quite invalid. Therefore, we
next performed a series of experiments to put these questions
to direct analysis (2).

a) Failure to reverse tolerance induced in vivo with
DNP-D-GL or DNP-L-GL by trypsinization of cells before
adoptive transfer.
The protocol of this experiment in mice is schematically
depicted in the left panel of Fig. 8. The anti-DNP antibody
responses of groups of primary recipients are summarized in
the top right panel of Fig. 8, where it is shown that recipients treated with either DNP-D-GL or DNP-L-GL were significantly unresponsive as compared to saline controls (98%
and 92% diminution by DNP-D-GL and DNP-L-GL, respectively).

The spleen cells from these groups of primary recipient
mice were obtained and then washed three times with medium.
Each pool was divided into two samples, one of which was
left untreated while the second sample was treated with trypsin prior to transfer into secondary recipient mice. All
mice were challenged with DNP-KLH intraperitoneally immediately after cell transfer and then bled 7 days later. As
shown in the lower right panel of Fig. 8, cells exposed to
saline in the initial recipients developed very good adop-

tive anti-DNP antibody responses in the final recipients; trypsinization slightly, but not significantly, improved these responses. In contrast, cells exposed to either DNP-D-GL or DNP-L-GL failed to respond in the final recipients, and this inability to respond was not appreciably reversed in either case by trypsinization. Failure of trypsinization to reverse tolerance induced in these in vivo conditions may, of course, reflect the possible loss of DNP-specific B cells by phagocytosis in the reticuloendothelial system or by other means, a possibility on which no data yet exists.

b) Failure to reverse tolerance induced by DNP-D-GL and reversal of tolerance induced by DNP-L-GL in vitro by trypsinization of cells before adoptive transfer.

In one experiment of this type, depicted in Fig. 9, spleen cells from DNP-KLH-primed A/J donor mice were incubated at 37°C in Mishell-Dutton conditions with either DNP-D-GL or DNP-L-GL or saline alone. After 48 hours the respective cell groups were harvested from the dishes and washed three times in MEM. Each pool was divided into two samples, one of which was left untreated while the second was trypsinized. The respective cell pools were then transferred to irradiated, syngeneic recipients which were challenged with DNP-KLH and then bled seven days later. As shown in Fig. 9, recipients of cells incubated with saline developed good adoptive secondary responses to DNP-KLH and, trypsinization of such cells resulted in a substantial increase in the magnitude of these responses. Recipients of cells incubated with DNP-D-GL were significantly diminished in their secondary responses (86% as compared with controls) and, moreover, treatment with trypsin did not abolish the unresponsive state. In striking contrast are the results obtained in recipients of cells incubated with DNP-L-GL. If such cells were transferred without trypsinization, a very significant level of suppression (88%) comparable to that induced by DNP-D-GL occurred. Treatment of such cells with trypsin, on the other hand, restored the adoptive secondary anti-DNP response to essentially normal levels. In other experiments (not shown) we observed that in vitro incubation with DNP-L-GL for as long as four days resulted in a tolerant state that could be reversed by trypsinization (2).

c) Reversal of tolerance induced by DNP-D-GL in vitro
at 4°C by trypsinization of cells before adoptive transfer.
The question of whether or not conditions could be
found whereby trypsin could be employed to reverse (or rather
prevent) the tolerance-inducing sequence of cellular events
was approached by taking advantage of the fact that tolerance induction readily occurs in this system by in vitro incubation of primed cells with DNP-D-GL even at low temperatures. We reasoned, therefore, that perhaps at low temperature the transduction of any tolerogenic signal might be
sufficiently delayed so that reversal by trypsinization
would be feasible if the cells were subjected to this
enzymatic treatment right away. The following experiment
demonstrates that, indeed, this is true (Fig. 10).

As shown in Fig. 10, recipients of saline-control cells
incubated at either 4°C or 37°C developed very good adoptive
secondary anti-DNP responses and, again, these responses
were improved by treatment with trypsin. Recipients of cells
exposed to DNP-D-GL, but not trypsinized prior to transfer,
displayed markedly depressed responses irrespective of the
temperature of incubation (91% and 95% diminished at 4°C and
37°C, respectively). However, treatment of these cells with
trypsin prior to transfer had a significant effect upon
their subsequent capacity to respond which was determined to
a great extent upon the temperature used for incubation with
DNP-D-GL. Thus, cells exposed to DNP-D-GL at 4°C developed
secondary responses after trypsinization that were not
statistically significantly different from those of saline-
control cells also treated with trypsin ($0.30 > P > 0.20$).
Indeed, the magnitude of the responses in this group was even
greater than that obtained with saline-control cells not
subjected to trypsin treatment. In the case of cells incubated with DNP-D-GL at 37°C, trypsinization markedly improved
the ultimate response by comparison with those of cells exposed to DNP-D-GL but not trypsinized (10 fold) but did not
abolish the statistically significant difference with respect to responses of saline-control cells incubated at that
temperature and then treated with trypsin ($0.005 > P > 0.001$).

These data indicate, therefore, that failure to reverse the tolerant state, once induced by trypsin, reflects
more complex consequences of receptor-tolerogen binding than
simply surface blockade. Moreover, as will be discussed
below, the capacity of trypsin to reverse a state of B cell
refractoriness is not merely reflective of the enzymatic
clearing of antigen-blocked surface receptors.

259

In summary, Fig. 11 illustrates very simply the situation we have described for DNP-D-GL at length and what is probably true for comparable molecules such as DNP-POL and perhaps DNP-Levan. The message here is that binding by specific cells of determinants on such structurally unique molecules in an appropriately high epitope density will result in rapid tolerance induction that is not amenable to reversal by usually employed procedures provided that: 1) The molecules are bound by B cells in the appropriate concentration range in free solution--i.e. not attached to macrophages or other cell surfaces, and 2) the antigen-binding event occurs in the absence of helper T cell participation. The tolerant state is characterized by its rapid irreversibility and it does not involve the participation of suppressor T cells. This form of tolerance induction is most probably the least physiologic in nature since it is not likely that such molecules are commonly, if ever, encountered by immunocompetent individuals. However, the mechanisms by which such substances induce a state of irreversible cell inactivation may well be germane to our understanding of these processes in a very general way. As will be pointed out later, recent studies by Ault and Unanue have demonstrated that DNP-D-GL tends to persist for relatively long periods on the cell surface, thereby resulting in inhibition of receptor resynthesis that ordinarily occurs in the case of metabolizable DNP-proteins (24). To what extent this inhibition alone or more complex intracellular events play important roles in the inactivation processes has yet to be determined.

REVERSIBLE B CELL INACTIVATION

A state of B cell refractoriness can be induced to a variety of antigens in a variety of ways. The most effective methods employed have the common feature of treating animals with haptenic determinants on molecules or substances that fail to stimulate T cells or do so very poorly. Thus, in addition to DNP-D-GL, such tolerance has been induced by administration of: 1) hapten on other non-immunogenic moieties such as the synthetic copolymer L-GL in poly-L-lysine (PLL) non-responder guinea pigs (5) or inbred mice (1-3); 2) haptenic derivatives of autologous proteins (16-20), autologous or syngeneic red cells (21); or 3) polysaccharides such as type III pneumococcal polysaccharide (22, 23) in the appropriate dose range. We have previously suggested that a possible explanation for the ease of tolerance induction with hapten conjugates of non- or weakly-immunogenic substances may be the relative lack of sufficient helper T cell function occurring under certain conditions of administering such compounds (5, 8). This reasoning predicts that the ease of tolerance induction in B cells by any molecule will be inversely related to the degree of helper T cell activity induced by the molecule, a prediction which, in general, appears to be borne out by experimental evidence (3, 5, 8, 23).

Indeed, as shown in some of the preceding experiments, exposure of DNP-specific B cells to normally immunogenic DNP-protein conjugates can under appropriate conditions result in B cell refractoriness. This was the case in Table I where DNP-OVA rendered DNP-KLH-primed B cells unresponsive. This was also the case in non-responder strain 13 guinea pigs treated with DNP-L-GL, a molecule which is immunogenic in strain 2 responder animals. However, an important distinction can be made concerning the nature of the unresponsive state induced by the latter molecules as compared to that induced by DNP-D-GL, namely, that the tolerant state induced by DNP-OVA and DNP-L-GL is more readily reversible. This has been shown in the experiment in Table I where DNP-OVA-induced responsiveness was quite readily reversed by exposure of the cells to trypsin prior to adoptive transfer. The same was true in the case of DNP-primed mouse spleen cells rendered tolerant by exposure to DNP-L-GL in vitro (Fig. 9); such treatment did not reverse the unresponsiveness induced by DNP-D-GL.

We have explored this phenomenology further by in vivo experiments in which two questions were asked. First, it is possible to induce unresponsiveness in vivo in DNP-primed populations by exposure to normally immunogenic DNP conjugates under conditions in which relative lack of helper T cell activity exists? Second, to what extent is unresponsiveness induced in this manner reversible?

The experiment shown in Fig. 12 illustrates that in an adoptive transfer model, DNP-KLH-primed spleen cells can be rendered relatively unresponsive to secondary challenge with DNP-KLH by prior exposure, in situ, to DNP conjugates of BGG, OVA, L-GL or D-GL for suitable time periods (3). The experiment in Fig. 13 is a modification of the preceding one in which DNP-KLH-primed donor spleen cells were adoptively transferred to recipients after being depleted of T cells by anti-Θ serum treatment. These cells were then exposed in vivo to the same conjugates (with the addition of DNP-KLH)

261

for a longer period of time (7 days) and then retrieved from the spleens of the first recipients. Upon transfer to new irradiated recipients together with an additional population of KLH-primed helper T cells, the inability to develop secondary anti-DNP antibody responses was substantially restored in the case of cells exposed to DNP-BGG and DNP-OVA but not in the case of cells exposed to DNP-D-GL or DNP-L-GL (3).

Two important points must be emphasized here. The first is that the ability to render B cells unresponsive in such experiments by exposure to normally immunogenic conjugates depends upon the fact that the cells are primed, hence of relatively high average affinity, and are exposed in the relative absence of helper T cell activity. The second point is that, for whatever reason(s) unresponsiveness occurs in these conditions, it is at least partially reversible for at least a finite period of time. This is contrasted clearly by the situation with cells exposed in vivo to DNP-D-GL or DNP-L-GL. It is by no means clear as to whether or not the unresponsiveness induced by DNP-BGG and DNP-OVA involves the participation of suppressor T cell functions and if so, to what extent, but the results of current experimentation in our laboratory should resolve this question. Indeed, although the tolerant state induced by DNP-D-GL in mice has been shown not to involve suppressor T cells, this is still an open possibility for tolerance induced by DNP-L-GL. However, the consistent irreversible nature of tolerance induced by DNP-L-GL in in vivo conditions argues somewhat against the latter possibility.

Figure 14 summarizes the alternatives that one may envisage are presented to specific cells when other means of receptor-substrate binding occur than is depicted in the earlier schematic figure (Fig. 11). The heading receptor blockade, which seemed quite appropriate when this scheme was prepared 1 1/2 years ago, is most likely incorrect in terms of actual cell surface events since recent evidence of Ault and Unanue indicates that B cells rapidly interiorize and catabolize conventional antigens and resynthesize surface immunoglobulin receptors even, apparently, in the absence of actual cell triggering (25). The important point of distinction here is that the unresponsiveness depicted in this figure is subject to reversal by various means for at least a finite period of time. The specific cell binding antigen of a common molecular structure in free solution and under conditions of moderate epitope density in the absence of T cell participation can probably undergo three alternative pathways: 1) (Top) The cell, because of avidity considerations among other things, may shed the antigen very rapidly, even before significant amounts are interiorized and remain normally responsive. This possibility is of trivial interest to considerations of tolerance mechanisms and is pointed out only for completeness of the alternatives. 2) (Bottom) The cell having completed the sequence of antigen binding with subsequent capping, interiorization and receptor resynthesis might encounter helper T cell activity of either a specific or non-specific nature induced within a critical time period after the B cell binding events have occurred. The element of time here seems to us to be of utmost and determining importance to either prevent or result in the final alternative. 3) (Middle) In the absence of T cell helper activity for a finite period of time, the B cell having undergone the first stages of cell-antigen interaction now realizes it is lost and slips into a state of irreversible tolerance.

The critical time during which a B cell is reversibly refractory most logically differs depending upon conditions of antigen concentration, etc., but has the common feature of inevitably resulting in irreversible tolerance if no appropriate intervention occurs. Precisely what intervention is appropriate is obscure but it is intriguing to consider that one of the important aspects of trypsin reversal is related to the effects of this enzyme on certain critical cell surface sites (other than immunoglobulin receptors) that might be the same or similar to the surface molecules involved in physiologic T-B cell interactions. If our recently postulated model for the role of histocompatibility gene products in such interactions is correct, then the B cell "acceptor" site would, indeed, be a likely candidate for the molecule crucially affected by trypsin.

The latter sequence (Fig. 14) is one more probably involved in physiologic mechanisms of tolerance. It is quite conceivable, for example, that B cells with specific receptors for autoantigens that may be constantly originating from the stem cell pool are rendered tolerant in the manner depicted by virtue of undergoing the antigen-binding sequence in absence of T cell helper functions. Likewise, the development of autoantibody production is understandable when conditions allowing for non-specific or cross-reactive T cell activation arise as, for example, with chronic infections.

Finally, although the sequence in Fig. 14 alludes to the consequences of antigen binding in the absence of T cell participation, it is not unlikely that the consequences of suppressor T functions are precisely the same, and perhaps for the same reasons--i.e. absence of helper T cell function. This reasoning is stimulated by the point emphasized by Tony Basten (this volume) that suppressor T cells, at least of the antigen-specific variety, might well act to a major degree by suppressing helper T cells of the same specificity. Since the obvious net effect of this balance should in some circumstances be the cancelling out of helper function, the B cell would, therefore, be in the predicament depicted as alternative 3 in Fig. 14. To what extent suppressor activity of T cells or macrophages may directly affect B cells, and if so, by what cellular mechanisms must await more detailed analysis.

CONCLUSIONS

The studies presented here serve to focus not only on two distinctive forms of B cell tolerance but also on certain of the fundamental issues to which investigations on the phenomenology of tolerance should be primarily directed, namely, potential applicability of the model systems employed to clinical use and relevance of what is learned to mechanisms of self tolerance.

The potential clinical applicability of tolerance systems such as that represented by DNP-D-GL could be enormous. The properties of the D-GL molecule and presumably other structurally similar substances that promote inactivation of specific B lymphocytes binding determinants attached to D-GL opens a wide area of deleterious antibody production to attack. Since studies thus far have delineated the potent tolerogenic properties of D-GL bearing small, well-defined determinants, the immediate practical possibilities include tolerization in patients with hypersensitivity to the benzylpenicilloyl determinants of penicillin and its analogues. More dramatic application would be the use of D-GL bearing nucleotide and nucleoside determinants to abolish anti-nuclear antibody production in patients with systemic lupus erythematosus (SLE). Indeed, preliminary studies in our laboratory have demonstrated that nucleoside-D-GL complexes can effectively abrogate anti-nuclear antibody production in mice, and long-term investigations of the effects of these molecules in the pathogenesis of autoimmune disease in NZB mice are currently being undertaken. In another area of

perhaps the largest potential usefulness, namely, treatment
of common immediate hypersensitivity disease states, the
groundwork is being laid but a vast amount of further research is essential. Thus, we have established the fact that
determinants coupled to D-GL will effectively tolerize B
cells of the IgE class as well as other antibody classes
(4). However, what is not yet determined is whether more
complex multi-determinant antigens will be tolerogenic to B
cells once coupled to D-GL. This will be absolutely necessary if one is to consider the possible induction of tolerance in patients with hay fever by administering purified
ragweed antigens coupled to D-GL. Studies currently underway
in our laboratory should resolve this issue in one way or
another in the not too distant future. Finally, of course,
if any of these possible therapeutic applications are to be
achieved, it will be essential to determine methods by which
these substances can be administered to the patient with
relative impunity to his or her health.

The issue of relevance of the various experimental
models of B cell tolerance to the mechanisms of self-tolerance remains highly conjectural, but a reasonably educated
framework of thought can be derived from the available systems being studied. If the assumption is made that T cells
specific for self-antigens capable of providing helper function for B cells do not exist (for reasons not to be considered here), then the functional inactivation of B cells
specific for auto-antigens may occur via the following pathway primarily in relation to the concentrations of the self-
antigens concerned. Thus, in the case of self-antigens in
high concentrations and ready accessibility--i.e. serum proteins, circulating histocompatibility antigen molecules,
etc.--specific B cells arising from the stem cell pool become virtually bathed in these antigens and are routinely
inactivated perhaps even very early in their differentiation
pathway. Cells possessing specific receptors for binding
these self-antigens would not, therefore, be expected to be
detected at least by the currently available techniques. On
the other hand, in the case of self-antigens that exist in
relatively low quantities sequestered perhaps in selected
tissue sites--i.e. thyroglobulin--, it would be understandable why B cells specific for such antigens might be rather
easily found, as indeed they have in recent years. The pre-
sumption follows, however, that the B cells detected have
not themselves been exposed to an appreciable extent to the
antigen--those which have contacted the antigen in sufficient
amounts and for a sufficient duration of time are either in-

activated or in the process of becoming so, provided helper T cell activity is lacking. In the event that some form of (e.g. non-specific) T cell help occurs--for example, during a chronic infectious process involving release of significant quantities of adjuvant substances--then autoantibody production may readily ensue and be of either transient or more prolonged duration depending on the circumstances.

How then does the inactivation sequence occur in such B cells following the binding of self-antigens in the absence of helper T cell function. If, as appears to be the case, B cells can bind, cap, interiorize or catabolize the antigen molecules and resynthesize their surface receptors in the absence of helper T cells (25), then it is possible to envisage that either after one or perhaps after several such cycles of antigen-binding receptor resynthesis the cell may be induced to undergo terminal blast transformation, thus, eliminating it from the available cell pool. The absence of a helper T cell influence, therefore, results in a normal pathway to this end result (terminal blastogenesis) with no capability for further differentiation into antibody-producing or memory cells. If the evidence becomes clear that suppressor T cells may be involved in the maintenance of some forms of self-tolerance and that such involvement is a direct effect on B lymphocytes, then the possibility must be considered that such suppressor T cells accomplish their functional effects likewise by stimulating B cells to undergo terminal differentiation. Definitive answers to these possibilities may be soon forthcoming.

ACKNOWLEDGMENTS

I am deeply indebted to all of our colleagues who participated in the studies described herein, in particular, Dr. Toshiyuki Hamaoka without whom many of these observations would not have been possible. I also am grateful to Ms. Candace Maher for excellent secretarial assistance in preparation of the manuscript. We also thank the publishers of the Journal of Experimental Medicine for permission to reproduce certain figures presented herein.

This work was supported in part by Grants AI-10630 and AI-09920 from the National Institutes of Health, U.S. Public Health Service.

REFERENCES

1. Katz, D.H., Hamaoka, T. and Benacerraf, B., J. Exp. Med. 136:1404, 1972.

2. Hamaoka, T. and Katz, D.H., J. Exp. Med. 139:000, 1974.

3. Katz, D.H., Hamaoka, T. and Benacerraf, B., J. Exp. Med. 139:000, 1974.

4. Katz, D.H., Hamaoka, T. and Benacerraf, B., Proc. Nat. Acad. Sci. 70:2776, 1973.

5. Katz, D.H., Davie, J.M., Paul, W.E. and Benacerraf, B., J. Exp. Med. 134:201, 1971.

6. Osborne, D.P., Jr. and Katz, D.H., J. Exp. Med. 136:439, 1973.

7. Osborne, D.P., Jr. and Katz, D.H., J. Exp. Med. 137:991, 1973.

8. Katz, D.H. and Benacerraf, B., Adv. Immunol. 15:1, 1972.

9. Katz, D.H., Transpl. Rev. 12:141, 1972.

10. Howard, J.G., Transpl. Rev. 8:50, 1972.

11. Sjöberg, O., J. Exp. Med. 135:850, 1972.

12. Möller, E. and Sjöberg, O., Transpl. Rev. 8:26, 1972.

13. Katz, D.H., Paul, W.E., Goidl, E.A. and Benacerraf, B., J. Exp. Med. 133:169, 1971.

14. Armerding, D. and Katz, D.H., J. Exp. Med. 140:000, 1974.

15. Mosier, D.E., Johnson, B.M., Paul, W.E. and McMaster, P.R.B., J. Exp. Med. 139:1354, 1974.

16. Havas, H.F., Immunology. 17:819, 1969.

17. Borel, Y., Nat. New Biol. 230:180, 1971.

18. Golan, D.T. and Borel, Y., J. Exp. Med. 134:1046, 1971.

19. Fidler, J.M. and Golub, E.S., J. Exp. Med. 137:42, 1973.

20. Walters, C.S., Moorhead, J.W. and Claman, H.N., J. Exp. Med. 136:542, 1972.

21. Hamilton, J.A. and Miller, J.F.A.P., Eur. J. Immunol. 3:457, 1973.

22. Mitchell, G.F., Humphrey, J.H. and Williamson, A.R., Eur. J. Immunol. 2:460, 1972.

23. Mitchell, G.F., In The Lymphocyte: Structure and Function, edited by J.J. Marchalonis, Marcel Dekker, Inc., New York, 1974.

24. Ault, K., Unanue, E.R., Katz, D.H. and Benacerraf, B., Proc. Nat. Acad. Sci. 71:000, 1974.

25. Ault, K. and Unanue, E.R., J. Exp. Med. 139:1110, 1974.

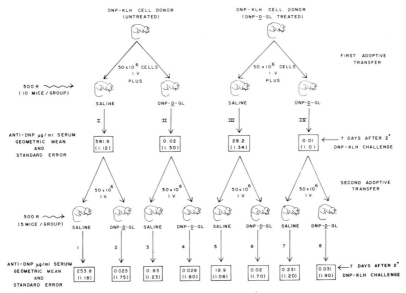

Fig. 1. Maintenance of DNP-specific tolerance after serial adoptive cell transfers. 50 x 10^6 spleen cells from A/J mice primed with DNP-KLH 46 days earlier were injected intravenously into two groups (I and II) of syngeneic, irradiated (500 R) recipients (10 mice per group). Two additional groups (III and IV) of recipients were injected with cells from identically primed donors which had been treated with 1.0 mg of DNP-D-GL intraperitoneally 7 days before transfer. Immediately after cell transfer recipients were treated with either DNP-D-GL (groups II and IV) or saline (groups I and III) and then challenged 3 days later with 100 µg of DNP-KLH i.p. in saline. Seven days after secondary challenge, mice in each group were bled and killed. Suspensions of their spleen cells were prepared and adoptively transferred (50 x 10^6 cells/recipient) to groups of new irradiated, syngeneic recipients who were then divided into subgroups (5 mice each) which were either subjected to DNP-D-GL treatment immediately after cell transfer (group 2, 4, 6 or 8) or not (groups 1, 3, 5 and 7). Three days after cell transfer, these new recipients were challenged with 100 µg of DNP-KLH i.p. in saline. Serum anti-DNP antibody levels of groups I-IV and groups 1-8 on day 7 after their respective secondary challenges are illustrated. Statistical comparisons of group I and groups II and III yielded P values of 0.001 > P in both cases. Comparison of group 1 with 5 yielded a P value of 0.005 > P > 0.001. Comparison of group 1 with groups 2, 3, 4, 6, 7 and 8 yielded P values of 0.001 > P in all cases (taken from Ref. 1).

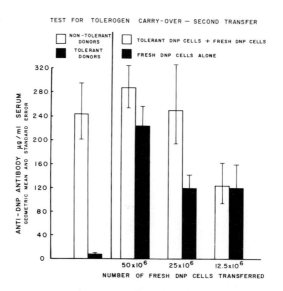

Fig. 2. Elimination of the possibility of carry-over
of tolerogen or activity of suppressor cells in serial adoptive cell transfers. The experimental groups I and II of
Fig. 1 were established using spleen cells from A/J donor
mice primed 51 days earlier with 100 µg of DNP-KLH in CFA.
The results obtained in these two adoptive transfer groups
were comparable to those shown in Fig. 1. Spleen cells from
these first transfer recipients were then adoptively transferred intravenously to new recipients (50 x 10^6 cells per
recipient). Certain groups of recipients of cells rendered
tolerant by DNP-D-GL in the first adoptive transfer were
also injected on the same day with varying numbers of spleen
cells from DNP-KLH-primed donor mice. Comparable groups of
mice which received only the respective numbers of these
"fresh" DNP-primed cells were established as controls. Three
days later all mice were secondarily challenged with 100 µg
of DNP-KLH and then bled 7 days thereafter. Mean serum anti-
DNP antibody levels of groups of 5 mice on day 7 after secondary challenge are shown (taken from Ref. 1).

270

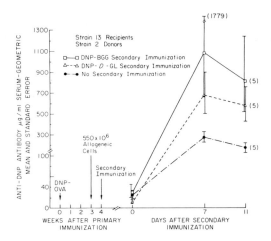

Fig. 3. Stimulation of anti-DNP antibody production as a result of transfer of immunocompetent strain 2 cells into primed strain 13 recipients: The effect of secondary antigenic challenge with DNP-BGG and DNP-D-GL. 550×10^6 strain 2 lymph node and spleen cells were injected intravenously into strain 13 recipients primed 3 weeks earlier with DNP-OVA. Recipients were either not boosted or boosted with 1.0 mg of DNP-BGG or DNP-D-GL in saline 6 days after transfer. Serum anti-DNP antibody concentrations just prior to secondary immunization and on days 7 and 11 are illustrated. The numbers in parentheses refer to the numbers of animals in the given groups (taken from Ref. 5).

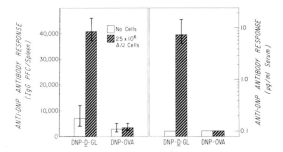

Fig. 4. The effect of allogeneic cell transfer on the primary responses to DNP-D-GL and DNP-OVA. Normal CAF_1 mice were injected intravenously with 25×10^6 parental A strain spleen cells and then challenged intraperitoneally with either 100 μg of DNP-D-GL or DNP-OVA. Control CAF_1 mice, which received no allogeneic cell transfer, were challenged with either 100 μg of DNP-D-GL or 100 μg of DNP-OVA. Ten days following cell transfer and challenge both serum anti-DNP antibody levels and IgM and IgG anti-DNP PFC were determined (taken from Ref. 7).

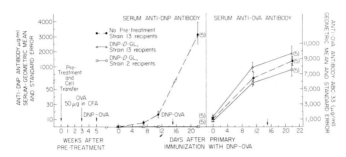

Fig. 5. Failure of "allogeneic effect" to modify DNP-specific tolerance induced by the administration of DNP-D-GL or DNP-L-GL 1 day before cell transfer. On week 0 strain 13 and strain 2 guinea pigs were injected intraperitoneally with 3.0 mg of either DNP-D-GL or DNP-L-GL in saline or saline alone; 24 hours later all guinea pigs received 200 x 10^6 lymph node and spleen cells from strain 2 donors; two or three weeks after cell transfer, all recipients were immunized with 50 μg of OVA emulsified in CFA. This was followed 2 weeks thereafter by primary immunization with 1.0 mg of DNP-OVA in saline (day 0). A final challenge with 1.0 mg of DNP-OVA in saline was carried out on day 14 or day 15. Serum anti-DNP and anti-OVA antibody concentrations just prior to primary DNP-OVA immunization and on days 7, 11 and 22 are illustrated. The numbers in parentheses refer to the numbers of animals in the given groups (taken from Ref. 5).

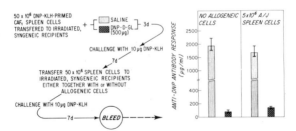

Fig. 6. Induction of DNP-specific tolerance by exposure of DNP-KLH-primed cells to DNP-D-GL in vivo in adoptive recipients. The protocol is depicted schematically on the left of the figure. Each group consists of 6 mice. Relevant statistical comparisons of antibody responses yielded the following P values: 1) Cells exposed to DNP-D-GL compared with saline-control cells, $0.001 > P$ when transferred either with or without allogeneic cells and 2) cells exposed to DNP-D-GL and transferred together with allogeneic cells as compared to DNP-D-GL-treated cells transferred without allogeneic cells - $0.10 > P > 0.05$ (taken from Ref. 2).

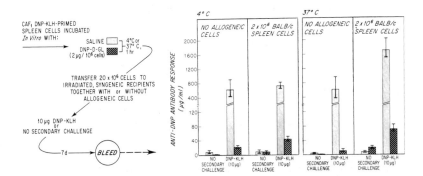

Fig. 7. Induction of DNP-specific tolerance by incubation of DNP-KLH-primed cells in vitro with DNP-D-GL before adoptive transfer. The protocol is depicted schematically on the left of the figure. Two experiments are shown. In one the temperature of in vitro incubation of cells with either saline or DNP-D-GL was 4°C while in the other it was 37°C, as indicated. Each group consists of 5 mice. Relevant statistical comparisons of secondary responses to DNP-KLH challenge yielded the following P values: 1) Cells incubated with DNP-D-GL compared with saline-treated cells, 0.001 > P at both 4°C and 37°C and when transferred either with or without allogeneic cells, and 2) cells incubated with DNP-D-GL and transferred together with allogeneic cells as compared to DNP-D-GL-treated cells transferred without allogeneic cells, 0.05 > P > 0.025 at 4°C and 0.01 > P > 0.005 at 37°C (taken from Ref. 2).

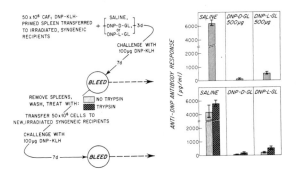

Fig. 8.

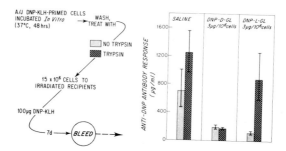

Fig. 9. Failure to reverse tolerance induced by DNP-D-GL and reversal of tolerance induced by DNP-L-GL _in vitro_ by trypsinization of cells before adoptive transfer. The protocol is schematically depicted on the left. Each group consists of 5 mice. Relevant statistical comparisons of responses yielded the following P values: Non-trypsinized vs. trypsinized saline-control cells - 0.20 > P > 0.10; Non-trypsinized vs. trypsinized DNP-D-GL-treated cells - 0.90 > P > 0.80; Non-trypsinized vs. trypsinized DNP-L-GL-treated cells - 0.05 > P > 0.025; Non-trypsinized saline-controls vs. non-trypsinized DNP-D-GL and DNP-L-GL-treated cells - 0.01 > P > 0.005 in both cases; Trypsinized saline-controls vs. trypsinized DNP-D-GL-treated cells and DNP-L-GL-treated cells - 0.001 > P > and 0.60 > P > 0.50, respectively (taken from Ref. 2).

Fig. 8. Failure to reverse tolerance induced _in vivo_ with DNP-D-GL or DNP-L-GL by trypsinization of cells before adoptive transfer. The protocol is schematically depicted on the left. Each group consists of 10 mice in the top panel, 5 mice in the bottom panel. Relevant statistical comparisons of responses yielded the following P values: 1) Top panel - comparison of saline-treated controls with DNP-D-GL-treated cells and DNP-L-GL-treated cells yielded 0.001 > P in both cases, and 2) Bottom panel - a) saline-treated control cells compared to DNP-D-GL or DNP-L-GL-treated cells, 0.001 > P, irrespective of whether or not cells were treated with trypsin, and b) non-trypsinized DNP-D-GL or DNP-L-GL-treated cells compared to their respective trypsinized counterparts - 0.10 >P > 0.05 in both cases (taken from Ref. 2).

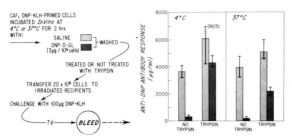

Fig. 10. Reversal of tolerance induced by DNP-D-GL in vitro at 4°C by trypsinization of cells before adoptive transfer. The protocol is depicted schematically on the left. Each group consists of 5-6 mice. Relevant statistical comparisons of responses yielded the following P values: 1) Non-trypsinized saline-controls vs. non-trypsinized DNP-D-GL-treated cells - 0.005 > P > 0.001 and 0.001 > P at 4°C and 37°C incubation temperatures, respectively; and b) Trypsinized saline-controls vs. trypsinized DNP-D-GL-treated cells - 0.30 > P > 0.20 and 0.005 > P > 0.001 at 4°C and 37°C incubation temperatures, respectively (taken from Ref. 2).

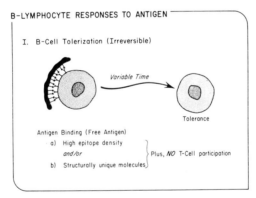

Fig. 11. Irreversible B cell tolerance induction.

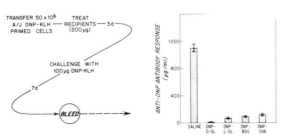

Fig. 12.

275

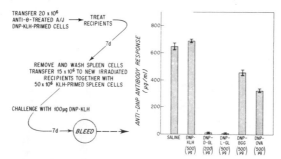

Fig. 13. Partial reversal of tolerance induced _in vivo_ with immunogenic DNP proteins by serial adoptive transfer. The protocol is schematically depicted on the left of the figure. Primary recipient groups were tested with saline or one of the DNP conjugates as indicated below the data bars. Each group consists of 5 mice. Relevant statistical comparisons of responses of the various recipient groups yielded the following P values: a) Saline vs. DNP-KLH - 0.90 > P > 0.80; b) Saline or DNP-KLH vs. DNP-D-GL or DNP-L-GL - 0.001 > P in every case; c) Saline or DNP-KLH vs. DNP-BGG - 0.40 > P > 0.30; d) Saline or DNP-KLH vs. DNP-OVA - 0.10 > P > 0.05; and e) DNP-BGG or DNP-OVA vs. DNP-D-GL or DNP-L-GL - 0.001 > P > in every case (taken from Ref. 3).

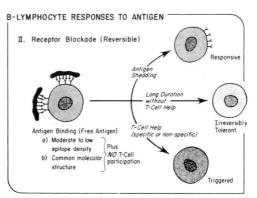

Fig. 14. Reversible B cell inactivation.

Fig. 12. Induction of tolerance in adoptively transferred DNP-specific B cells by exposure of such cells to nonimmunogenic or unrelated immunogenic DNP-carrier conjugates. The protocol is schematically depicted on the left of the figure. Recipient groups were treated with saline or one of the DNP conjugates as indicated below the data bars. Each group consists of 6 mice. Statistical comparison of antibody responses of recipient groups treated with the various DNP-carrier conjugates prior to secondary challenge to those of saline-control recipients yielded the P values of 0.001 > P in all cases (taken from Ref. 3).

DISCUSSION FOLLOWING DAVID KATZ

MITCHELL: How do you view the nature of "T cell help" - the absence of which facilitate tolerance induction?

KATZ: Obviously, you are trapping me into getting into the questions of mechanism(s) of T-B cell interactions about which this conference is only indirectly related. Clearly, our views on this matter are based in large measure on the observations we have recently published elsewhere (J. Exp. Med. 137:1405, 1973 and Proc. Nat. Acad. Sci. 70:2624, 1973.) concerning the genetic restrictions for optimal T-B cell interactions. As you are all aware, we believe that the interactions occur via B cell surface sites, which we have called "acceptor" molecules and appropriate molecules either on or secreted by T lymphocytes. I am glad, in fact, that you raise this question because it is germane to possible alternative explanations of the effect of trypsin on lymphocyte surfaces. For example, trypsin may exert its reversing effects on refractory B cells by either altering, appropriately exposing and/or removing and inducing resynthesis of the acceptor molecules that for some reason have been rendered inactive by prior encounter of B cells with antigen under either absent or suppressor T cell conditions. It is conceivable that activation or excitation of this surface acceptor site is essential not only for B cell triggering but also for prevention of the cell becoming refractory. Normally, the B cell is programmed to not proliferate, etc, - if activation of the acceptor site does not occur within a given time after the antigen-binding event--release from the ensuing state of refractoriness would therefore necessitate the involvement of the acceptor molecule somehow. I bring these possibilities out merely as intuitive speculations on the issue; certainly, no hard data exists to either support or rule out these possibilities.

E. MÖLLER: When you "rescue" cells from tolerance with the allogeneic effect, have you studied the affinity distribution of those producing cells compared to a normal distribution? It is probable that most of those cells in that situation are producing low affinity antibody and not really the truly "tolerant" cells which are reverted from tolerance.

KATZ: I agree fully with the possibility that you have raised. Indeed, it is our feeling that the "subpopulation" of B cells apparently stimulated in these circumstances of an allogeneic effect could be low affinity cells that were not actually rendered irreversibly tolerant under conditions of exposure to DNP-D-GL. We have not, however, analyzed the affinity distribution in these responses. I would like to add that we do not believe that truly tolerant cells in this model can be "rescued"--rather, the partial response we might observe under certain conditions probably reflects the escape of certain cells from the tolerance-inducing process.

SCOTT: As you mentioned, trypsin may not reverse tolerance induced by DNP-D-GL because D-GL is not trypsin sensitive and it may also block the receptor. It also is likely that trypsin may act on other structural membrane proteins. My questions are firstly, do you know whether the B cell receptor is, in fact, trypsin-sensitive? Secondly, would you comment on the possible analogy between trypsin-reversal of tolerance and the known effects of this enzyme on the Con A agglutination, where trypsin may alter membrane fluidity?

KATZ: I would prefer that Emil Unanue comment on the effects of trypsin on B cell membrane receptors and the response to your second point is that the possible analogy exists and may indeed be relevant but, in what way, I do not as yet know.

UNANUE: In our hands trypsin doesn't remove all surface Ig. The total amount of surface Ig removed by trypsin is approximately 50%, as judged by immunochemical quantitation. By immunofluorescence one can find three groups of lymphocytes--one where all surface Ig is removed, a second where most surface Ig remains, and a third where a part of it is removed.

BACH: Could you point out the differences in conditions between those required to induce tolerance for IgG production by DNP-D-GL as compared to the conditions under which you induced tolerance in the IgE system? (time, dose, etc.)

KATZ: The conditions employed were essentially identical for both antibody classes.

GERSHON: Do you see reversible and irreversible tolerance as different entities or two points on a spectrum and why?

KATZ: I am inclined to consider reversible and irreversible tolerance to be different points on a continuous spectrum, in general, although the rapid irreversible state induced by certain molecules such as DNP-D-GL may never manifest itself as any recognizable spectrum. The reason why I feel this way is again more intuitive than factual since hard evidence in this regard must certainly await more definitive technology than exists at present.

G. MÖLLER: In your last slide you indicate that B cells with antigen on the surface can develop in three different ways. One of these resulted in a paralyzed cell without further events being introduced after the intital antigen binding. The production of a paralyzed cell is most likely an active event. Therefore, binding of antigen to B cells can by itself not cause deletion of the cell, because it can be activated by e.g., a T cell. Something other than binding to the Ig receptor must therefore be responsible for tolerance. What are your thoughts on the nature of the signal?

KATZ: Obviously, we are all striving to understand the nature of the signals generated at cell surface membranes and we are still quite unaware in this regard. However, I am not quite in agreement with your assumption that the binding of antigen alone to B cells is insufficient to result in tolerance. This premise excludes the equally valid possibility that the "off-signal" to a given cell is programmed into the functional repertoire of the cell if and when the cell receives less than its necessary complement of "on-signals". For those of us who subscribe to the general belief that antigen-binding per se may not be a sufficient "on-signal", then the absence of, for example, acceptor site activation may within a finite time result in a refractory cell. Such a state of refractoriness would not have occurred in the absence of an initial antigen-binding event and therefore the latter event alone, in these conditions, results in tolerance or refractoriness.

DIENER: Did you say that DNP-D-GL is shed from the cell? Is it internalized? If internalized it could be suicidal since catabolism would fail to occur.

KATZ: No, DNP-D-GL is not shed from the cell surface very well. As Emil Unanue will describe a little later, a major portion remains on the cell membrane for a fairly long time. Some, however, does get into the cytoplasm but it is not yet possible to say whether or not it is the internalized material that induces tolerance. We are inclined to believe that the tolerogenic signal is initiated at the cell surface. We can say that whatever else may result from early internalization of DNP-D-GL, death of the cell is not one since these cells remain viable in culture for several days after exposure to DNP-D-GL.

BASTEN: I would like to comment on the use of trypsin. We find that trypsin is less satisfactory than chymotrypsin in treatment of cells for the following reasons: (1) It does not strip immunoglobulin from B cells as effectively. (2) It results in greater cell loss. (3) It may produce a delayed redistribution particularly of T cells from spleen to liver as measured by Chromium 51 tracer studies. Abrogation of an effect by trypsin treatment requires stringent controls, particularly in view of disparate effects of trypsin on T cells and B cells.

BOREL: To maintain the B cell tolerance, the possibility exists that it is an active process mediated by hapten-specific suppressor T cells. Whether suppressor T cells are T cells with their receptors occupied by the antigenic determinant or maintain the antigenic determinant on the B cell surface, or both, is an open question.

SMITH: What is the maximum interval in which T-helper cells can "rescue" potentially "irreversibly tolerant" cells, i.e., when does reversible become irreversible through T-helper function?

KATZ: That is a difficult question to answer in a single, finite manner. It appears that for matabolizable antigens, such as the DNP-carrier conjugates used in the present studies, an interval of around 3 days may be sufficient in the proper conditions.

BENACERRAF: This discussion will be much more informative
after Emil Unanue has presented his data on the fate of
the tolerogen after it is bound to the B. cell. Then it
will appear that we can distinguish the types of B cell
tolerance as stated by David Katz: (1) An irreversible type seen with poorly metabolizable materials such
as DNP-DGL and Levan. (2) The reversible types observed in the absence of T-cell helper effect with such
molecules as DNP-OVA or DNP-L-GL. In this latter case,
it must be determined whether a) suppressor T cells
have been generated, or b) whether tolerance results
for a finite period of time from the injection with
antigen in excess in the absence of T cell helper function.

HIGH-DOSE TOLERANCE IN MICE DEFICIENT IN REACTIVE T CELLS

Graham F. Mitchell

Walter and Eliza Hall Institute
P.O. Royal Melbourne Hospital
Victoria, 3050, Australia

INTRODUCTION

The two antigen-reactive lymphocyte types, T cells and B cells, are believed to be sensitive to certain "signals" upon contact with antigen: a) "on signals" which initiate the transformation of B cells into antibody-secreting cells and B memory cells, and T cells into sensitized lymphocytes and T memory cells, and b) "off signals" resulting in tolerance (cell paralysis, functional silence) and probably cell death. In the course of most antibody responses, T cells influence (often markedly) the activities of B cells, and one popular belief is that T cells modify, either directly or indirectly, the antigen-initiated "signals" at the surface of B cells.

The finding that animals depleted of T cells respond well to some antigens but poorly to others has led to the division of antibody (i.e. B cell) responses into T cell independent and T cell dependent. Several general statements can be made about T cell dependence/independence in vivo (reviewed in 1,2):- a) secondary antibody responses are usually T cell dependent whereas many primary responses are not; b) in keeping with a) most IgG antibody responses are highly T cell dependent whereas many IgM responses are not; c) in keeping with b), but not widely confirmed, high combining-site affinity antibodies are more T cell dependent than low affinity antibodies; and d) the antigens which elicit comparable antibody (IgM) responses in intact and T cell-deficient mice are highly persistent, polymeric and apparently do not stimulate T cells. Conceivably, therefore antigens generate "on signals", quite independently of T cells, in the majority of B cell precursors of IgM-secreting cells which are of low antigen-binding capacity (ABC) because of the low combining-site affinity of the antigen receptors on such B cells. By contrast, "on signals" are not generated in the majority of B cell precursors of IgG-secreting cells of high ABC unless activated T cells are also present. The two types of B cells have been referred to as B^μ and B^γ cells, respectively. This paper presents evidence in favor of the notion that the absence of activated T cells, and thus the failure to generate "on signals" in B^γ cells, leads to "off signals" provided the amount of antigen available to the B^γ cells is high.

Three Experimental Systems in which Tolerance is Induced in Mice Suspected or Known to be Deficient in Reactive T Cells.

In several laboratories over the past few years, I have been interested in the fate of B cells after contact with relatively large amounts of antigen in the absence of reactive T cells. The following are three systems in which B cell tolerance appears to follow from the interaction between antigen and B cells (in particular, B^γ cells) when few, if any, T cells are activated. This outcome was predicted by Bretscher and Cohn (3-5) although the general idea had been raised earlier that an encounter between antigen and reactive (immuno-competent) cell leads to tolerance unless another influence is brought to bear on that cell.

System 1: Inhibition of anti-DNP antibody responses to DNP-protein with DNP-(H,G)-A--L in genetic low responders to (H,G)-A--L (6).

The evidence is compelling that T cells are functionally silent in H-linked genetic low responsiveness to synthetic polypeptide antigens such as (T,G)-A--L and (H,G)-A--L in mice (discussed in 7). Specifically reactive T cells are either absent, readily tolerized or unable to interact with antigen-binding B cells. C3H.SW(H-2^b) mice are low responders to (H,G)-A--L whereas C3H(H-2^k) mice are high responders. C3H.SW mice pretreated with DNP-(H,G)-A--L show a marked but transient reduction in the anti-DNP antibody response to DNP-ovalbumin relative to the response in H-2 congenic C3H mice (Table I). Ordal and Grumet (8) have studied this type of inhibition much more extensively.

System 2: Inhibition of IgG anti-DNP antibody responses to DNP-protein with DNP-lysine-SIII (9-11).

Pneumococcal polysaccharide (SIII) is an apparently non T cell stimulating antigen in mice which elicits T cell independent IgM responses (e.g. 12-14). Conjugates of DNP-lysine-SIII inhibit primary, secondary, and adoptive anti-DNP responses to strong antigens such as DNP-hemocyanin from <u>Maia squinada</u> and DNP-chicken gamma globulin. IgG anti-DNP responses are more susceptible to inhibition than IgM anti-DNP response (Table II), low doses of DNP-lysine-SIII itself eliciting IgM anti-DNP responses (15). The system is similar to that of Katz and colleagues (this volume), using DNP-D-GL.

TABLE I

ABILITY OF DNP-(H,G)-A--L TO INDUCE A TRANSIENT HYPO-
RESPONSIVENESS TO DNP-OVA IN (H,G)-A--L
"NONRESPONDER"MICE

Strain	Pretreatment*	Percent antigen bound**	
		day 7	day 13
C3H/HeJ ("responder", H-2^k)	-	56 ± 3	73 ± 3
	+	48 ± 5	60 ± 3
C3H.SW ("nonresponder", H-2^b)	-	61 ± 3	83 ± 2
	+	<10	49 ± 13

*Eight two month old male mice per group, half pretreated with 1 mgm aqueous dinitrophenylated-(H,G)-A--L i.v. and all injected the next day with 30µg DNP-ovalbumin (OVA) in Freund's complete adjuvant into the footpads. All mice boosted 24 days later with aqueous DNP-OVA and bled 7 and 13 days after challenge.

**Percent antigen bound at 1/100 serum dilution using a Farr test with labelled DNP-human serum albumin ($\pm$SE of mean). (H,G)-A--L = synthetic polypeptide, poly-L(His, Glu)-poly D L-Ala--poly-L-Lys.

System 3: Inhibition of IgG anti-sheep erythrocyte antibody responses in athymic mice (16).

This system provides good evidence that B cells which would normally differentiate into IgG-secreting cells under T cell influence are inhibited by contact with antigen in T cell deficient mice; in this case the putatively athymic "nude" (nu/nu) mice. If nu/nu mice are injected with high doses (10^8 - 10^9) of sheep erythrocytes (SRBC), they respond by producing substantial numbers of direct (IgM) plaque-forming cells (PFC) in the spleen and very few, if any, indirect (allotypic IgG) PFC. If such mice are injected later with T cells and 10^8 SRBC, they fail to respond by producing significant numbers of direct or indirect PFC. Nu/nu mice injected previously with HRBC, or not pretreated, respond well by producing anti-SRBC PFC to an inoculum of T cells and SRBC. Nu/nu mice injected previously with SRBC produce anti-TNP, but not anti-SRBC, PFC when injected with T cells and TNP-SRBC. This type of tolerance in nu/nu mice has been also studied by Schrader (17), using chicken gamma globulin (CGG).

TABLE II

INHIBITION OF A PRIMARY ANTI-DNP RESPONSE TO DNP-CGG
USING DNP-lys-SIII

Injections		No. of mice (C3H/HeJ)	PFC per spleen (day 14)			
			Anti-DNP		Anti-CGG	
day 0	day 7		Direct	Indirect	Direct	Indirect
DNP-lys-SIII	DNP-CGG	4	2370 (1.3)	0	1520 (1.3)	27,660 (1.5)
—	DNP-CGG	4	1740 (1.9)	10,260 (1.3)	1890 (1.5)	47,230 (1.4)

DNP-lys-SIII = DNP-lysine conjugated to type III pneumococcal polysaccharide (9), 200µg aqueous antigen i.v. DNP-CGG = dinitrophenylated chicken gamma globulin, 200µg alum precipitated plus 10^9 pertussis organisms i.p. Indirect PFC developed with a rabbit anti-mouse IgG serum. SRBC used in PFC assay were coated with DNP-Fab prepared from rabbit anti-SRBC globulins or with CGG from chickens immunized against SRBC. Geometric mean PFC responses, limits of standard error of mean obtained by dividing and multiplying by the number in brackets. PFC assays performed according to the method of Cunningham. PFC = plaque-forming cell, SRBC = sheep erythrocytes.

TABLE III

REDUCED ABILITY OF SPLEEN CELLS FROM HIGH DOSE SRBC-PRETREATED NU/NU MICE TO TRANSFER AN ADOPTIVE ANTI-SRBC RESPONSE WHEN INJECTED INTO IRRADIATED RECIPIENTS TOGETHER WITH T CELLS AND SRBC.

Experimental nu/nu: 10^9 SRBC $\xrightarrow{\text{7 days}}$ Spleen Cells →

Control nu/nu: 10^9 HRBC ⟶ Spleen Cells →

Irradiated recipients* + T cells* + 10^8 SRBC

	Percent reduction in average number of anti-SRBC PFC per spleen at 6-7 days. (Experimental/Control)	
	Direct PFC	Indirect PFC**
	0	98
	0	93
	9	99

*nu/+ hydrocortisone-resistant thymocytes or "educated" thymocytes (16).
**Indirect PFC developed with an anti "a" (BALB/c type) Ig allotype serum.
Nu/nu and nu/+ derived from the 3rd to 5th backcross to BALB/c. Irradiated recipients were BALB/c.Ig^b (BAB/14), total of 33 mice in these three experiments. SRBC = sheep erythrocytes, HRBC = horse erythrocytes, PFC = plaque-forming cells.

On adoptive transfer spleen cells from 10^9 SRBC-injected nu/nu mice elicit IgM responses but not IgG responses when injected with T cells and 10^8 SRBC (Table III). Since direct PFC are observed on transfer, the lack of expression by B^μ cells in the one-host system above (c.f. 18 and 19) requires explanation. The most likely is that circulating antibody (i.e., T cell independent antibody) is inhibiting B cells of low ABC simply by competition for antigen. Such antibody is presumably not present in sufficient amounts, or is not present early enough, to inhibit the IgM response in the adoptive transfer system. No evidence has been obtained in Systems 2 and 3 for a delayed appearance of antibodies in tolerant mice (c.f. System 1).

An extension of System 3 provides good evidence that T cell independent antigen recognition by B cells occurs within 24 hours of injection using SRBC as antigen. Sprent and Miller (20) observed a transient unresponsiveness of spleen cells from very recently primed mice in standard adoptive transfer systems in irradiated recipients. When spleen cells are taken from nu/nu mice injected 1 day previously with 10^9 SRBC and injected into irradiated recipients together with T cells and 10^8 SRBC, neither an IgM nor an IgG anti-SRBC PFC response is observed (16). Thus, B cells not only "see" antigen shortly after injection of high doses but (at least the B^γ cells) are rendered tolerant by this antigen.

Recent experiments in collaboration with J.F.A.P. Miller have demonstrated that spleen cells from SRBC-injected nu/nu mice, which had been further injected with T cells and SRBC, are able to increase the response of other nu/nu mice to SRBC. These experiments are quite preliminary, but results of two experiments are pooled in Table IV. The potency of spleen cells from T cell-injected SRBC-tolerant nu/nu mice is increased slightly over that of a comparable low number of spleen cells from T cell injected, nontolerant nu/nu mice. This increased activity may or may not be significant, but it is clear from the data that "helper" T cell activity can be detected in spleen cell suspensions from both groups of T cell-injected nu/nu mice. We are pursuing this line in an effort to determine whether T cell dependent antibodies normally limit the presumed antigen-induced proliferation of helper T cells in reconstituted athymic mice.

TABLE IV

ASSAY FOR T CELL ACTIVITY IN SPLEENS FROM SRBC-TOLERANT NU/NU MICE INJECTED WITH T CELLS AND SRBC.

Injection to nu/nu spleen cell donors		No. of nu/nu recipients of 10^7 spleen cells + 10^8 SRBC (day 13)	PFC per spleen in recipients at day 19**	
day 0	day 9		Direct	Indirect
10^9 SRBC	T cells* + 10^8 SRBC	5	7150	7980
-	T cells + 10^8 SRBC	5	2100	2820
-	-	3	650	100
		4	520***	0

*Hydrocortisone-resistant thymocytes ($1^1/2$ BALB/c donors per 1 BALB/c nu/nu).
**Geometric mean PFC
***PFC response in 4 nu/nu mice injected intravenously with 10^8 SRBC only.

DISCUSSION AND SPECULATION

The observations in the three systems above lead to the conclusion that B cell precursors of IgG antibody-secreting cells (B^γ cells) are far more susceptible to "T cell-independent tolerance induction" than B cell precursors of IgM antibody-secreting cells (B^μ cells). Since large amounts of antigen (or highly persistent antigen) are required in these systems, the tolerance must be a form of "high dose" or "high zone" tolerance. The absence of responding T cells seems to render B^γ cells, presumably of high ABC, preferentially susceptible to tolerance induction. It must be remembered that all virgin B cells may well be expressing μ rather than γC_H genes at the time of initial contact with antigen. With antigen alone providing the signal for switch in C_H gene expression, IgG antibodies will always be of higher affinity than IgM antibodies for the particular determinant which effected the switch. This switched B cell requires the T cell dependent "second signal" in order to differentiate into IgG antibody-secreting cells. These considerations apply in particular to IgG_1 antibody production, this Ig class being highly T cell dependent and one which is markedly susceptible to tolerance induction (21). Conceivably, IgG_1 antibodies make up the bulk of high affinity antibodies in the mouse. [Of the Ig classes, IgG_1 and IgE are believed to be the most highly T cell dependent. Since these are the skin-fixing Igs, their actual T cell dependence relative to IgG_{2a} and IgA, for example, may be much less. In athymic nu/nu mice, for example, reduced levels of circulating IgG_1 and IgE antibodies may simply reflect the affinity of these (sub) classes for mast cells, etc. (which, incidentially, may be increased in number in nu/nu mice (22)).]

The antigen dose requirements in the type of tolerance discussed here, together with the known effects of T cell products (or at least T cell-dependent "lymphokines") or macrophage activities, lead to the hypothesis that T cells effect judicious removal of antigen from the milieu of antigen-binding B cells of high ABC by attracting and activating phagocytes in the immediate vicinity of these B cells. (T cell products could effect antigen digestion without phagocyte participation by activating digestive enzymes (e.g., proteases) from serum components or inactivating the serum protease inhibitors (e.g., $\propto 2$ macroglobulin, $\propto 1$ anti-trypsin)). This postulated role of T cells in T cell-B cell interactions in vivo has been discussed at length elsewhere (1,2). Figure 1 highlights the features of the hypothesis in which the antigen dependent "first signal" plays a dominant role in the triggering of B cells and the T cell dependent "second signal" is, in point of fact, a discontinuation of the "first signal", or a reduction in the frequency of the "first signal", in B cells of high ABC. The B^{μ} cells which "see" low amounts of antigen because of their low ABC do not require this "second signal" in order to differentiate into IgM antibody-secreting cells. Hence, the relative T cell dependence of high affinity antibodies and the T cell independence of low affinity antibodies.

It is predicted that B cells of high ABC which present antigen to T cells will be the actual B cells which are influenced preferentially by the nearby activated T cells. Any cell surface moieties which interfere with the access of T cells to antigen-binding B cells will reduce the efficiency of B cell triggering. Thus, Ig allotypic determinants and H or H-linked specificities may prejudice but should not absolutely preclude T cell-B cell interactions in the response to certain antigens (discussed in 2). This emphasis on B cell-associated antigen is not meant to infer that antigen supported in this location is the only means of activating T cells. Antigen on macrophage surfaces may well induce T cell activation (23), but this will have little effect on antigen-binding B cells unless the latter are in the vicinity of the activated T cells. Of course, an increased number of specifically-reactive T cells generated in this manner will alter late or booster responses.

There are two observations using hapten-carrier antigens in rabbits which appear not to fit with the predictions of the above hypothesis. Rabbits primed with hapten-carrier X respond by producing high affinity anti-hapten antibody on challenge with hapten-carrier Y. Moreover, preimmunization with carrier X leads to relatively low affinity antibody in response to hapten-carrier X challenge (24,25). Both observations have been made in one host systems. Thus, in the case of hapten-carrier X-primed rabbits responding to hapten-carrier Y challenge, preexisting anti-hapten antibodies may well be reducing the availability and tolerogenicity of antigen for B cells of high ABC (26). In vitro challenge of hapten-primed cells with high doses of the hapten on a heterologous carrier leads to inhibition (27-29). Low dose antigen challenge results in anti-hapten antibody, even in the absence of T cells - the dose of antigen is

presumably not high enough to induce tolerance in primed
B cells of high ABC and T cells are, therefore, not required
to protect from tolerance induction. On the carrier preimmunization effect, one is here presumably looking at
antibody production of unprimed B cells of low ABC which
must be in vast excess over B cells of high ABC in the
primary response to the hapten. T cell dependent high
affinity antibodies may well go undetected in analysis of
primary response sera unless analyses involving plaque-
forming cells are used. (30)

Antigen dose effects are known to influence profoundly
the outcome of the interaction between antigen, T cells,
B cells and the various ancillary cells. According to the
present hypothesis, low doses of antigen will elicit small
amounts of high affinity antibodies quite independently of
T cells (29). The antibody may be either IgG (from primed
B^γ cells) or IgM (from unprimed, "nonswitched" B^μ cells).
In the early studies on T cell-B cell interactions, the idea
was popular that increased antigen dose could overcome the
requirement for T cells in the induction of a B cell
response. There is by now much evidence against the notion
(as it applies to B^γ cells, reference 2) although it was
implicit that T cells do not provide an obligatory "second
signal" for B cell triggering. The present hypothesis goes
along with the latter (31 c.f. 4,5) but takes the Bretscher
and Cohn position (4,5) on the fate of B cells (B^γ cells)
responding to large amounts of antigen or persistent antigen in the absence of the "second signal".

On the point of T cell dependence of Ig classes in
antibody responses, it must be emphasized that the primary
IgM response to sheep erythrocytes (SRBC) is clearly T cell
dependent, whereas that to many other antigens including
(T,G)-A--L, is not. The number of T cells reactive to the
complex antigen SRBC in unprimed mice is likely to be high,
whereas the number reactive to (T,G)-A--L is likely to be
very low. Perhaps substantial T cell involvement in the
primary response to SRBC c.f. (T,G)-A--L in normal c.f.
athymic mice, ensures that the majority of B cells binding
antigen are recruited regardless of whether these cells are
B^γ cells of high ABC or B^μ cells of intermediate ABC. These
latter cells bind insufficient antigen to switch to γC_H
gene expression but bind enough to be susceptible to "high
dose" tolerance in T cell deficient mice (Fig.1). Such
cells would not be recruited into antibody production in the
primary response of either normal or T cell deficient mice

to (T,G)-A--L or T cell deficient mice to SRBC. These same cells (B$^\mu$ cells of intermediate ABC) may be the cells recruited (over and above the B$^\mu$ cells of low ABC) into antibody production by "extraneous" T cell involvement and/ or phagocyte stimulation in the IgM response to SIII in mice (13,32,33). Clearly antibody affinity (or cross-reactivity) measurements become important in these and related systems.

Finally, with respect to two aspects of tolerance of specific importance to this Conference, namely, "suppressor T cells" and "blocking factors", it is perhaps worth mentioning that suppressor T cells may well be hyperactive "helper" T cells which, by eliminating antigen as discussed above, reduce the number of B cells receiving the "first signal". If the end result of T cell + phagocyte activity is antigen elimination, there is presumably little reason to produce antibodies. Regarding "blocking factors", it is clear that if tolerance induction in B cells of high ABC is facilitated by a lack of reactive T cells, then "blocking factors" (e.g., antigen antibody complexes) need only operate at the level of T cells in order for B cell tolerance to be inducible by antigen. Thus, in many circumstances the presence of "blocking factors" for T cells may be a prelude to the deletion of B cells of high ABC. Sustained T cell "silence" will ensure that new B cells of high ABC, generated from the bursal equivalent, will be highly susceptible to tolerance induction, a situation which may also apply in the maintenance of tolerance to some self antigens.

REFERENCES

1. Mitchell, G.F., In Contemporary Topics in Immuno-biology, edited by M.D. Cooper and N.L. Warner, Plenum Press, New York, Volume 3. In press.

2. Mitchell, G.F., In The lymphocyte: Structure and Function., edited by J.J. Marchalonis, Marcel Dekker Inc., New York. In press.

3. Bretscher, P. and Cohn, M., Science. 169:1042, 1970.

4. Bretscher, P., Transplant. Revs. 11:217, 1972.

5. Cohn, M., In Genetic Control of Immune Responsiveness, edited by H.O. McDevitt and M. Landy, Academic Press, New York, p. 367, 1972.

6. Mitchell, G.F. and McDevitt, H.O., (unpublished observation), 1972.

7. Genetic Control of Immune Responsiveness, edited by H.O. McDevitt and M. Landy, Academic Press, New York, 1972.

8. Ordal, J. and Grumet, F.C., personal communication, 1973.

9. Mitchell, G.F., Humphrey, J.H. and Williamson, A.R., Eur. J. Immunol. 2:460, 1972.

10. Mitchell, G.F. and Humphrey, J.H., In Microenvironmental Aspects of Immunity, edited by B.D. Jankovic and K. Isakovic, Plenum Press, New York, Vol. 29, p. 125, 1973.

11. Mitchell, G.F., Humphrey, J.H. and Hamilton, J.A., (unpublished observations).

12. Howard, J.G., Transplant. Rev. 8:50, 1972.

13. Byfield, P., Cell. Immunol. 3:616, 1972.

14. Manning, J.K., Reed, N.D. and Jutila, J.W., J. Immunol. 108:1470, 1972.

15. Klaus, G.G.B. and Humphrey, J.H., personal communication, 1974.

16. Mitchell, G.F., Lafleur, L. and Andersson, K., Scand. J. Immunol. 3:39, 1974.

17. Schrader, J.W., J. Exp. Med. In press.

18. Klein, J., Livnat, S., Hauptfeld, V., Jerabek, L. and Weissman, I., Eur. J. Immunol. 4:41, 1974.

19. Ordal, J.C. and Grumet, F.C., Transplant. Proc. 5:175, 1973.

20. Sprent, J. and Miller, J.F.A.P., J. Exp. Med. 138:143, 1973.

21. Hay, F.C. and Torrigiani, G., Eur. J. Immunol. 4:5, 1974.

22. Viklicky, V., Sima, P. and Pritchard, H., Folia Biol. 19:247, 1973.

23. Rosenthal, A.S. and Shevach, E.M., J. Exp. Med. 138: 1194, 1973.

24. Steiner, L.A. and Eisen, H.N., J. Exp. Med. 126:1161, 1967.

25. Paul, W.E., Siskind, G.W., Benacerraf, B. and Ovary, Z., J. Immunol. 99:760, 1967.

26. Kontiainen, S. and Mäkelä, O., Immunology. 20:101, 1971.

27. Klinman, N.R., J. Exp. Med. 133:963, 1971.

28. Doughty, R.A. and Klinman, N.R., J. Immunol. 111: 1140, 1973.

29. Klinman, N.R. and Doughty, R.A., J. Exp. Med. 138: 473, 1973.

30. Claflin, L. and Merchant, B., J. Immunol. 110:252, 1973.

31. Mitchison, N.A., Rajewsky, K. and Taylor, R.B., In Developmental Aspects of Antibody Formation and Structure, edited by J. Sterzl and I. Riha, Academia, Prague, Vol. 2, p. 547, 1970.

32. Byfield, P., Christie, G.H. and Howard, J.G., J. Immunol. 111:72, 1973.

33. Howard, J.G., Christie, G.H. and Scott, M.T., Cell. Immunol. 7:290, 1973.

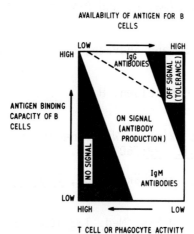

Fig. 1. Proposed influences of antigen on virgin B cells of various antigen-binding capacities (ABC) responding in the presence of large or small numbers of activated T cells. As examples, when the availability of antigen is high, virgin B cells of low ABC are triggered and produce IgM antibodies of low affinity, whereas B cells of high ABC are rendered tolerant. Conversely, when the availability of antigen is low, B cells of ABC receive no signals, whereas most B cells of high ABC switch from μ(IgM) to γ(IgG) C$_H$ gene expression and are triggered into IgG antibody production (of high affinity). The availability of antigen is reduced directly and indirectly by phagocytes and activated T cells, respectively. The scheme also applies to non virgin, primed B cells (of B$^\gamma$ type) other than that "on signals" result invariably in IgG antibodies again of various affinities.

DISCUSSION FOLLOWING GRAHAM MITCHELL

G. MÖLLER: You showed that DNP-SIII induced non-responsive-
ness of IgG antibodies following a challenge with DNP-
protein. Since this type of unresponsiveness is found
with DNP coupled to protein carriers, it seems likely
that the carrier rather than the hapten is responsible.
To my thinking it is the polyclonal B cell activating
property of the carrier which is responsible, but I
would be interested to hear your explanation.

MITCHELL: I would certainly agree that it is the carrier
which is of importance in this system of carrier-depen-
dent hapten-specific tolerance. I have been emphasizing
the persistence and the apparently non-T cell-activating
properties of the carrier rather than any polyclonal
B cell-activating property. In the system of Klinman,
large but not small amounts of hapten-heterologous
protein carrier and no amount of hapten-homologous
protein carrier will induce tolerance in anti-hapten B
cells. David Katz mentioned a similar observation in
his presentation. Thus for the moment I would stress
the combination--high availability of antigen for B
cells and lack of helper T cells--for tolerance induction in B cells of high antigen-binding capacity.

TAYLOR: Graham's hypothesis of the action of helper T-cells
as being to protect B cells from tolerance, would in
fact explain my results quite well. We might assume
that thymectomized-irradiated mice have a few helpers,
but lack suppressor T-cells. Their B cells would thus
be protected from tolerance (the results suggest they
were slightly primed). The injection of normal lymph
node cells would then supply suppressor T cells. One
would then have to make the assumption that suppressor
cells act only on helpers, and not directly on B-cells.

MITCHELL: I agree. One way to account for the difference
between the nudes and B mice is that T cell-dependent
suppression in the Gershon and Taylor systems acts
against injected helper T cells. We have not found
evidence for suppressor effects in spleen cells from
T cell-injected, B cell tolerant nude mice, (Table IV).
I am worried about the specificity in Dick Gershon's
system and the possibility that in Roger Taylor's system, reactive B cells are being recruited out of lymph

nodes by a T cell-dependent immune response occurring
in the spleen. Transferred lymph node cells unlike
spleen cells would then have a reduced capacity to
collaborate with helper T cells in antibody production.

I have long been in the "suppressor T cell = excess
help" school. Hyperactive T cells or phagocytes remove
antigen and thereby compete with B cells of antigen-
binding capacity for antigen. I think the Basten data
now speaks against this and is in line with the notion
that the suppressor effect is directed against helper
T cells rather than B cells. The question now arises,
does T cell-dependent high affinity antibody divert
helper T cells from the immediate environment of many
of the antigen-binding B cells? Interestingly, skin-
fixing antibodies are highly T cell-dependent (i.e. IgG
and IgE). Such antibody, when fixed to a mast cell for
example, may lure T cells away from B cells. The
relevant activation of T cells for a particular B cell
involves the T cells in the immediate vicinity of that
B cell. Chiller cannot find T cell-dependent suppressor
effects when he looks at the IgG1 response to HGG whereas Basten does find them when he looks at the presumably
mixed (IgG1 & IgG2a) anti-DNP response to DNP-HGG.
Anti-HGG titrations would be of interest in the Basten
system.

BRITTON: The T cell-independence of induction of B cell
    tolerance is reflecting the T cell-dependence of syn-
    thesis of the antibody which will combine with the
    antigen in such a form that it becomes tolerogenic. In
    the case of Roger Taylor's experiments, where T cell-
    dependence of induction of B cell tolerance to HGG was
    demonstrated, the synthesis of this antibody is thymus-
    dependent. In the case of Bγ cell tolerance to SRBC
    the synthesis of antibody is thymus-independent which
    was indicated by the data of Graham Mitchell obtained in
    the nude mouse. I emphasize that the existence of such
    antibody is hypothetical.

MITCHELL: There is an interesting point here. We do not
    know whether the presence of T cell-independent anti-
    body is required for tolerance induction in the T cell-
    dependent antibody classes. Is high affinity B cell
    tolerance facilitated by the presence of T cell-inde-
    pendent antibody as well as the absence of helper T

cells? Chiller and Weigle have looked for concomitant
antibody production in the course of HGG tolerance
induction but have not found it.

PAUL: Graham, your theory will have to deal with the heterogeneity of precursor cells in regard to affinity.
Thus, when you speak of high doses of antigen tolerizing
high affinity B_γ cells, do you not envisage that for a
class of B cells of somewhat lower affinity that dose
should be stimulatory. I would anticipate a shifting
down in affinity rather than an ablation of the IgG
response.

MITCHELL: A reduction in the amount of IgG would certainly
be expected to result with a shifting down in average
affinity. I believe the central point of the hypothesis
is that it takes into account the heterogeneity of B
cells with regard to affinity. A B cell of low antigen-
binding capacity requires a high dose of antigen to be
stimulated; this same dose of antigen will tolerize a B
cell of high antigen-binding capacity. The postulate
is that T cells reduce the availability of antigen for
the former cells at some critical time point after signal
one (antigen) has been "read" by the cell. Failure to
do this leads to B cell tolerance. It could be achieved
by promoting phagocytosis of antigen or by activation
of proteolytic enzymes. With low doses of antigen, B
cells of high antigen-binding capacity will not require
T cells to protect from tolerance induction and will be
induced into antibody production; this antibody, of
course, being of high affinity.

FELDMANN: Antigen persistence is one point you emphasize
strongly as a prerequisite for tolerance in vivo. In
vitro antigens persist, regardless of their chemical
nature. In the SRC tolerance system in the nude mouse,
it would be easy to test if persistence per se (long
access of antigen) is of major importance, or whether
accessibility of high concentrations of antigen to cells
is the critical feature by using fixed red cells (eg.
[glutaraldehyde]) in this tolerance system. Have you
used fixed red cells?

MITCHELL: The persistence of antigens in vitro may well contribute to the difficulty of inducing IgG (high affinity)
antibodies in vitro. Any mechanism which increases the
availability of antigen for B cells in vitro will

promote <u>low</u> affinity (IgM) antibody production. I did
actually try at one time to induce a normal IgM response
in nude mice by mixing SRBC with gluteraldehyde or
heavy trinitrophenylation. The attempts were unsuccessful. There are presumably far more appropriate antigens
of the type Sela uses which would enable one to answer
this particular question. I don't know whether a small
number of antigen signals over a long period of time
with low doses of persistent antigen will affect a B
cell in the same manner as a large number of antigen
signals over a short period of time with high doses of
metabolizable antigen.

FUNCTIONAL RELATIONSHIPS IN
ANTIGEN-RECEPTOR INTERACTIONS IN B LYMPHOCYTES

Emil R. Unanue
Kenneth A. Ault

Department of Pathology
Harvard Medical School
Boston, Massachusetts 02115

We have been studying the events that transpire in B lymphocytes upon interaction of their surface Ig with an appropriate ligand. Our objectives are to establish the reaction of the cell to ligand-receptors complexing in the absence of any cooperative signal from the thymic helper cells. By knowing precisely the reactions that a ligand to the receptor by itself can or cannot induce, one may then be able to place in a better perspective some immunological phenomena such as tolerance or the cellular cooperative interactions. Our studies have used as ligand either anti-Ig or specific antigen. The general results with both have been comparable. The studies with specific antigen are more difficult to carry out because of the paucity of cells binding a given antigen molecule.

The general design of the experiments is to treat lymphocytes in vitro with a rabbit IgG having antibody activity against various classes of Ig and then to follow the interaction by various immunocytochemical or biochemical procedures. The IgG can be labelled with fluorescein, radioiodine or ferritin and followed by immunofluorescence, by autoradiography or by electron microscopy, respectively.

Surface Ig, the receptor of antigen in the B lymphocyte, is distributed throughout the cell membrane. In the mouse, using freeze etch as the method to visualize the membrane, surface Ig form a continuous lattice with small microaggregates (reviewed in 1); in man the tendency is for microaggregation to be more prominent, leaving large areas of bare membrane (2). Microaggregation of receptor Ig is not the result of the technical procedure used for mapping. In studies with Drs. Abbas and Karnovsky, we have shown that such microaggregation occurs even in conditions where the surface topography was studied using monovalent ferritin-labelled antibodies. Monovalent antibodies are not expected to distort or change the original distribution of the surface Ig. The reason for the microaggregation is not known but may result from protein-to-protein interactions at the cell membrane. Upon interaction of anti-Ig with surface Ig, the complex readily redistributes into aggregates that flow to one pole of the cell. This is the phenomenon called capping first reported by Taylor et al. (3). Capping is a clear demonstration that the Ig molecules are not fixed rigidly on the cell surface but are free to translate themselves within the plane of the membrane in accordance with the fluid mosaic model of membrane structure proposed by Singer and Nicholson (4). One important condition for redistribution is that the anti-Ig be bivalent, that is to say, that cross-linking of adjacent sites take place; monovalent antibody will not initiate the process (1, 3). Capping is not a passive phemenon but involves an energy-dependent step. Treatment of lymphocytes with inhibitors of glycolysis or of oxidative phosphorylation will stop capping but will not prevent the focal aggregation of complexes on the membrane (3, 5).

What is the importance and function of receptor redistribution? The redistribution of complexes on the membrane is not sufficient to stimulate most lymphocytes to proliferate and differentiate into plasma cells (6). However, receptor redistribution appears to play a role in binding an antigen molecule with higher avidity. Indeed, in unpublished experiments we have shown that the amount of antigen bound to lymphocytes under conditions where capping is suppressed is reduced by about 75%. Furthermore, aggregation of receptors on purpose--by the use of critical amounts of anti-Ig-- increases immune responsiveness probably because this aggregation brings into play lymphocytes with low affinity receptors (6).

At the same time the lymphocyte is capping its receptors, it also begins to move (7) (Fig. 1). The increase in translational motility is clearly evidenced by examining cells under the microscope at 37^{0}C. The increase in translational motility is conditioned to a cross-linking ligand, like capping, and involves energy and a biochemical step sensitive to disopropylfluorophosphate--DFP, an irreversible inhibitor of serine esterases. The results suggest that the ligand-receptor interaction activates a proenzyme that is in some way involved in the process of cell movement.

Capping and translational movement can be dissociated from each other. For example, the microfilament-disrupting drug cytochalasin B stops movement completely, although it will not greatly affect the capping of receptors. Likewise,

302

cells treated with DFP still cap but are reduced in their translation. We have concluded that capping involves some membrane perturbation produced by a signal from a cross-linking ligand and perhaps involves membrane flow. Translational motility is a part of the chain reaction initiated by the ligand and serves to orient the cap to the trailing edge of the cell, although by itself the translational process is not essential for capping. We speculate that the stimulation of cell motility is an important facet in immune induction having to do with the association of the specific lymphocyte with antigen in lymphoid tissues.

At the time that complexes are being capped, the lymphocyte starts interiorizing them in an energy-dependent process (2, 3, 8). The interiorized complexes with time are digested and eliminated. The capacity of lymphocytes to degrade the interiorized complexes was studied by labelling the anti-Ig with ^{125}I and determining the fate of the ^{125}I after its binding to the B cell. Such an experiment is depicted in Fig. 2. With time the ^{125}I label is eliminated from the lymphocyte and appears in the culture fluid. Analysis of the culture fluids discloses that the bulk of the ^{125}I is bound to amino acids and to partially digested products of IgG. It should be noted that a small amount of the ligand-receptor complex is eliminated as a whole complex from the lymphocyte. This shedding of complexes doesn't involve interiorization nor metabolic energy.

Following the elimination of the complex, the lymphocyte starts resynthesizing new receptors to the extent that by 6 to 18 hours the cell surface has a full complement of receptor molecules on its membrane. In fact, ligand-receptor interaction stimulates the lymphocyte for an increased rate in protein synthesis. As expected, the reexpression of surface receptors requires protein synthesis. Indeed, if following capping lymphocytes are cultured in the presence of inhibitors of protein synthesis, reexpression of new surface Ig is prevented. Two points are worth stressing. First, in order for the lymphocyte to have full receptors on its surface, one must eliminate the ligand (anti-Ig) from the culture. It is our thought that, as long as the ligand is present, the receptors are in a constant cycle of reexpression--complexing to ligand-pinocytosis-catabolism. However, we have no proof of this point. The second point is that the amounts of newly synthesized receptors is the same as in the cell that has not gone through a cycle of capping; in other words, the lymphocyte maintains a control in the amount of receptor that it displays on its surface.

In summary, the ligand-receptor interaction triggers a series of reactions that start at the cell membrane and interconnect by unknown ways with intracellular organelles. The result is stimulation of membrane movement, clearance of the membrane, initiation of cell movement, increased protein synthesis, reexpression of surface Ig and probably other as yet unidentified cellular changes. Clearly, the lymphocyte has a remarkable ability to clean itself of surface complexes and then to reexpress new surface Ig, which is of great functional importance. The series of events are summarized in Table I.

TABLE I

CONSEQUENCES OF LIGAND-RECEPTOR INTERACTION IN B LYMPHOCYTES

Effect	Requirements	Postulated Function
1. Redistribution of ligand-receptor complex	Capping involves an energy-dependent step. Focal membrane aggregation is energy dependent.	High avidity for binding antigen
2. Translational mobility	Motion depends on metabolic energy, on the activation of a serine esterase and on integrity of microfilaments.	Increased random motility may favor the meeting of lymphocytes with other immune cells
3. Interiorization of complex	Energy dependent	
4. Shedding of complexes	Energy dependent	Could bind macrophage and serve as a means for concentrating antigen.

In order to study the interaction of lymphocytes with labelled antigen, we have followed the protocols depicted in Fig. 3, using lymphocytes from mice immunized to dinitrophenylated (DNP) proteins. The essence of the procedure is to label the DNP specific lymphocytes with DNP on various carriers to which no helper T cells are available. The lymphocytes then are placed in culture, and the elimination of the labelled material from the cell is determined; alternatively, the lymphocytes are incubated with labelled DNP proteins, and at different time intervals their capacity to bind for a second time new labelled DNP guinea pig albumin (GPA) is determined.

We have carried out studies using DNP bound to globular proteins (9), many of which induce tolerance such as autologous albumins, or Ig or ovalbumin. The main results are as follows: Initially, the number of lymphocytes binding DNP varies from 30 to 150 per 10^5 lymphocytes examined. The binding is totally blocked by 10^{-3}M DNP lysine and anti-Ig but not by unrelated proteins. After binding of the labelled material, the lymphocytes rapidly eliminate it. Lightly conjugated DNP proteins interact weakly with the lymphocyte, rapidly dissociating and leaving the receptors on the cell. Multivalent DNP proteins are likewise eliminated, but the process is slower and is accompanied by the loss of the receptor. Indeed, as early as one-half hour and no later than four hours, the bulk of radioactivity has disappeared from the cell. Coincident with the loss of the labelled antigen, the receptors are likewise lost as evidenced by the inability to label lymphocytes again with new, freshly labelled antigen. We have surmised that the lymphocyte is eliminating the ligand-receptor complex in the same way as it was eliminating the anti-Ig-Ig complex, that is, by a combination of interiorization and degradation plus shedding from the cell surface. The exact process with antigen is not known because of the limitation imposed by the experimental assay (autoradiography). As with anti-Ig, new receptors reappear after several hours of culture. Indeed, by about one day a normal number of lymphocytes binding DNP proteins are found again in cultures. The B lymphocytes that bind DNP proteins are not triggered to differentiate and proliferate. However, we have observed certain changes in cell density of DNP cells after 24 hours, suggesting some early abortive changes in the cell. Representative experiments are shown in Fig. 4. In summary, as with anti-Ig, B lymphocytes eliminate antigen-receptor complexes and then go on to synthesize a full complement of new receptors.

We have been particularly interested in studying the interaction of DNP bound to a synthetic polymer made up of d amino acids. Such polymers, such as the d-glutamic acid and d-lysine copolymer (60:40 ratio, D-GL) studied intensively by Katz, Benacerraf and co-workers, are very potent tolerogens (see their papers in this Symposium). Brief exposure of lymphocytes from DNP-primed mice to DNP-D-GL in vitro leads to a state of irreversible DNP tolerance. We labelled lymphocytes from mice primed with DNP-hemocyanin with radio-iodinated DNP-D-GL to which we had bound tyramine groups. Such labelled cells were placed into cultures and followed for several days. In contrast to the rapid elimination of DNP bound to globular proteins, DNP-D-GL was poorly eliminated from a great many B lymphocytes. Indeed, by 24 or 48 hours after a brief pulse with DNP-D-GL, a great many of the B lymphocytes still maintained this compound (Fig. 4).

It was of no surprise that a lymphocyte would fail to eliminate an undigestible polymer made of d amino acids. What surprises us were two results: one that a great part of the compound was on the cell surface; and secondly, that free anti-DNP receptors were not reexpressed by the cell. Indeed, with the use of a purified anti-DNP antibody, we have been able to show that cells exposed to DNP-D-GL had DNP-reactive material on their surface. Also, cells exposed briefly to DNP-D-GL would never bind DNP-GPA to their surface. In contrast to DNP-D-GL lymphocytes eliminated DNP-L-GL and expressed new anti-DNP receptors.

These results with DNP-D-GL raise a series of important issues. One issue concerns the interiorization process and its interruption by a carrier molecule made up of d amino acids. So far, the interiorization has been thought of as a process initiated by a cross-linking ligand where the carrier portion of the molecule played no important role. The present result implies that interiorization is a process that involves some biochemical step with the carrier molecule which can be blocked by a compound that is nondigestible by normal protcolytic enzymes. The second issue is the incapacity of the DNP-D-GL-treated cell to reexpress new receptors. The actual process in question is not clear. Perhaps new anti-DNP receptors are resynthesized, but they are either displayed on the surface and immediately become bound in the complexes, or they are secreted instead of being fixed to the surface; or perhaps receptor synthesis is blocked. This is an important point to clear up since it would seem that the inability to reexpress new DNP receptors is in great part responsible for the prolonged state of tolerance.

Studies like this with DNP-D-GL must now be carried out with other nonmetabolizable antigens in order to establish whether this is a general phenomenon or one peculiar to this compound.

The relevance of these studies with DNP on hapten specific tolerance is obvious. DNP compounds that do not bring into play specific helper T lymphocytes can produce, under appropriate circumstances, a state of tolerance. However, on the basis of how the B lymphocytes handle them, one must postulate two distinct forms of tolerogens: one represented by the metabolizable compounds (such as autologous albumin or Ig) and the other represented by nondigestible material. The result suggest that with the former the B lymphocyte can eliminate the antigen and acquire fresh receptors; hence, the tolerant state should depend either on some suppressive function perhaps of hapten specific T lymphocytes in the absence of carrier specific T lymphocytes or on some functional intrinsic defect of the B lymphocytes since they are able to reexpress receptors. On the other hand, with nondigestible antigen, the B lymphocyte seems definitely altered as a result of its inability to complete the normal cycle of clearance. Further studies should help us in the understanding of the molecular basis of tolerance.

REFERENCES

1. Unanue, E.R. and Karnovsky, M.J., Transpl. Proc. 14: 184, 1973.

2. Ault, K.A., Karnovsky, M.J. and Unanue, E.R., J. Clin. Invest. 52:2507, 1973.

3. Taylor, R.B., Duffus, P.H., Raff, M.C. and de Petris, S., Nat. New Biol. 233:225, 1971.

4. Singer, S.G. and Nicholson, G.L., Science. 175:720, 1972.

5. Unanue, E.R., Karnovsky, M.J. and Engers, H.D., J. Exp. Med. 137:675, 1973.

6. Katz, D.H. and Unanue, E.R., J. Immunol. 109:1022, 1972.

7. Unanue, E.R., Ault, K.A. and Karnovsky, M.J., J. Exp. Med. 139:295, 1974.

8. Engers, H.D. and Unanue, E.R., J. Immunol. 110:465, 1973.

9. Ault, K.A. and Unanue, E.R., J. Exp. Med. Volume 139, 1974. In press.

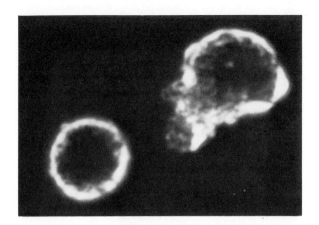

Fig. 1. This is a darkfield photomicrograph of lymphocytes after incubation with anti-Ig. The lymphocyte to the
right is in the process of translation and exhibits the
typical ameboid, hand-mirror shape. The lymphocyte to the
left is stationary. Anti-Ig stimulates movement of B cells
only (from: Unanue et al, J. Exp. Med. 139:295, 1974).

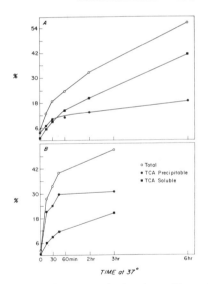

Fig. 2. Two experiments that show the elimination of
degraded ^{125}I-IgG anti-Ig from human peripheral blood lymphocytes were incubated with the ^{125}I-labelled antibody, then
washed and placed in culture. Curves represent elimination
of total ^{125}I, of ^{125}I bound to protein (thrichloroacetic--
TCA--precipitable) or ^{125}I bound to amino acids (TCA-soluble).
Note the progressive elimination with time of TCA-soluble
material (from: Ault et al, J. Clin. Invest. 52:2507,
1973).

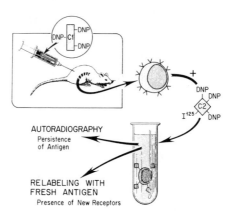

Fig. 3. This graph demonstrates the protocol used for studying fate of antigen bound to B lymphocytes. Lymphocytes were harvested from mice immunized with DNP-hemocyanin, incubated briefly _in vitro_ with DNP on different carriers and studied as represented (9).

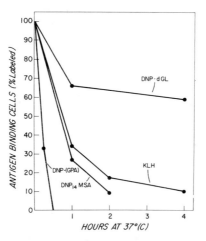

Fig. 4. This is a summary of various experiments showing the fate of various DNP compounds from lymphocytes. Vertical axis represents number of cells with autoradiographic grains. The number of cells at time 0, after a brief exposure, is 100%. (Published in part by Ault and Unanue, J. Exp. Med. Volume 139, 1974. In press.)

B CELL TOLERANCE IN VITRO
THE FATE OF THE TOLERANT CELL AND ITS CONTROL BY HORMONES

E. Diener and K-C Lee

The MRC Transplantation Group
Departments of Immunology and Biochemistry
The University of Alberta, Edmonton, Alberta, Canada

The tolerant cell is defined as a lymphocyte which carries the genetic information for a specific antigen recognition pattern but has temporarily or permanently ceased to express its competence to become an effector cell (antibody-forming cell, killer cell, helper cell) upon further contact with the relevant antigen. Since the life span of a tolerant cell may be a matter of a few days only, proof in functional terms for its existence is difficult. Tolerant cells may be recognized experimentally by reversing their state of unresponsiveness to one of immunocompetence at various time intervals after tolerance has been induced. The usefulness of such an exercise is obvious: If we knew how to reverse tolerance, we might be able to reveal retrospectively tolerance-inducing mechanisms at the biochemical level. Some time ago, we were able to demonstrate that in vitro tolerance could be reversed by means of proteolysis within one to two days after induction but not later (1). This we have taken as evidence in support of the hypothesis that under tolerogenic conditions, antigen remains attached to the immunocompetent cell's surface in concentrations high enough to cause paralysis by long-term blocking of receptors. This was further supported by the subsequent observation that under such conditions the cell is, indeed, unable to remove the antigen from its surface by the capping mechanism in contrast to cells maintained under immunogenic conditions (2).

We are now going to present evidence which suggests a tolerance-inducing mechanism operating at the intracellular level. Furthermore, we shall describe experiments which indicate that susceptibility of lymphocytes to the induction of unresponsiveness may be controlled by glucocorticosteroid hormones. All experiments have been carried out in vitro using polymerized flagellin (POL) at either immunogenic or tolerogenic concentrations. These studies were exclusively concerned with B cell tolerance, as tested by measuring numbers of antibody-forming cells (AFC) produced by CBA mouse spleen cells during 4 days of culture.

311

The first of the above conclusions has emerged from experiments in which we attempted to establish an in vitro antigen dose response curve for tolerance induction in spleen cell suspensions from mice injected 24 hours previously with 10 mg of cortisone; a dose conventionally regarded as immunosuppressive. We had already learned from earlier experiments by Lee and Langman (3) that cortisone-suppressed spleen cells become totally response in vitro when given 2-mercaptoethanol (2ME) at a concentration of 5×10^{-5} molar. This suggests that at least a proportion of immunocompetent cells must have escaped destruction by the hormone. However, without the addition of 2ME, we have shown that the cortisone-induced immune suppression was related to the antigen dose. The optimally immunogenic concentration for cortisone-treated cells was 200 fold lower than that for normal control cells (Fig. 1). The question we address ourselves to in this presentation is whether the shift in the antigen dose threshold for immune induction in cortisone-treated cell populations is paralleled by a similar shift in the antigen threshold concentration for tolerance induction. In normal spleen cells tolerance may be induced in vitro by preincubating them for 6 hours in the presence of 10 to 20 µg/ml of POL followed by washing and culturing them for 4 days in the presence of an optimally immunogenic antigen dose of 250 ng/ml. Similarily, cortisone-treated spleen cells were, thus, incubated with an otherwise immunogenic concentration of POL (250 ng/ml) for 6 hours, washed and challenged for 4 days in vitro with 1 ng/ml of POL. The results (see Table I) indicate that for in vivo cortisone-treated cells, tolerance was, indeed, induced with an antigen dose which for normal spleen cultures is considered immunogenic. This suggests the possibility that unresponsiveness could be the result of some intracellular process triggered by the antigen rather than by receptor blocking alone. Alternatively, cortisone at cytotoxic concentrations may selectively have killed off part of the immunocompetent cells, the remaining ones being those cells which are normally rendered tolerant by immunogenic doses of antigen. Essentially, similar findings were made when cortisone treatment of spleen cells was carried out in vitro at concentrations of 1 and 0.1 µg/ml of Prednisolone. However, at a dose of 0.01 µg/ml, the hormone had hardly any effect on the antigen dose response curve except for high antigen concentrations. In the presence of Prednisolone, an antigen dose which was tolerogenic for normal cells, was now immunogenic (Fig. 2). This phenomenon was further investigated by comparing the influence of different concentrations of Prednisolone on the induction of tolerance in vitro. Groups

of cultures were set up with normal mouse spleen cells in
the presence of Prednisolone from 10 μg/ml to 1 ng/ml. POL
at a dose of 10 μg/ml was added to each group and the ensuing
immune response measured 4 days later. This dose of antigen
is tolerogenic for normal cells. To account for antigen
specificity of tolerance, sheep red cells (SRC) were added to
each culture along with POL at a dose of 3×10^6 cells/ml.
The results obtained (Fig. 3) show that a dose of 10 ng/ml
of Prednisolone completely prevented the induction of tolerance to POL while it had no effect on the immune response to
the immunogenic concentration of SRC. The fact that the
concentration of Prednisolone, causing this phenomenon, is
close to the physiological concentration of glucocorticosteroids in vivo adds further interest to this finding.
It is important to note that lymphocytes that had already
become tolerant during exposure to supraimmunogenic concentrations of POL for 6 hours failed to reverse their state of
unresponsiveness when treated with Prednisolone. Thus, the
drug had to exert its influence on the cells at a time of
antigen encounter. This, however, was not true when 2-mer-
captoethanol (2ME) was also added together with Prednisolone
at a concentration of 5×10^{-5} molar (Table II). 2ME, when
added alone, was without effect. Reversibility of tolerance
by treatment with the drug and 2ME was possible within a
time interval of 48 hours following induction (Table III).

TABLE I

EFFECT OF CORTISONE ON THE ANTIGEN DOSE RESPONSE

Spleen cells from mice injected 24 hours previously with
10 mg of cortisone are rendered tolerant by an otherwise
immunogenic concentration of POL (i.e. 250 ng/ml).

Cortisone Treatment 10 mg in vivo	POL for 6 hrs	Challenge for 4 days	AFC/culture ± SEM	
			POL	SRC*
+	1 ng	1 ng	1410 + 246	18 + 16
+	250 ng	1 ng	185 + 54	43 + 31
-	1 ng	1 ng	1945 + 166	3393 + 340
-	250 ng	1 ng	2690 + 185	2750 + 88
-	20 μg	250 ng	50 + 17	1175 + 168

*SRC were added along with POL at a concentration of
3×10^6 cells/culture.

TABLE II

EFFECT OF PREDNISOLONE TOGETHER WITH 2-MERCAPTOETHANOL ON TOLERANT MOUSE SPLEEN CELLS

Tolerance was induced by incubating normal spleen cells in vitro for 6 hours with 20 μg POL/ml. After washing the cells were cultured for 4 days in the presence of 250 ng/ml of POL + Prednisolone (P) and 2-mercaptoethanol (2ME).

Preincubation with POL for 6 hrs	Challenge with POL	AFC/culture ± SEM	
		POL	SRC*
20 μg/ml	250 ng/ml	405 ± 27	1231 ± 116
250 ng/ml	250 ng/ml	9940 ± 605	2725 ± 488
20 μg/ml	250 ng/ml + P + 2ME	13795 ± 323	3631 ± 205
20 μg/ml	250 ng/ml + 2ME	95 ± 12	2412 ± 125

*SRC were added along with POL at a concentration of 3×10^6 cells/culture.

The above experiments have demonstrated that certain corticosteroids such as hydrocortisone and its analogue Prednisolone exert a profound immuno-regulatory function in vitro with respect to tolerance. It is of particular interest that such hormones were also effective at concentrations that may occur under physiological conditions in vivo. This raises the distinct possibility that in vivo the immune system is partially under regulatory control by glucocorticosteroids. In fact, the apparent association of certain immunological disorders with either cortisone deficiency (Addison's disease) or cortisone hyper-production (Cushing's disease) (4) may point in this direction. Our data do not elucidate the mechanisms by which the hormones affect immune performance. They suggest, however, that glucocorticosteroids, at least in part, influence immunocompetent cells metabolically by setting the triggering thresholds with respect to the antigen dose required for induction of immunity and tolerance.

TABLE III

EFFECT OF PREDNISOLONE (P) TOGETHER WITH 2-MERCAPTOETHANOL (2ME) ON TOLERANT MOUSE SPLEEN CELLS

Treatment groups day 0 and day 1 were cultured for a total of 4 days. Treatment groups day 2 and day 3 were cultured for a total of 6 and 7 days, respectively, to allow for a full 4 day response post treatment.

Treatment of Cells				AFC/culture $\pm$ SEM	
Day 0	Day 1	Day 2	Day 3	POL	SRC*
250 ng POL				7030 $\pm$ 202	4462 $\pm$ 150
20 µg POL				115 $\pm$ 15	2012 $\pm$ 117
20 µg POL + P + 2ME				3120 $\pm$ 122	5612 $\pm$ 207
20 µg POL + P + 2 ME				3730 $\pm$ 400	4656 $\pm$ 43
20 µg POL		+ P + 2 ME		1896 $\pm$ 550	1925 $\pm$ 525
250 ng POL		+ P + 2 ME		5496 $\pm$ 420	1390 $\pm$ 570
20 µg POL			+ P + 2 ME	228 $\pm$ 75	1140 $\pm$ 231
250 ng POL			+ P + 2 ME	4972 $\pm$ 360	995 $\pm$ 145

*Sheep red cells (SRC) were added along with POL at a concentration of 3 x 10^6 cells/ml.

SUMMARY

The effect of glucocorticosteroids on the antigen dose response curve and on tolerance induction in vitro have been investigated. It was found that cortisone in vivo or its water soluble analogue Prednisolone in vitro at concentrations which were immunosuppressive for reactivity to sheep erythrocytes caused a shift in the dose response curve to polymerized flagellin as measured in vitro. Thus, cortisone-induced immunosuppression to otherwise immunogenic doses of the antigen was found to be due to tolerance, while lower antigen concentrations were immunogenic. Prednisolone at low, non-immunosuppressive concentrations, however, prevented the induction of unresponsiveness in vitro with otherwise tolerance-inducing concentrations of antigen.

Tolerance, once induced in vitro, could be reversed by Prednisolone together with 2-mercaptoethanol but not by either of the two agents alone. Some of these data suggest that: a) Tolerance results from metabolic events induced by interaction of antigen with surface receptors, and b) Corticosteroids may control immunocompetence by setting the triggering thresholds with respect to the antigen dose required for induction of immunity and tolerance.

ACKNOWLEDGMENTS

This work was supported by the Canadian Medical Research Council, the National Cancer Institute of Canada # 55-45021 and the National Institute of Health, U.S.A. # 1 RO1 AI11595-01.

REFERENCES

1. Diener, E. and Feldmann, M., Cell. Immunol. 5:130, 1972.

2. Lee, K-C, Langman, R.E., Paetkau, V.H. and Diener, E., Eur. J. Immunol. 3:306, 1973.

3. Lee, K-C and Langman, R.E. In preparation.

4. Irvine, W.J., Chan, M.M.W. and Scarth, L., Clin. Exp. Immunol. 4:489, 1969.

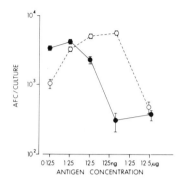

Fig. 1.   Antigen dose response curve in vitro of spleen cells from CBA/CaJ mice injected 24 hours previously with 10 mg of cortisone.

    -●- = cortisone-treated spleen cells
    -o- = untreated control cells
    AFC = antibody-forming cells/culture ± SEM

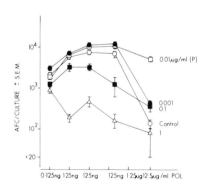

Fig. 2.   Antigen dose response curve in vitro of mouse spleen cells in the presence of different concentrations of Prednisolone (P).

    AFC = antibody-forming cells to POL ± SEM control
          cultures had no P added.

317

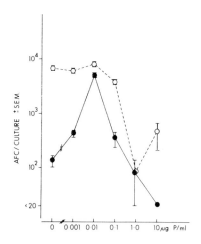

Fig. 3.   Effect of Prednisolone on the induction of tolerance.   Spleen cells were cultured with a tolerogenic concentration of POL in the presence of different amounts of Prednisolone (P) as indicated on the abscissa.   Sheep erythrocytes (SRC) at a concentration of 3×10^6/ml were added along with POL.

-o- = response to sheep erythrocytes (SRC)
-●- = response to polymerized flagellin (POL) at tolerogenic concentrations of 5 μg/ml.

GRAFT-VERSUS-HOST REACTIONS,
TUMOR SPECIFIC IMMUNITY AND SELF TOLERANCE

Sven Britton

Division of Immunobiology, Karolinska Institutet
Wallenberglaboratory, Lilla Freskati
104 05 Stockholm 50, Sweden

INTRODUCTION

Injection of immunocompetent lymphoid cells into allogeneic hosts incapable of rejecting the inocula (graft-
versus-host, GVH) results in gross distrubances of, primarily, the host's lymphoreticular system to which the injected cells home (1). One of the many features of these
reactions is that the immunocompetence of the host as regards
antibody formation is transiently enhanced. During other
phases of the GVH reaction the antibody-forming ability is
markedly reduced (2). The immunoenhancing effect of the GVH
reaction has lately been coined "the allogeneic effect" (3).
Not only B cell functions such as antibody formation but
also claimed T cell properties such as rejection of transplanted leukemic cells has been announced to be enhanced by
GVH reactions (4). From these latter experiments (4), it
has actually been stated that "the potential promise of such
an approach to the immunotherapy of human cancer is considered" (5).

I, as many others, for better (5) or for worse (6),
want to join the cancer-curing craze. I have studied the in
vitro cellular immune response to a lymphoma tumor in lymphocytes of mice undergoing a graft-versus-host reaction with
special reference to the effector cell taking part in the
reaction. As I arrive to the tentative conclusion that a
considerable part of this anti-tumor response is directed
against self-antigens on the tumor cells, the reaction thus
possibly constituting an example of breakdown of self-tolerance, I think the data have relevance for this conference.
Somewhat beyond the scope of this conference, though, I shall
report on the protective effects of GVH reactions on the in
vivo growth of the lymphoma tumor tested.

MATERIALS AND METHODS

Animals. Parental A/Sn (H-2^a) mice and their F$_1$ hybrids
A x CBA (H-2^a/H-2^k), A x C57B (H-2^a/H-2^b), A x 5M (H-2^a/H-2^b)

were used as hosts and cell donors in the tumor experiments. CBA (H-2^k) and AKR (H-2^k) mice were used for raising allo-anti-θ sera. New Zealand white rabbits were used for raising heterologous mouse bone marrow lymphocyte antiserum (MBLA).

Tumor. A Moloney virus-induced lymphoma (YAC), adapted for growth in an ascites form in a A/Sn mice by George Klein, Department of Tumor Biology, Karolinska Institutet, and carried by serial passage in our mouse colony, was used as test tumor. In these experiments it was used during its 234th to 272nd passage. The in vivo growth behavior of this tumor both in its parental host as well as in F$_1$ hybrids and allogeneic hosts has been described in much detail elsewhere (6).

Labelling of tumor cells and cytotoxic assay. These techniques have been described in much detail previously (7, 8). In brief, tumor cells were taken out aseptically from the abdomen of tumor-bearing mice and after washing were labelled in vitro with ^{125}I-iodo-deoxyuridine (^{125}IUdR) obtained from Amersham, England. 10^5-labelled tumor cells were placed together with 10^7 spleen cells in a 35 mm plastic petri dish (Falcon) in a 1 ml volume of tissue culture medium plus 10% heat-inactivated fetal calf serum. The dishes were then placed in a 10% CO_2 atmosphere at 37ºC and rocked for 16 hours. The test was harvested at that time and the percent release of isotope was calculated (7). In each experimental group spleen cells from three mice were pooled.

Antisera. Allo-anti-θ (C3H) sera was produced as described before (9) by repeatingly injecting AKR mice with CBA thymus cells. AKR normal serum was used for control. Sera were heat-inactivated and ultrafiltrated before use in the in vitro assays. Guinea pig serum absorbed with agarose and diluted 1/2 was the source of complement. Mouse bone marrow lymphocyte heterologous antiserum (MBLA) was produced as described before (10) essentially by twice intravenous injections of lymphocytes from thymectomized bone marrow protected mice into rabbits. Such antiserum was thereafter absorbed with mouse thymocytes and erythrocytes until no more antibodies against these cell elements could be detected by means of cytotoxic or agglutination tests. The retained bone marrow specific antibody of the antiserum used in these experiments amounted to a cytotoxic titre of 1/32 where 100% dead cells were the end point in a vital dye cytotoxic test.

Production of selectively purified cell preparations.
Splenic lymphocytes deprived of thymus-derived lymphocytes
were produced either by exposing normal spleen cells to an
allo-anti-θ serum plus guinea pig complement , diluted 1/2
in a balanced salt solution. Each reaction step took place
at 37° for 30´. Control cells were treated as above but
with normal AKR serum.

Thymus cell-deprived spleen cells were also obtained
by harvesting the spleen cells from animals that had thymectomized, lethally irradiated (750 r) and repopulated with
10^7 anti-θ-treated syngeneic bone marrow cells. Spleen cells
from such treated animals were used within two weeks after
repopulation.

Spleen cell suspensions deprived of cells carrying the
MBLA marker were obtained by treating normal spleen cells
with heat-inactivated anti-MBLA serum and guinea pig complement diluted 1/2. Control spleen cells were treated with
heat-inactivated normal rabbit serum and complement.

Spleen cells deprived of adherent cells were obtained
by twice exposing the cells to carbonyl iron powder and
each time extracting the cells attaching to the iron particles by means of a magnet. The details and efficiency of
this procedure has been described before (11).

RESULTS

Kinetic of appearance of cytotoxic cells in spleen cells
from animals undergoing a GVH reaction. When F_1 hybrid mice
such as A x C57BL are injected with parental A/Sn spleen
cells, cytotoxic cells develop which kill YAC lymphoma target cells carrying the same histocompatibility antigens as
the injected parental cells as well as the host cells. The
kinetics of this reaction is not very dose dependent, but
the intensity of the reaction is markedly dose dependent
(Fig. 1). When a more detailed analysis of the appearance
of cytotoxic cells in GVH spleens was performed, a two-peak
response was observed (Fig. 2). This was true in F_1 animals
injected with the optimal dose of 20 x 10^6 parental (A/Sn)
spleen cells. The peak responses were obtained at days 2
and 14 after injection of the parental cells; the former
peak being less reproducible than the latter.

The effect of graft-versus-reaction on tumor-specific immunity. Utilizing the above cytotoxic system, it is difficult to demonstrate tumor-specific cytotoxic immunity. In our hands this normally requires at least three injections of 10^7 heavily in vitro irradiated (10,000 r) syngeneic tumor cells. When tumor-specific immunity (i.e. cytotoxic spleen cells against I^{125}-labelled YAC appearing in A/Sn or its F_1 hybrids injected in vivo with YAC killed tumor cells) finally develops, the cytotoxic spleen cells are always highly sensitive to anti-θ serum plus complement (Fig. 3).

In several experiments it was studied whether tumor-specific cytotoxicity could be increased and accelerated by interposing a GVH reaction during the immunizing regimen against the TSTA of the tumor cells. The time schedule proposed by Katz (3) for enhancing an anti-hapten response by means of a GVH reaction was followed in principle, and 10^7-irradiated YAC tumor cells were injected into various A/Sn F_1 hybrids whereafter they were given 2 x 10^7 parental (A/Sn) spleen cells 10 days later. One week after injection of the parental spleen cells, they were given a further challenge of 10^7-irradiated YAC tumor cells, and their spleen cells tested against I^{125}-labelled YAC 4-7 days after the last tumor inoculation. Figure 4 summarizes 14 such experiments using various F_1 hosts as spleen cells from mice receiving only parental lymphoid cells as compared with that of mice receiving repeated injections of tumor cells and in addition parental spleen cells (Fig. 4). In order to find out whether an immunoenhancing effect against TSTA of the GVH reaction was shielded due to the possibility that the cytotoxic potential was at maximum already in the spleen cells receiving 2 x 10^7 parental spleen cells, a suboptimal dose (Fig. 5) of parental spleen cells was injected during the course of immunization against TSTA with irradiated tumor cells. Using a dose of only 1 x 10^6 parental spleen cells interposed between two injections of irradiated tumor cells, it can be seen that the cytotoxic effect was considerably increased as compared to the one in spleen cells from animals receiving twice injections of irradiated tumor cells plus injection of 1 x 10^6 syngeneic spleen cells in between (Fig. 5).

On the origin of the effector cytotoxic cell in spleens from animals undergoing a graft-versus-host reaction. It has been claimed before (12, 13) that the cytotoxic cell in the host organ in which a graft-versus-host reaction is going on is, indeed, of host origin. This cell is displaying a non-specificcytotoxicity against both the injected parental cells as well as the surrounding host cells. We have tried to analyze this in our experimental system, but, using otherwise highly effective and specific anti-H-2 antisera, we have so far been unable (S. Britton, unpublished experiments) to identify the origin (host or parental) of the cytotoxic cell. When we have exposed spleen cells from animals undergoing a GVH reaction to pretreatment with allo-anti-⊖, anti-MBLA and iron, respectively, (Fig. 6 and 7), we were also unable to depict the organ origin of the effector cytotoxic cell. It is clear though that it is distinct from the one found in spleen cells of animals specifically immunized against TSTA as that cell was found to be highly sensitive to all anti-⊖ serum (Fig. 3).

   The protective effects of GVH reactions on in vivo growth of YAC lymphoma cells. It has been claimed with considerable emphasis that the GVH reactions have a tumor protective effect in vivo and that such a reaction can even interfere with an already growing leukemia (4,5). We find no such evidences (Figs. 8 and 9). Mice injected three times with irradiated syngeneic tumor cells and in between the last injections, in addition, injected with either parental or syngeneic (2×10^7) spleen cells show a delayed outgrowth of a subsequent challenge of 10^4 live lymphoma cells (Fig. 8). However, there is no difference in between the two groups. Animals receiving only parental spleen cells do not resist the challenge of live tumor cells (Fig.8). If instead the survival time after similar treatments is determined, it can be seen that only animals preimmunized with irradiated tumor cells and injected with syngeneic spleen cells will resist a subsequent challenge of living tumor cells, whereas animals pretreated with irradiated tumor cells plus parental spleen cells or parental spleen cells alone display no protective effects (Fig. 9).

CONCLUSIONS

   Using a virus-induced lymphoma cell carrying tumor-associated antigens as labelled target cell in a cytotoxic assay, it has been clearly shown that in the GVH spleen cytotoxic spleen cells appear with reactivity against epitopes on the lymphoma cell. As the target lymphoma cell carries no transplantation antigens, but the TSTA, foreign to either the parental or the host cells, one could assume that cytotoxicity was, indeed, directed towards the TSTA.

The in vivo experiments of Katz et al (4) would support such an idea. My experiments tend to exclude this possibility. The experimentally induced tumor-specific immunoreactivity of spleen cells against these TSTA is highly sensitive to anti-Θ serum treatment whereas the GVH-induced cytotoxicity is completely resistant to this serum. Also, the kinetics of the appearance of the GVH-induced cytotoxicity tends to argue against reactivity being directed against TSTA since reactivity in the spleen is detectable already two days after injection of parental cells. This would be too early for an anti-TSTA cellular immune response to develop. We are presently analyzing whether the two peaks of cytotoxicity in GVH spleen reflects traffic of effector cells and whether the origin of the effector cells in the two peaks is the same.

Although the data in this paper clearly support the previous notion that a GVH reaction can also influence T cell performances (14, 15), the author is mostly inclined to believe that the cytotoxicity recovered in the GVH spleen is directed against self-antigens and that at least the latter peak response, recoverable fourteen days after an optimal dose of parental spleen cells, is mediated by the same type of cell which is effector cell in the antibody-induced cell-mediated cytotoxic reaction (8,11).

The author, as well as others(4,5),have been unable to detect any antibodies in the serum of GVH animals with properties of inducing cellular autocytotoxicity (S. Britton, unpublished experiments), but this is most probably due to immediate absorption of such antibodies to host tissues.

In these experiments,I find no protective effects of the GVH reaction against in vivo growth of lymphoma cells, albeit the spleen cells of the same animals showed a very strong cytotoxicity in vitro. There is still a possibility that I have been unlucky in picking somewhat wrong doses or slightly wrong time schedules of immunizations for tumor protection to be evident. It is evident from these experiments, though, that whatever effects a GVH reaction has on a tumor-specific immune response, it is going to be difficult to monitor, thus calling for great precaution before announcing it as a mean of curing human cancers.

ACKNOWLEDGMENTS

My American colleague, Dr. James Forman, took part in the initiation of this work. Erna Möller kindly supplied me with the anti-θ and anti-MBLA sera, and Ulla Claeson and Gun Stenman did, as always, all the experimental work. Goran Möller revised the manuscript for me and for you. Ulla Persson proposed the experiment outlined in Fig. 5. These studies were supported by grants from the Swedish Cancer Society.

REFERENCES

1. Simonsen, M., Act. Path. Microbiol. Scand. 40:480, 1957.

2. Lawrence, W. and Simonsen, M., Transplantation. 5:1304, 1967.

3. Katz, D., Transplantation Rev. 12:141, 1972.

4. Katz, D., Ellman, L., Paul, W., Green, I. and Benacerraf, B., Cancer Res. 32:133, 1972.

5. Ellman, L., Katz, D., Green, I., Paul, W. and Benacerraf, B., Cancer Res. 32:141, 1972.

6. Britton, S., Transplant. Rev. 7:1, 1971.

7. Forman, J. and Britton, S., J. Exp. Med. 137:369, 1972.

8. Britton, S. and Forman, J., Transplantation. 17:180, 1974.

9. Greaves, M. and Möller, E., Cell. Immunol. 1:372, 1970.

10. Niederhuber, J. and Möller, E., Cell. Immunol. 3:559, 1972.

11. Britton, S., Perlmann, H. and Perlmann, P., Cell. Immunol. 8:420, 1973.

12. Volkman, A., J. Exp. Med. 136:21, 1972.

13. Singh, J., Sabbadini, E. and Sehon, A., J. Exp. Med. 136:39, 1972.

14. Osborne, D. and Katz, D., J. Exp. Med. 138:825, 1973.

15. Lindholm, L. and Strannegård, Ö., _Int. Arch. Imm_.
In press, 1974.

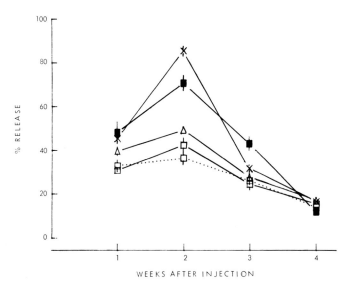

Fig. 1. Kinetic appearance of cytotoxic spleen cells in A $\overline{\text{x C57BL}}$ mice injected with varying doses of A/Sn spleen cell. Target cells YAC (H-2^{a}) lymphoma cells. x————x 20 x 10^6 cells injected. ■————■ 200 x 10^6 △————△ 2 x 10^6 □————□ 0.2 x 10^6 ☐········☐ uninjected.

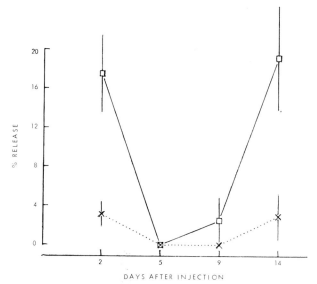

Fig. 2. Kinetic appearance of cytotoxic spleen cells in A $\overline{\text{x 5M}}$ and A x C57BL mice injected with 20 x 10^6 A/Sn spleen cells at day 0. Data are mean + SE of four experiments. Background release of tumor cells alone is deduced. ☐————☐ injected with 20 x 10^6 cells. A/Sn cells ☐·····☐ injected with 20 x 10^6 syngeneic (A x 5M or A x C57BL, respectively) spleen cells.

327

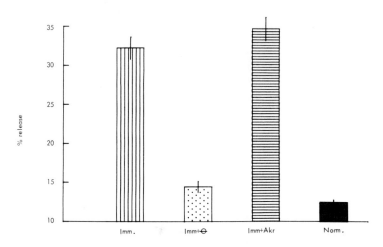

Fig. 3.   Cytotoxicity in spleen cells of A x CBA mice
injected three times one week apart with 10^7 heavily irradiated (10,000 r) YAC tumor cells.   Tested one week after
last injection against I^{125}-labelled YAC target cells.
Imm. = Immunized spleen cells.   Imm. + ⊖ = Immunized spleen
cells treated with anti-⊖ serum plus C´.   Imm. + AKR =
Immunized spleen cells treated with normal AKR serum plus
complement.   Norm. = Normal A x CBA spleen cells.

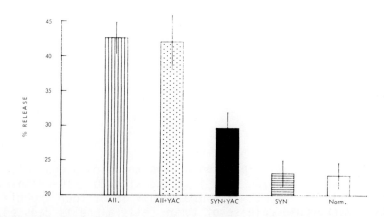

Fig. 4.

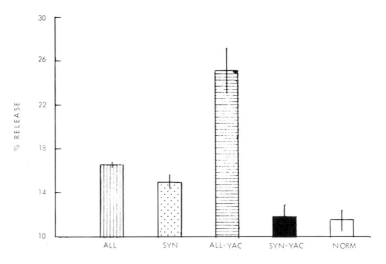

Fig. 5. Cytotoxicity of spleen cells from animals
(A x C57BL) receiving a suboptimal dose of parental spleen
cells. Target cell I^{125}-labelled YAC. ALL. + YAC = Spleen
cells from animals receiving twice injections of 10^7
irradiated YAC tumor cells and one week before last injection
1 x 10^6 parental (A/Sn) spleen cells. Tested 12 days after
injection of parental cells only and tested 12 days later.
Syn. + YAC = Injected twice with irradiated YAC and 1 x 10^6
syngeneic spleen cells 12 days before test. Syn. = injected
with 1 x 10^6 syngeneic spleen cells 12 days before test.
Norm. = Spleen cells from untreated A x C57BL mice.

Fig. 4. Mean percent release + SE of spleen cells from
fourteen experiments with similar experimental approach.
Effector cell donors of strains A x CBA, A x C57BL, A x 5M.
Target cell I^{125}-labelled YAC. All. = Spleen cells from F_1
mice injected with 2 x 10^7 A/Sn spleen cells 9-12 days
before test. All. + YAC = Spleen cells from animals in
addition injected with 10^7-irradiated YAC tumor cells fourteen days before and one week after injection of parental
cells. Syn. + YAC as previous group but injected with 2 x
10^7 syngeneic spleen cells 9-12 days before test. Syn. =
Injected with 2 x 10^7 syngeneic spleen cells 9-12 days
before test. Norm. = Spleen cells from uninjected F_1
controls.

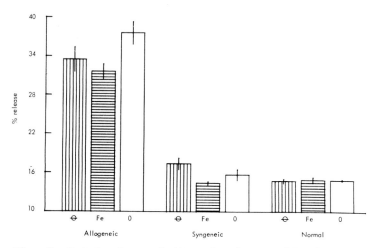

Fig. 6. Cytotoxic activity of spleen cells from animals (A x CBA) receiving 20 x 10⁶ parental spleen cells (allogeneic). 20 x 10⁶ syngeneic spleen cells (syngeneic) and untreated, respectively. Tested 12 days after injection of cells. Θ = pretreated with anti-Θ plus C´. Fe = Pretreated with iron powder. 0 = untreated.

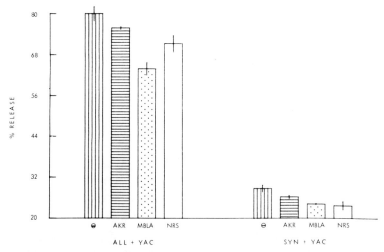

Fig. 7. Cytotoxic activity of spleen cells from animals (A x 5M) injected 20 x 10⁶ parental (A/Sn) spleen cells (ALL + YAC) or 20 x 10⁶ syngeneic spleen cells (Syn. + YAC) and one week later injected with 10⁷ irradiated YAC tumor cells. Θ = spleen cells pretreated with allo-anti-Θ plus C´. AKR = Pretreated with normal AKR serum plus C´. MBLA = Pretreated with anti-MBLA plus C´. NRS = Pretreated with normal rabbit serum plus C´.

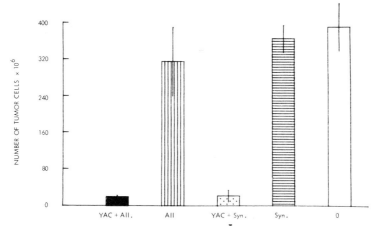

Fig. 8. Number of YAC tumor cells harvested from A x
5M animals injected i.p. with 10^4 live YAC tumor cells fourteen days before harvest. Values are means + SE from 8
animals. YAC + ALL = Animals pretreated with two weekly i.p.
injections of 10^7-irradiated YAC tumor cells plus 20 x 10^6
parental (A/Sn) spleen cells i.v. one week before challenge
with 10^4 live YAC tumor cells. ALL = Animals injected with
20 x 10^6 parental spleen cells one week before challenge
with 10^4 live YAC cells. YAC + Syn. = Injected with two
weekly i.p. injections of 10^7-irradiated YAC tumor cells
followed by one i.v. injection of 20 x 10^6 syngeneic spleen
cells one week before challenge with 10^4 live YAC cells.
Syn. = Animals injected with 20 x 10^6 syngeneic spleen cells
one week before challenge. 0 = Animals only challenged with
10^4 live YAC i.p.

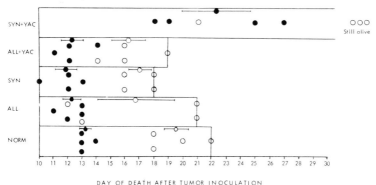

Fig. 9. Groups of animals (A x C57BL) treated as in
Fig. 8 with exception that immunization with irradiated
tumor cells in groups Syn. + YAC and ALL. + YAC was done
with 10^7 cells twice before and one one week after injection
of spleen cells. Challenge with live tumor cells done
5 days after last injection with irradiated cells thus 12
days after injection of spleen cells.

RECEPTOR BLOCKADE BY TOLEROGEN: ONE EXPLANATION OF TOLERANCE

Yves Borel, M.D. and Marlene Aldo-Benson, M.D.

From the New England Medical Center Hospital
and Tufts University School of Medicine,
Boston, Massachusetts.

INTRODUCTION

According to the clonal selection theory, natural tolerance to self antigens is due to the elimination of clones of lymphoid cells which recognize "self" (1). This idea was challenged by the demonstration in normal adults of lymphoid cells capable of recognizing auto antigens (2). Furthermore, studies on the number of antigen-binding cells (ABC) in tolerant animals brought conflicting results: ABC were found to be increased (3,4), unchanged (5-7) or, in most instances, decreased (8,9). A decrease in the number of ABC is consistent with Burnet's hypothesis that tolerance involves their elimination. However, there are alternative explanations. For example, the receptors of ABC could have been internalized or shed into the serum, or tolerizing antigen on the cell surface interfered with the detection of the ABC.

We have approached this problem using the system of carrier-determined tolerance (10,11). This experimental model closely resembles natural tolerance because the carrier (isogeneic IgG) is a self protein and the hapten (dinitrophenyl, DNP) by itself is neither immunogenic nor tolerogenic. Moreover, DNP-isogeneic IgG induces tolerance in a number of strains of mice regardless of their capacity to respond to the immunogen (DNP-KLH) (12). The practical implications of this system are indicated by the F_1 mice by the induction of immunologic tolerance to nucleic acid antigens using conjugates of nucleosides bound to syngeneic IgG (13).

In this paper we review the evidence that ABC are not eliminated in tolerant animals. Instead, they bind the tolerogen thereby blocking their receptors for antigen. We call these cells tolerant cells and propose that blockade of their receptors accounts not only for many phenomena observed in acquired tolerance but may very well be the mechanism of natural tolerance.

The tolerant cell.

Autoradiography, using either DNP-KLH-I^{125} (the tolerogen) or purified I^{125} murine anti-DNP antibody, was done with spleen cell suspensions from normal or tolerant animals. Six to eight week old BDF$_1$ mice were made tolerant of DNP either by a single injection of 0.2 mg of DNP$_7$-isogeneic IgG. The animals were either injected with tolerogen alone or were also challenged with the antigen. (In the latter case, 0.2 mg of DNP-KLH was given in complete Freund's adjuvant immediately after the single or the last tolerogen injection). Control groups include normal untreated animals and animals treated with the antigen (DNP-KLH) given in the same dose and by the same route (i.v.) as the tolerogen. Five days after the last injection autoradiographic studies were done.

The number of spleen lymphoid cells which bound the antigen (DNP-KLH-I^{125}) or tolerogen (DNP-MGG-I^{125}) was the same in both normal animals and in animals tolerant for one week (14). Blocking studies showed that the binding of antigen or tolerogen by lymphocytes was hapten-specific (14). Thus, there is no evidence that the specificity of the receptor on the ABC has changed in tolerant animals. In contrast to the results obtained in animals tolerant for one week, the number of cells binding the antigen or the tolerogen in animals tolerant for four weeks was markedly reduced (14).

To investigate whether this reduction was apparent or real, autoradiography was done using purified I^{125}-labelled anti-DNP antibody to determine whether DNP was present on the cell surface. This indirect method revealed that in animals tolerant for one week there was a significant increase in the number of hapten-bearing cells as compared to normal untreated animals (Fig. 1). Of special importance is the fact that this increase was not observed in animals treated with the antigen. In animals tolerant for four weeks, the number of hapten-bearing cells was also markedly increased (Fig. 2). This was the case whether the animals were treated with tolerogen alone or treated with tolerogen and challenged i.p. with the antigen. In sharp contrast in animals treated only with the antigen, hapten-binding cells were not found in numbers exceeding the background.

The specificity of the binding of anti-DNP to the tolerant cells was determined by inhibition studies. These were done on spleen cell suspensions from mice tolerant for four weeks. The results show that the binding of anti-DNP to these cells is hapten specific. Unlabelled anti-DNP (which was shown to be only IgG1) blocked 80% of the binding above the background level, whereas unlabelled IgG1 gave only a small amount of nonspecific blocking (29%) (Fig. 3). In all these autoradiographic studies only labelled intact lymphocytes were enumerated; macrophages were excluded from the calculations.

Are the results due to binding of the hapten (DNP) or the carrier (IgG) to lymphocytes? Three lines of evidence favor the former: a) DNP-binding cells can be specifically deleted by either highly labelled DNP-MGG-I^{125} (antigen suicide technique)(15); b) using different fluorescent conjugates (DNP-MGG conjugated to fluorescein and DNP-KLH conjugated to rhodamine), we found that over 95% of ABC's had double fluorescence (16); and c) autoradiographic data show that the number of cells in normal animals which bind DNP-MGG-I^{125} is the same and that the binding is specific (14), not for the protein carrier, but for the hapten moiety.

Nevertheless, the question remains whether, in addition to cells binding the hapten because of receptors specific for DNP, other cells have DNP on their surface because they bound the IgG carrier. This could occur either specifically (monocytes have a receptor for the Fc fragment of IgG1 (17) and B cells have a receptor for aggregated IgG)(18), or nonspecifically. A small number of spleen lymphoid binds I^{125}-anti-DNP antibody (about 20 per 10^5) nonspecifically. Binding cannot be blocked by unlabelled anti-DNP antibody or by IgG1. In contrast, the increased number of cells with DNP on their surface observed in tolerant animals can be specifically inhibited by unlabelled anti-DNP antibody but not by IgG. We, therefore, carried out further experiments.

In the first, we took advantage of our recent observations that the induction of tolerance to DNP-MGG requires that the carrier be of the IgG1 or IgG2a classes (19). It was found that animals treated with DNP bound to IgG1 had increased numbers of DNP-bearing cells as compared to normal. In contrast, in mice treated with DNP bound to Ig2b and IgG3 (which are ineffective in the induction of tolerance), there was no significant increase in the number of DNP-binding cells (Fig. 4).

In the second experiment we varied the conjugation site of DNP on mouse IgG1 because it was found that not only the immunoglobulin class, but the manner of binding of the hapten to it was critical in the induction of tolerance (20). (DNP-ε-lysine-IgG1 is tolerogenic, whereas DNP-azo which binds to histidine or arginine of IgG1, and DNP-mustard, which binds to carboxyl groups of IgG1, are not tolerogenic.) Only in animals treated with DNP-ε-lysine-IgG1 was the number of DNP-bearing cells increased (Table I).

These data demonstrate that receptor blockade occurs only when the determinant induces tolerance. Thus, a functional divergence in the tolerogenic and immunogenic forms of the same antigenic determinant (DNP) is demonstrated. On the one hand, the tolerogen occupies membrane receptors of the ABC.

TABLE I

Treatment	Tolerance Induction	Hapten Bearing Cells	Receptor Blockade
DNP-ε-lysine-IgG1	+	49 ± 10	+
DNP-azo-IgG1	−	0	−
DNP-mustard-IgG1	−	0	−

Table I. Mice injected with DNP-ε-lysine γ1 or DNP-mustard γ1 were immune. The number of hapten-bearing cells listed is that number of cells binding I^{125}-anti-DNP in excess of the nonspecific normal background (20 ± 1). The tolerant animals receiving DNP-ε-lysine γ1 were the only animals having hapten-bearing cells above background. This value was significantly different from the nontolerant animals ($p < .001$).

Receptor Blockade: One explanation of acquired and self tolerance.
Receptor blockade is a plausible explanation of many phenomena related to acquired tolerance. For example, lymphoid cells from tolerant animals do not undergo antigen-specific proliferation in vitro (21, 22). In addition, receptor blockade is an attractive explanation of self tolerance. It is known that lymphocytes with surface receptors for autologous antigens exist (2). Direct interaction

between self antigens and these receptors may cause receptor blockade. The idea of receptor blockade also explains why the presence of the antigen is necessary for both the induction and maintainance of tolerance (23).

Alternatively, it is possible that small amounts of antibody to self antigens are produced. These antigen-antibody complexes might remain on the cell surface in vivo, as described by Diener and Feldmann (24). These explanations of self tolerance are also consistent with the blocking factors of the Hellströms (25). Whether the blocking factor is an antigen-antibody complex (26), antigen receptor complex, or the tolerogen itself (27), the end result is the same: occupation of receptors on potentially self-reactive lymphocytes. Thus, the delicate balance between natural tolerance and autoimmunity would depend upon the balance between lymphoid cells with receptors occupied by the antigen and lymphoid cells with free receptors. Autoimmune disease would be the result of a preponderance of lymphoid cells with available receptors.

ACKNOWLEDGEMENTS

This study was supported by NIH Grant #AI-09825 and the Damon Runyon Foundation, Grant #1262.

Dr. Benson is a Fellow of the Massachusetts Arthritis Foundation.

REFERENCES

1. Burnet, F.M., Vanderbilt Univ. Press, Nashville, Tenn., 1959.

2. Bankhurst, A.D., Torrigiani, G., and Allison, A.C., Lancet.

3. Howard, J.G., Elson, J., and Christie, G.H., J. Exp. Immunol. 4:41, 1969.

4. Sjöberg, O., and Möller, E., Nature. 228:780, 1970.

5. Humphrey, J.H., and Keller, H.U., In Developmental Aspects of Antibody Formation and Structure, edited by J Sterzl and I. Riha, Academia Prague, 2:485, 1970.

6. Ada, G.L., Byrt, P., Mandell, T., and Warner, N., In Developmental Aspects of Antibody Formation and Structure, edited by J. Sterzl and I. Riha, Academia Prague, 2:485, 1970.

7. Cooper, H.G., Ada, G.L., and Langman, R.E., Cell. Immunol. 4:289, 1972.

8. Katz, D.H., Davie, J.M., Paul, W.E., and Benacerraf, B., J. Exp. Med. 134:201, 1971.

9. Louis, J., Chiller, J.M., and Weigle, W.O., J. Exp. Med. 137:461, 1973.

10. Borel, Y., Nature New Biology. 130:180, 1971.

11. Golan, T.D., and Borel, Y., J. Exp. Med. 134:1046, 1971.

12. Borel, Y., and Kilham, L., Proc. Soc. Exp. Biol. Med. 145:470, 1974.

13. Borel, Y., Lewis, R.M., and Stollar, B.D., Science. 182:76, 1973.

14. Aldo-Benson, M., and Borel, Y., J. Immunol. In press.

15. Golan, D.T., and Borel, Y., J. Exp. Med. 136:305, 1972.

16. Lewis, R.M., and Borel, Y., (unpublished observation).

17. Basten, A., Miller, J.F.A.P., Sprent, J., and Pye, J., J. Exp. Med. 135:610, 1972.

18. Anderson, C.L., Grey, H.M., Fed. Proc. 33:802, 1974.

19. Borel, Y., and Kilham, L., Fed. Proc. 5:4408, 1973.

20. Palley, R., Leskowitz, S., and Borel, Y., In preparation.

21. Dutton, R.W., J. Immunol. 93:814, 1964.

22. Borel, Y., and Schlossman, S., J. Immunol. 106:397, 1971.

23. Triplett, E.L., J. Immunol. 89:505, 1962.

24. Diener, E., and Feldmann, M., J. Exp. Med. 31:132, 1970.

25. Hellström, I., and Hellström, K.E., _Nature._ _230_:49, 1971.

26. Sjögren, H.O., Hellström, I., Bansal, S.O., and Hellström, K.E., _Proc. Nat. Acad. Sci._ _68_:1372, 1971.

27. Wekerle, H., Cohen, I.R., and Feldmann, M., _Nature New Biology._ _241_:25, 1973.

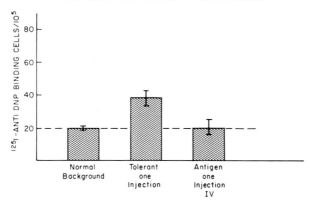

Fig. 1. Determination of hapten-binding cells in one week tolerant mice. Results are expressed as number of labelled cells per 100,000 lymphocytes. Group one consists of 6 normal mice, assayed separately. Group two consists of 4 mice receiving one i.v. injection of DNP_7MGG. Group three consists of 4 mice receiving one i.v. injection of DNP_{83}-KLH. The number of labelled cells in the tolerant group is significantly higher than in the normal or the antigen injected group ($p < .001$).

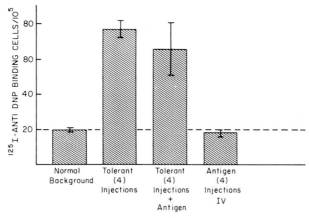

Fig. 2. Determination of DNP on the surface of splenic lymphocytes in 4 week tolerant mice. The groups consist of 6 normal mice; 4 mice receiving 4 injections of DNP_8-MGG i.v. weekly; mice treated exactly as the second group but also receiving one dose of DNP_{83}-KLH; and mice receiving DNP_{83}-KLH i.v. in four weekly injections. There was no significant difference between the normal group and the DNP-KLH injected group ($p > .2$). However, there is a significantly higher number of cells which bind anti-DNP antibody in the two tolerant groups than in either the normal or the antigen-injected group ($p < .001$).

340

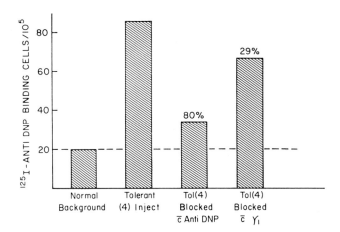

Fig. 3. Specificity of labelling of DNP on cell surface in four week tolerant animals. The first group of 3 normal mice has a non-specific labelling. The second group of three animals has received four weekly i.v. injections of DNP_{10}-MGG. When these same tolerant lymphocytes were preincubated with unlabelled anti-DNP antibody, 80% of the labelling above background was blocked. When unlabelled $\gamma 1$ immunoglobulin was pre-incubated with the tolerant cells, only a small percent (29%) of nonspecific blocking is noted.

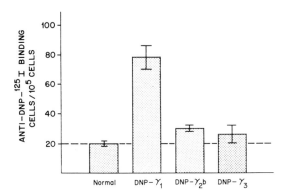

Fig. 4. Relationship of hapten-bearing cells to induction of tolerance. Groups of four mice were injected with either tolerogenic DNP_{12}-IgG1 or non tolerogenic DNP-IgG2b or DNP-IgG3. Labelling of spleen cells from DNP-IgG1 injected mice was significantly higher than normal controls (p< .001), while both the DNP-Ig2b and DNP-Ig3 were similar to normals and significantly lower than the tolerant animals (p < .005).

GENERAL DISCUSSION - SESSION III

MECHANISMS OF B CELL TOLERANCE

Hugh McDevitt, Chairman

NOSSAL: My comments relate chiefly to Dr. Borel's concept of
retained antigen on B cell receptors as a mechanism for
tolerance. Over the period 1963-1968, Ada, Mitchell
and I spent much time searching for the distribution
and persistence of tolerogen after _in vivo_ injection of
^{125}I-labeled tolerogen. We never obtained evidence of
blocked B cells. Admittedly, most of our work was on
flagellar antigens, which cause a different type of
tolerance. However, we did study antigens such as rat
or bovine serum albumin, hemoglobin and other monomeric
proteins. I suggest that Dr. Borel should test his
theory by injecting into his mice a tolerogenic dose of
DNP-^{125}-IgGl, and simply study the distribution and
persistence of the antigen. I believe he will _not_ find
persistence on B cell receptors for four weeks.

McDEVITT: Dr. Nossal's studies were done on _sections_ of
lymph nodes, and it would have been quite easy to miss
antigen-binding cells with 10-15 grains carried by the
entire cell. I was seeking information as to whether
anyone had induced tolerance with highly-labeled anti-
gens-either metabolizable antigens such as HGG, or non-
metabolizable antigens such as DNP-D-GLT labeled with
I^{125}, and then studied cell suspensions from lymph nodes
for the persistence of antigen-binding cells.

BOREL: We are very well aware of Nossal's studies on the
fate of antigen in tolerant animals. However, I do not
think that the methods used (autoradiographic studies
using tissue section and complex antigen) were able to
resolve the issue as to whether small numbers of antigenic determinants would stay on the surface of the
specific antigen-binding cell.

UNANUE: Drs. Paul and Davie found no DNP-D-GL binding cells
in tolerant mice-We find DNP-D-GL persisting _in vitro_.
Both results can be explained by saying that _in vivo_
the DNP-D-GL cells are "opsonized" and taken up by the
reticuloendothelial system.

Insofar as Borel's studies - his results do not

support his conclusion since in no control has he shown that the DNP-IgG is bound to the cloned lymphocyte-the observations that DNP tolerogen is found but not the DNP - immunogen is expected since the former is retained and the latter is eliminated by the immune response. To establish that he has receptor blockade he should transfer lymphocytes depleted of the specific cloned anti-DNP cell.

ADA: I think there are two very important questions arising from Yves' work! 1) Is he, in fact, measuring the per-sistence of DNP-IgG on the cells he examines? 2) If so, are the cells which he observes those cells which were rendered tolerant? This is more difficult to answer.

PAUL: One difficulty in the use of labeled antigen as tolerogen is the amount of radioactivity which one would have to administer. Thus, if a dose of 1 mg of tolerogen is required and a specific activity of $20\mu Ci/\mu g$ is desired, each mouse would have to be given 20 mCi of ^{125}I.

BENACERRAF: I would like to ask Yves Borel: 1) How much antigen did you use to establish tolerance and what is the 1/2 life of the antigen? 2) Do you have any data indicating the participation of suppressor T cells in your system?

BOREL: The dose we used to induce tolerance is 0.2 mg of DNP isogeneic IgG. I agree with the possibility that after receptor blockade did occur on the hapten-binding cell, the tolerogen might leave this cell and bind to another lymphoid cell. On the one hand it raises the question of the relevance of our finding, or, on the other, it might be the mechanism by which tolerance is maintained.

[Editor's Note: Dr. Borel felt that data on the possibility of suppressor cells in his system were too preliminary to comment upon]

FELDMANN: I'd like to come to Yves's defense. Various people have been surprised that in Yves's DNP IgG toler-ance model there is receptor blockade four weeks after the injection of tolerogen. Basically, Yves pointed out that his form of tolerance is reversible in vitro by culturing spleen cells from tolerant mice for two days.

Thus, his is a reversible tolerance system, and thus, it should not surprise us that antigen-binding cells are still present, even in large numbers in his animals.

Just a point of philosophy about basic mechanisms of tolerance in mature B cell. We have had presented in the last two days various systems of tolerance, some of which are reversible but others are not. Conceptually, they can be fitted into a model of tolerance as a differentiation sequence, with different stages such as:

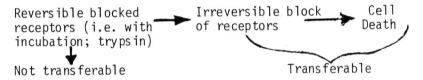

Reversible blocked receptors (i.e. with incubation; trypsin) ⟶ Irreversible block of receptors ⟶ Cell Death

Not transferable   Transferable

It seems important in different models of tolerance to know the level of suppression, for both T or B cell tolerance, as a preliminary step to understanding the different stages of tolerance induction.

G. MÖLLER: I think the body of evidence strongly favors Borel's conclusion. The missing link to show that the binding cells are actually the tolerant cells is very difficult to demonstrate. The important question is what happens. Do you figure tolerance in this system to be an entirely passive event (blocking) or is a signal generated by binding?

BOREL: I agree that the fact that the class of IgG (IgG$_1$, Ig2a) which are tolerogenic have an Fc fragment which binds to cells raises the question of the role of these cells in the induction of tolerance to the hapten. Although this question is still open, we were unable to prevent tolerance to DNP-IgG$_1$ by treating the host with large doses of IgG$_1$ prior to and during the induction of tolerance to DNP-IgG$_1$. Thus, so far, we have no evidence which indicates that Fc binding of the carrier plays a role in the induction of tolerance to DNP bound to this carrier.

HERZENBERG: Michael Julius has been using fluorescent-labeled DNP-MGG to stain spleen cells from unprimed mice. He finds he can substantially reduce the number of binding cells by including aggregated immunoglobulin in the

staining medium to block Fc receptor binding of the
DNP-MGG.

PAUL: The fluorescence activated cell sorter should provide
a way to determine whether the antigen-bearing cells
which Borel has described are indeed blocked, and
DNP-specific immunocompetent lymphocytes. If fluorescent anti-DNP is used to label these cells, they could
be purified. Borel points out that tolerance is ablated
in vitro; thus, incubation of purified cells in the
presence of cells congenic at the allotype locus followed by in vivo or in vitro challenge and a determination of whether anti-DNP of the allotype of the tolerized mouse is produced should determine the potential
competence of the blocked cells.

BASTEN: I should like to comment on the concept of receptor
"blockade" with particular reference to Dr. Borel's
observations with various DNP-MGG preparations. The
"Fc receptor" on murine B cells is known to bind IgG_1
preferentially. Selective uptake of $DNP-IgG_1$ onto B
cells as detected by anti-DNP antibody binding could,
therefore, be due to attachment to the membrane via Fc
as well as Ig receptors. Since $DNP-IgG_1$, but not DNP-
IgG_{2a}, or $DNP-IgG_{2b}$ tends to be tolerogenic, it is
tempting to speculate that tolerance induction at the
level of the B cell depends on Fc receptor dependent
formation of an antigen antibody lattice on the cell
membrane. Perhaps the role of suppressor T cells is to
"distract" carrier-reactive cells, thereby creating
optional conditions for tolerogenesis and protecting the
B cell from activation.

KATZ: As this session is closing, I would just like to expand on the issues raised by Marc Feldmann a few minutes ago. I think we are all in agreement with the
premise that there are multiple mechanisms of cell
unresponsiveness. However, I believe too much emphasis
is being placed on the yet unsolved technical questions
involved in demonstrating the presence or absence of
"blocked" cells in vivo. I would like to draw attention
to what appears to me to be the real question here -
and that is, what need is there for the cell to maintain the presence of antigen on its surface to remain
refractory? In other words, shouldn't we be concentra-
ting on the fact that it is entirely possible, indeed
quite likely, that B cells can be expressing receptors

capable of binding antigen but not be functional? Erna
Möller's data indeed says this, in that even in animals
tolerized by NNP-Cap there are specific NNP-binding
cells, but no response.

MECHANISMS OF T CELL TOLERANCE

WILLIAM WEIGLE, CHAIRMAN

UNIFYING CONCEPTS IN TOLERANCE INDUCTION FOR VARIOUS T AND B CELL SUB-POPULATIONS

G.J.V. Nossal and Beverley L. Pike

The Walter and Eliza Hall Institute of Medical Research
Melbourne, Victoria 3050, Australia

In the six short years that have elapsed since the first
Brook Lodge Conference on Immunological Tolerance (1), so
much has happened in cellular immunology that parts of that
volume now have a quaintly old-fashioned ring. Though T-B
cell collaboration was discussed from the tolerance viewpoint, and though suppressor effects were cursorily mentioned, a dominant impression emerging from a re-reading is
a desire to ascribe tolerance induction to one, unique causal
mechanism. At the present conference we are vying with each
other to be pluralistic, having realized that there are certainly numerous ways of achieving tolerance. We are offering
so many different causative mechanisms for the various model
systems under consideration that we risk committing the
opposite error of losing our precious raft of tolerance, the
acquired capacity for "self-non-self" discrimination, in the
vast sea of immune regulation. There may be some merit in
retaining the hope that one of the many models elucidates
principles of particular value for self-tolerance. The present paper is intended to offer three speculations: first,
that mechanisms of tolerization of T and B cells will be
essentially similar; secondly, that the tolerance by multivalent antigen complexes, including antibody-mediated tolerance, which has been the chief preoccupation of our laboratory for a decade, rests on a mechanism quite distinct from
that for soluble, monomeric antigens, but of great importance
in certain specialized situations; and thirdly, that the
currently unpopular notion of "clonal abortion" (2) represents a valid and physiologically relevant pathway of tolerance induction.

Background to and nature of the phenomenon of effector
cell blockade.
 Of the many model antigens that have been used to study
tolerance, two types have been especially popular. The first
type includes heterologous serum proteins or more recently,
such proteins substituted with a small number of hapten residues. These antigens, if rendered free of aggregates, diffuse widely through the extracellular fluid after intravenous
injection and, in the absence of significant quantities of

natural antibody, show little localization to either dendritic cells or macrophages in lymphoid tissue. Molecules of
this type preferentially cause tolerance in adult animals,
affecting both T and B cells at appropriate dosage and are
poorly immunogenic. The second group of antigens have predominantly been used as B cell tolerogens. They are antigens
with multiple identical antigenic determinants, frequently of
high molecular weight. This group includes antigens such as
pneumococcal polysaccharide, bacterial endotoxins, polymerized bacterial flagellins or haptens coupled to these antigens acting as carriers. These antigens are B cell tolerogens in vitro but only at certain doses; at other doses being
good immunogens both in vivo and in vitro. They stimulate
antibody formation with at least a degree of independence
from T cells, being able to trigger B cells from nu/nu mice
into antibody formation in vivo and in vitro. This capacity
of multivalent antigens may, in part, be due to their ability
to cause aggregation and "capping" of B cell immunoglobulin
(Ig) receptors (3). It is now clear that capping is followed
by cycles of receptor regeneration and re-capping. It is
tempting to speculate that an excessively high rate of this
sequence of events could eventually depress the function of
that cell, thus, causing tolerance.

Recently, our group has studied the effect of multivalent antigens, not on the B cell precursors of antibody-
forming cells (AFC), but rather on the AFC themselves. While
it is generally assumed that tolerance involves some effect
on the initial event of transformation of small lymphocytes
into immunological effector cells, certain phenomena such as
"antibody formation on a treadmill", or the presence of
serum-blocking factors capable of antagonizing cytotoxic effects of lymphocytes, suggests that the final end result of
immunologic non-reactivity can also be achieved in other ways.
To our surprise, we were able to show that hyporeactivity
can be induced in B cells even at the latest stage of differentiation when a cell is engaged in maximal antibody production (4). In other words the antibody-secreting rate of a
single cell can be sharply reduced by attaching multivalent
antigen to it. This occurs with concentrations of antigen
in the same range as those which induce tolerance, and moreover, can be demonstrated both in vivo and in vitro. The
phenomenon appears to involve a true reduction in secretion
and not just a temporary adsorption of secreted antibody to
cell-attached antigen. We have called this new and surprising effect of antigen effector cell blockade.

A typical example of an antigen capable of causing ef-
fector cell blockade is dinitrophenylated <u>Salmonella</u> <u>adelaide</u>
flagella (DNP-FLA). This antigen consists of small particles
made up largely of flagellin polymerized into strands with
the DNP hapten present as multiple determinants on the protein backbone. High molecular weight is not obligatory,
however, as DNP_{20}-HGG and DNP_{37}-D-GL are also effective. In
contrast, DNP-caproic acid or lightly substituted proteins
such as $DNP_{4.5}HGG$ are ineffective. The phenomenon is illustrated in the following way. Hapten-specific AFC are generated in any standard fashion, either <u>in vivo</u> or <u>in vitro</u>,
and of either IgM or IgG-producing class. For example, mice
can be immunized with a small dose of 0.1 µg of DNP-FLA and
the spleen harvested 4 days later. Then, a spleen cell suspension containing AFC is held at 37^0 for 30 minutes either
in tissue culture medium alone (or with free hapten or an
irrelevant antigen) or in medium containing 100 µg/ml of DNP-
FLA. Then the cells are carefully washed and assayed for
antibody production by standard plaque procedures capable of
detecting DNP-specific AFC. It is found that the number of
plaques in the suspension that had been held with DNP-FLA
is considerably reduced, down to 20% - 50% of control values
depending on exact experimental conditions. More careful
examination shows that this is due to a reduction in the
antibody secretion rate by each single AFC. Thus, the experimental cell suspension yields plaques that are smaller and
which appear later after incubation. The end result is that
cells which would have made small or turbid plaques, if left
untreated, fail altogether to make plaques after DNP-FLA
blockade. The kinetics of blockade can be worked out by
binding DNP-FLA to the surface of cells at 0^0, washing them
and then incubating at 37^0 in the absence of further added
antigen. If the cells that have bound DNP-FLA in the cold
are immediately placed into a plaque-revealing erythrocyte
monolayer, no blockade is observed. After 20 minutes at 37^0
between antigen-binding and plaque revelation, a specific
AFC loss is seen, and the effect increases in magnitude over
the next hour. Clearly some active process is induced by the
antigen that has attached in the cold, which progressively
reduces antibody secretion rate. No effect is seen on AFC
present in the same suspension but directed towards an irrelevant antigen, showing that is is not a non-specific toxic
phenomenon.

A simple method of demonstrating effector cell blockade
is to take a group of animals at the height of an immune response and to inject half of them with DNP-FLA. If the

spleens are harvested 4 hours later, the blockaded group of animals yield fewer and smaller plaques. The effect is far too rapid for it to be due to any effect at the level of antigen-reactive B lymphocytes.

The most direct proof of the nature of effector cell blockade has come from our single cell studies. In these, spleens have been harvested from DNP-FLA immunized animals, and single AFC have been removed from the center of hemolytic plaques by micromanipulation. They were then placed for 30 minutes at 37^0 into coded microdrops containing either 100 µg/ml DNP-FLA or medium alone. The cells were then washed carefully by micromanipulation and placed, one by one, into plaque-revealing microdrops, and the rate of plaque growth was measured by repeated readings with an eye piece vernier. A three to four-fold reduction in rate of plaque growth as a result of blockade was noted.

Micromanipulation has also resolved the question of whether the blockade is due solely to antibody being held up or trapped by cell-associated antigen. Single AFC that had been subjected to blockade were micromanipulated into droplets containing ^{125}I-labelled antiglobulin, held there for 30 minutes at 0^0 and then manipulated on to glass slides, dried and subjected to radioautography. It was shown that the blockaded cells demonstrated no more antibody on their surface than did control AFC. This finding demonstrates in a direct way something that could have been inferred from the bulk experiments in which cells were first held with blockading antigen in the cold and then incubated at 37^0 without antigen. Those cells that were immediately placed into plaque-revealing monolayers performed normally. Had blockade been due simply to secreted antibody being held up at the cell surface by the multivalent, attached antigen, they should have demonstrated full inhibition immediately.

Experiments cited in other portions of this conference have shown that highly multivalent antigens can directly tolerize B cells and probably T cells. Now we see that antigens of the same type can slow down antibody secretion by AFC. One must obviously ask whether the two phenomena depend on a similar mechanism. It is even pertinent to wonder whether some examples previously believed to represent tolerance in the sense of inhibition of B cell conversion to AFC may not represent AFC blockade. The rapid reversibility of pneumococcal polysaccharide paralysis suggests that at least part of the effect could be due to blockade. We know little about the regulation of secretion rate by single cells. It is not too fanciful to suppose the following sequence. Most AFC retain surface Ig (5) as an integral part of their membrane. Though direct evidence is not yet available, it seems likely that the attachment of multivalent antigen to the surface of the single AFC could initiate the formation of patches and caps, as in non-secreting B lymphocytes, and finally, result in pinocytosis of immune complexes. This receptor rearrangement and endocytotic activity could interfere with the regulation of secretion at many levels. For example, in B lymphocytes, endocytosed Ig-anti-Ig complexes reach the Golgi apparatus (6), which is believed to be important in pre-secretion packaging. One can only speculate as to the influences which the surface receptor rearrangements could have on microfibrils and microtubules, but they may well be of a subtle and profound nature (7). The developing molecular biology of membrane function may well reveal important similarities between B cell tolerogenesis and effector cell blockade.

Our work on the question of effector cell blockade at the level of T cells is not yet so far advanced, but we are heartened by the fact that antigen-antibody complexes are powerful inducers of B cell effector cell blockade (Schrader, unpublished). It is likely that antigen-antibody complexes represent at least one form of blocking factor in the reaction of cytotoxic lymphocytes and tumor cells, which may, in some experimental models, be a T cell effect. We are currently pursuing the question of blockade of effector T cells by multivalent antigens both in alloantigenic ("killer" cell) and "helper" cell systems.

The question remains whether either true tolerance induction or effector cell blockade by multivalent antigens is a phenomenon of any physiological relevance. We do not know, for example, how an animal acquires tolerance to its own histocompatibility antigens. This could be through encounters between lymphocytes and soluble molecules of histocompatibility, material shed from cell surfaces and entering the serum. Alternatively, it could be through encounters between the potentially self-reactive cell and a multivalent matrix of antigen present on an adjacent cell surface. Perhaps a more plausible physiological role is that of antigen-antibody complexes. It could well be that these, in the zone of antigen excess, limit antibody production in many responses, including those against gut commensal microorganisms and certain auto-antigens.

Nevertheless, it is difficult to conceive that the dominant mechanism in the acquisition of self-tolerance depends on the formation of highly clustered aggregates of "self" antigens. For this reason we attach great importance to the experiments to be described in the next section.

Background to the concept of clonal abortion.
The elimination of clones of self-reactive lymphocytes was central to Burnet's (8) early thinking as the clonal selection theory was developed. Lederberg (9) refined the notion, stressing that lymphocytes might mature in stages. The first postulated differentiation state was one where the immature lymphocyte could react to antigen only by tolerance, i.e. irreversible blockade or elimination. If the cell did not encounter antigen at that stage, it progressed to a mature lymphocyte, which on meeting appropriate antigen, would be triggered into antibody production. Cohn (10) has termed this a maturation from paralyzable to inducible state. The elegance of the postulate lies in the fact that "self" antigens, present at all times, would "catch" all self-reactive clones during their paralyzable stage, leading to their functional elimination. Foreign antigens, pulsed in unexpectedly, would encounter some cells in the paralyzable state but far more in the inducible state. The immune induction of the latter cells would be the dominant end result. This idea, which is more appropriately termed clonal abortion (to distinguish it from clonal deletion, the removal of competent immunocytes) has been unpopular recently. The chief point against it is the observation that cell populations, e.g. from adult mouse spleen, containing mature immunocytes can be tolerized within one or a few days (11) by certain antigens. This clearly indicates that clonal abortion is not the only mechanism of tolerogenesis, a point already made through the studies with multivalent antigens. However, there are some indications in the past literature (reviewed in 12) which are consistent with clonal abortion. First, the dose of antigen needed to maintain tolerance, onee induced, is considerably less than that needed to induce it; a finding which becomes readily understandable if one assumes the need for one set of rather extreme conditions to achieve paralysis in mature cells, and a second set of conditions for preventing the neogenesis of lymphocytes competent to react against the tolerogen. Then there is the finding that cells from central lymphoid organs such as the thymus may be rendered tolerant more readily than those from secondary lymphoid organs (13). Finally, there are our own results (2) showing that lethally irradiated, fetal liver

reconstituted animals are rendered tolerant with antigens which immunize normal animals. This background provided us with encouragement to explore the possibility of clonal abortion in more definitive systems.

Adult mouse bone marrow as a source of maturing B cells. Stimulated by the prior work of Osmond and colleagues (14), we examined the potential of adult CBA mouse bone marrow as a source of immature B cells and "pre-B" cells to test the clonal abortion theory directly. This required first a detailed examination of the marrow lymphocyte population from the viewpoint of its immunoglobulin receptors and its functional capacity in B cell specific assays. It was noted (15) that organs such as spleen and lymph node contained lymphocytes that could readily be divided into two populations, namely, those which bound dilute ^{125}I-labelled rabbit anti-mouse globulin antibody and those which did not. With increasing concentrations of the labelling reagent, the percentage of labelled cells reached well-defined plateau levels. In contrast, bone marrow small lymphocytes failed to show this clear-cut bimodality. The percentage of labelled cells showed a linear increment throughout a 200-fold range of concentration, and the labelling intensity varied widely. Approximately one half remained unlabelled at the highest practicable antiglobulin concentration. These cells were not sensitive to treatment with anti-Θ serum plus complement, and an equivalent proportion of these Θ^{-ve} Ig^{-ve} cells were present in congenitally athymic (nu/nu) mice.

It was next decided to study the kinetics of maturation and renewal of Ig^{+ve} cells in the marrow (16). To do this, a double-labelling technique was used in which mice were injected each 8 hours with ^{3}H-thymidine for periods up to 84 hours, and then marrow cells were exposed in vitro to ^{131}I-labelled rabbit anti-mouse globulin. Radioautographic study readily distinguished the two isotopes. The total population of marrow small lymphocytes showed a rapid exponential increase, 50% being ^{3}H-thymidine-labelled by 32 hours and 80% by three days. However, small lymphocytes capable of binding "standard" amounts of anti-Ig became labelled with ^{3}H-thymidine only after a lag of about 1.5 days, and those small lymphocytes with the highest surface Ig density were delayed a further 12 hours in ^{3}H-thymidine labelling. The results strongly suggested a continuous, rapid renewal of bone marrow small lymphocytes, with lymphocytes emerging from the mitotic cycle lacking an Ig receptor coat, but acquiring this during a non-mitotic maturation phase lasting approximately two days. This suggestion was supported by tissue culture studies in which it was shown that the proportion of Ig^{+ve} small lymphocytes increased from about 40 percent to about 70 percent during three days of culture in the case of marrow, while decreasing from 40 percent to 20 percent in the case of spleen. The proportionate marrow increase was not affected by mitomycin-treatment, stressing the non-mitotic nature of the maturation.

The capacity of bone marrow cells to give an adoptive immune response to the T independent antigen, dinitrophenylated polymer of flagellin (DNP-POL) was next investigated (17). Bone marrow cells gave a somewhat lower response than would have been expected from their content of Ig^{+ve} lymphocytes. When time was allowed for the marrow cells to mature in the adoptive host, i.e. when the antigen challenge was delayed, the performance improved, whereas that of a spleen cell population similarly handled fell off. Similarly, when marrow cells were cultured in vitro and then adoptively transferred and challenged, their capacity to yield AFC increased, whereas that of spleen cells decreased.

These studies suggested that the postulated critical stage during which clonal abortion might be expected in the B cell population was during the non-mitotic maturation phase of Ig receptor appearance. The experiments to be reported in the next section aimed to test this postulate.

Tolerogenesis of B cells in vitro by low concentrations of oligovalent antigens.

In order to demarcate the phenomena to be described as clearly as possible from those in the preceding section on effector cell blockade, an antigen was chosen as being oligomeric and poorly immunogenic. This was $DNP_{0.9}$-HGG. Studies to be reported elsewhere (18) have shown this antigen to be a good tolerogen of DNP-specific B cells in vivo at doses approaching 1 mg per mouse. The functional capacity of B cells after varying periods of culture was tested by injecting cells intravenously into lethally irradiated mice which were immediately challenged with 5 µg DNP-POL. Nine days later, a time chosen because of the linearity of the cell dose, AFC response curve (17), the adoptive hosts were killed and spleens examined for anti-DNP AFC using standard hemolytic plaque tests. Though direct and enhanced plaques were always measured, in this system there were virtually no enhanced plaques. The culture system used was our standard Marbrook system modified so as to allow 60×10^6 cells to reside in the inner well in 4 ml of medium.

Figure 1 shows the results of culturing spleen or bone marrow cells for various times in the absence of antigens other than those contained in fetal calf serum. After two hours of culture, the adoptive immune potential of spleen is considerably higher than that of marrow, but as time progresses, marrow potential-nucleated cell improves, whereas spleen potential deteriorates.

Figure 2 gives the results of culturing cells in the presence of 4 µg/ml (2.5×10^{-8}M) $DNP_{0.9}$-HGG. The protocol of these experiments was that all cultures were maintained in vitro for three days, and each adoptive host received the cells from one culture, usually about 1.5×10^7 viable cells. Control cultures had 4 µg/ml of HGG (unconjugated with DNP) present throughout; such cultures behaved no differently from ones which had no antigen present. Experimental cultures had $DNP_{0.9}$-HGG present either throughout the three days of culture or else just for the last day. It can be seen that the presence of the DNP conjugate at this low concentration did not significantly affect spleen B cells. In contrast, its presence for the full culture period reduced the adoptive immune performance of bone marrow cells down to 21 percent of control values. Its presence over the last 24 hours only of culture was much less effective. The effect was immunologically specific. When cultures that had been incubated for three days with 4 µg $DNP_{0.9}$-HGG were injected into hosts that were challenged with either DNP-POL or NIP-POL, the NIP-POL challenged group made a normal number of anti-NIP PFC (1080 $\pm$ 209), whereas the DNP-POL group made only 128 $\pm$ 48 anti-DNP PFC. Other experiments (not shown) demonstrated that simple binding on of $DNP_{0.9}$-HGG to bone marrow cells, without a culture period, could not achieve the effect.

Figure 3 shows what very low doses of antigen can be instrumental in achieving the effect. This figure represents a pool of two separate sets of experiments. The spleen curve refers to experiments in which spleen cells were held in culture for one day with $DNP_{0.9}$-HGG, and were then washed, adoptively transferred and challenged. No tolerization was noted. In other experiments (not shown) the concentration of $DNP_{0.9}$-HGG was raised up to 1 mg/ml, but still no tolerance was achieved in the spleen B cells as judged by the adoptive transfer assay. Nor did prolonging the culture period to three days allow the demonstration of tolerance induction in spleen cells. In contrast, the bone marrow curve refers to experiments in which bone marrow cells were held for three days in culture with $DNP_{0.9}$-HGG at various concentrations. At 0.05 μg/ml no effect was noted, but maximal depression was already achieved with 0.4 μg/ml of antigen. In other experiments (not shown) the concentration of $DNP_{0.9}$-HGG was raised progressively to 400 μg/ml without increasing the degree of tolerance any further.

The poor capacity of this antigen to tolerize spleen cells in vitro was not expected; it is, in fact, in line with the experience that many investigators have had with oligo-valent antigens, though we believe that experimental circumstances can be found using still higher antigen concentrations in which mature B cells can also be rendered non-reactive in vitro with oligovalent antigens (e.g. 19). The new, and to us exciting finding, is that surprisingly low concentrations can tolerize B cells from bone marrow. In this regard we find the residuum of non-tolerizable cells of particular interest. About 20 percent of the adoptive immune capacity remains after culture with antigen. This could represent activity due to that sub-set of bone marrow B cells which had passed through the critical maturation phase before killing of the animal and which survives culture. Ex hypothesi, these should retain the capacity to react to DNP-POL. The other B cells may represent ones that had differentiated in culture, perhaps largely through non-mitotic maturation of Ig^{-ve} small lymphocytes to Ig^{+ve} small lymphocytes. Ex hypothesi, DNP-reactive B cells should be clonally eliminated during this phase in the presence of antigen. The antigen-specific and time-dependent effects of $DNP_{0.9}$-HGG (Figs. 2 and 3) appear to fit in completely with the predictions of the theory.

Much remains to be done in this experimental model. On the one hand, it would be important to remove from the bone marrow population at the start of culture those cells representing mature, Ig^{+ve} B cells, thus, removing one possible source of non-tolerizable cells. On the other hand, bone marrow contains more primitive cells, both stem cells and various categories of pre-B cells, which, given sufficient time, could mature in the adoptive host. These, receptor-free during the culture period, would have escaped tolerogenesis and could obscure clonal abortion under some circumstances. In view of the controversy that surrounds the concept of bone marrow as a bursal analogue, it would be advantageous to perform analogous experiments with thymus in some model capable of measuring T cell tolerogenesis. These endeavors are currently in progress in our laboratory.

While we feel that our results presented here strongly favor the concept of clonal abortion of B cells, we stress that this may not be the only mechanism of reaching B cell tolerance with monomeric antigens. For example, in some models straight receptor blockade may be at work. In others, it may be that mature B cells, coated with a sufficient amount of a monomeric antigen, become palatable to phagocytic cells and are thus eliminated. The possibility remains that "Signal 1 only", received over a sufficient length of time by a cell, leads to irreversible inactivation or death. With some antigens suppressor T cells are clearly involved in B cell tolerogenesis (20). We wish to propose, however, that clonal abortion as suggested by the present experiments is the mechanism of greatest physiologic significance. Acting at such low molarity, it would allow tolerance of high af-finity B cells towards a far greater range of self-antigens. The other processes may well relate more to "fail-safe" and negative feedback mechanisms. Definitive proof of clonal abortion must await cell separation methodologies that allow the different maturation stages to be isolated in vitro.

SUMMARY

This paper deals with two new series of experiments from our laboratory that, while performed on B cells, we believe to illustrate principles applicable to both T and B cells.

The first phenomenon is one that has been termed effec-tor cell blockade (4). It deals with the short-term effects of highly multivalent antigens on cells actively engaged in antibody synthesis against such antigens. A typical example is the dinitrophenyl (DNP) hapten coupled to polymerized flagellin or intact flagella of Salmonella adelaide (DNP-POL and DNP-FLA). This antigen, added to populations of anti-DNP plaque-forming cells (PFC), can severely impair their capacity to secrete antibody. If antigen is bound on to cells at 0^0 and then the suspension is washed, it exerts no effect for 15 minutes or so after warming the cells up, but then antibody secretion rate diminishes severely. The effect is dependent on concentration and valency of antigen, is immunologically specific, is not due to antigen carry-over into the plaque-revealing monolayer, is equal for direct and indirect PFC, is not due to progressive accumulation of secreted product at the cell surface and can be documented by micromanipulation. It is possible that a similar blockade mechanism could impair the function of the B cell precursors of PFC, thus, providing an explanation for B cell tolerogenesis by highly multivalent antigens and even for antibody-mediated tolerance.

The second phenomenon deals with the mechanism of tolerance induction by soluble, monomeric antigens. Evidence is presented consistent with the view that B cells mature through a stage during which they are exquisitely sensitive to tolerogenesis. This stage is after they exit from mitotic cycles in the bone marrow, as yet lacking an Ig receptor coat, and sometime during the next two to three days, while progressively larger amounts of Ig appear on the cell surface. If cultures of bone marrow are exposed to as little as 0.4 μg/ml of $DNP_{0.9}$-HGG (2.5×10^{-9}M) for three days, a specific tolerance develops in the maturing B cell pool such that, on adoptive transfer and challenge with a T-independent antigen, the anti-DNP PFC response is diminished five fold. In contrast, mature spleen B cells exposed to up to 2500 fold more antigen are not rendered tolerant. The phenomenon has been termed clonal abortion and is speculatively cast as the chief physiological mechanism of self-tolerance at both T and B cell levels.

ACKNOWLEDGMENTS

Original work included in this review was supported by grants from the National Health and Medical Research Council and the Australian Research Grants Committe, Canberra, Australia; by NIH Grant AI-0-3958, United States Public Health Service and by Contract N01-CB-23889 with the National Cancer Institute, National Institutes of Health, Department of Health, Education and Welfare, U.S.A., and by Volkswagen Foundation, Grant No. 112147. This is Publication No. 2011 from the Walter and Eliza Hall Institute.
We thank Misses K. Davern and L. Strzelecki for excellent technical assistance.

REFERENCES

1. Immunological Tolerance, edited by M. Landy and W. Braun, Academic Press, New York and London, 1969.

2. Nossal, G.J.V. and Pike, Beverley, L., In Immunological Aspects of Neoplasia, edited by E.M. Hersh and M. Schlamowitz, 1974.

3. Diener, E. and Paetkau, V.H., Proc. Nat. Acad. Sci. (U.S.). 69:2364, 1972.

4. Schrader, J.W. and Nossal, G.J.V., J. Exp. Med. In press, 1974.

5. Nossal, G.J.V. and Lewis, Heather, J. Exp. Med. 135: 1416, 1972.

6. Santer, V., Aust. J. Exp. Biol. Med. Sci. In press, 1974.

7. Yahara, I. and Edelman, G.M., Exp. Cell. Res. In press.

8. Burnet, F.M., In The Clonal Selection Theory of Acquired Immunity, Cambridge University Press, 1959.

9. Lederberg, J., Science. 129:1649, 1959.

10. Cohn, M., Ann. N.Y. Acad. Sci. 190:529, 1971.

11. Chiller, J.M. and Weigle, W.O., J. Exp. Med. 137:740, 1973.

12. Dresser, D.W. and Mitchison, N.A., Advan. Immunol. 8: 129, 1968.

13. Scott, D.W. and Waksman, B.H., J. Immunol. 102:347, 1969.

14. Osmond, D.G., Miller, S.C. and Yoshida, Y., In Haemopoietic Stem Cells, CIBA Foundation Symposium 13, p. 131, Churchill, London.

15. Osmond, D.G. and Nossal, G.J.V., Cell. Immunol. In press.

16. Osmond. D.G. and Nossal, G.J.V., Cell. Immunol. In press.

17. Stocker, J.W., Osmond, D.G. and Nossal, G.J.V., Immunol. In press.

18. Stocker, J.W. and Nossal, G.J.V., Cell. Immunol. In press.

19. Schrader, J.W., J. Exp. Med. In press, 1974.

20. Basten, A., Miller, J.F.A.P., Sprent, J. and Cheers, C.,
     J. Exp. Med. In press, 1974.

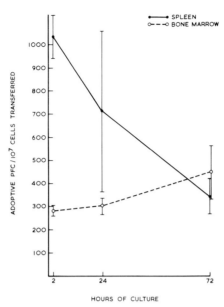

Fig. 1. The effect of varying periods of tissue culture on the capacity of spleen or bone marrow cell suspensions to mediate an anti-DNP response when transferred to lethally irradiated hosts and challenged with a T cell independent antigen. Vertical bars represent standard errors of the mean.

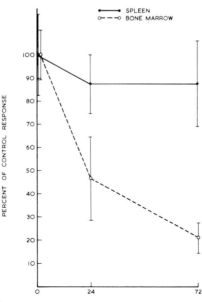

Fig. 2.   HOURS OF EXPOSURE TO ANTIGEN

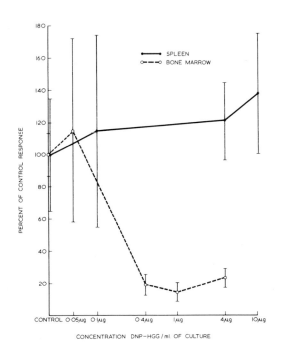

Fig. 3. Dose-response relationships in tolerance induction. Spleen cultures maintained for one day, bone marrow cultures for three days, in the continuous presence of the antigen doses indicated.

Fig. 2. The effect of 4 µg/ml of $DNP_{0.9}$-HGG on the adoptive immune performance of cultured spleen or bone marrow cells. All samples underwent three days tissue culture. Antigen was present either: a) throughout; b) for the terminal 24 hours of culture; or c) not at all, unconjugated HGG being present instead. Pool of a large number of experiments, results normalized to control values.

DISCUSSION FOLLOWING G. J. V. NOSSAL

HUMPHREY: Point one: Gerry Klaus and I completely confirm
what you call effector cell blockade in spleen cells
from mice given DNP-Levan in vivo. Anti-DNP anti-LE
plaque were smaller than expected, and this was shown
to be due to the presence of antigen in or on the cells
apparently preventing antibody secretion. Normal
plaque forming cells incubated with polymeric DNP antigens in vitro were also inhibited, and this was not reversible by washing. Have you any explanation how this
inhibition by antigen of an established antibody secreting mechanism is brought about?

Point two: John Owen and his colleagues have
been studying 12-13 day fetal liver cells cultured in
vitro. These start with no Ig+ cells, but after two
or three days in culture quite large numbers of Ig+
cells appear. This suggests that the fetal liver is
at least as likely to be the bursal analogue as is bone
marrow in ontogeny.

NOSSAL: I am very happy to have Dr. Humphrey confirm the
validity of effector cell blockade because Schrader and
I truly believe it to be an important regulatory process at both B and T cell level. As to mechanism, we
can only speculate. It is probable that the surface-
attached multivalent antigen activates the patching-
capping-endocytosis mechanism. If the endocytosed
antigen goes to the Golgi apparatus, it could interfere
with antibody packaging and secretion. In reply to the
second point, we too have evidence for emergence of B
cells in fetal liver, and this could well be the bursal
analogue in the embryo. I am referring more to the
gross enlargement of the pre-B cell pool as a "primary
lymphoid organ" type function for adult marrow. This
is what gives marrow characteristics resembling adult
thymus. One would not wish to press the analogue too
far, however.

KATZ: I would like to extend what John Humphrey just said
in that we also agree fully with the effector cell
blockade concept, and in this context we are planning
to use DNP- -GL to eliminate DNP-specific myelomas.
Of course, if this potentially clinically applicable
model is to be very useful it would be helpful to know
what the ultimate fate of such "blocked" cells may be

other than the diminished protein secretory capacity.
Do you have any information on this?

NOSSAL: No, operationally, it is very difficult to discrim-
inate in vivo between recovery of PFC from blockade and
replacement by newly-formed PFC. In vitro, unfortunately, isolated PFC do not live long enough in microdrops to allow study of unblocking. I would expect a
good chance of functional recovery, however, in the in
vivo situation.

DIENER: Lily Yung in my laboratory has obtained data which
supplement Nossal's data. Miss Yung used a model
whereby she repopulated irradiated syngeneic recipients
with a chromosome marker-controlled single clone of
hemopoietic cells. Such an animal would develop clonal
diversity of its antigen recognition potential within
20 days. Miss Yung has used this model to determine
the time during immune-ontogeny at which tolerance induction is first observed. It was found that parental
cells in an F_1 recipient would acquire tolerance to the
opposite parent well before they became immunocompetent
to extrinsic antigens.

NOSSAL: This goes in the same general direction; we attempted to use lethally irradiated, fetal liver-restored
mice to test the "clonal abortion" notion, but found
the model operationally rather clumsy. Nevertheless,
quite small doses of several antigens caused B cell
tolerance.

SCOTT: You have demonstrated specificity in these tolerance
experiments with bone marrow in the apparent absence of
receptors. In view of that, what is the lower limit of
detection in your system of Ig-bearing cells? That is,
how many Ig molecules must a cell have to be regarded
as positive? Secondly, if these cells are indeed Ig
negative, what does trypsin do to tolerance induction
in this model?

NOSSAL: When we call a bone marrow lymphocyte Ig negative,
i.e., not able to be labelled by 50 times the concentration of ^{125}I-anti-Ig that labels a major proportion
of mature peripheral B cells, we suspect it possesses
less than 1000 accessible Ig receptors at its surface.
Of course, it could still have a few hundred. The

point we wish to make is that there is a continuum--a continuous flowering-out of increased amounts of receptor material as the bone marrow small lymphocyte goes through its non-mitotic maturation.

We have not investigated the effects of trypsin in the model. It stands to reason, however, that if the emerging, tolerizable lymphocyte were deprived of its receptors, it would not see the antigen and thus could not be tolerized.

PAUL: Gelfand, Asofsky and I have examined the appearance of immunoglobulin bearing-cells in the spleen of BALB/c mice in the immediate neonatal period. In mice less than 8 hours of age the percent of cells bearing detectable Ig is 4% or less. If these cells are cultured for 24 hours a substantial increase in Ig-bearing cells occurs which can be very largely blocked by pretreatment with anti-kappa without complement. This suggests an interesting analogy to your work. However, our blockade was achieved by pretreatment suggesting that receptors existed on these cells, probably in low numbers, prior to the culture. Can you achieve tolerance in your in vitro bone marrow system by pretreatment with DNP-HGG, rather than by continuous presence of these antigen?

NOSSAL: The rather small amount of work that we have done on this so far has not achieved tolerogenesis, but I recognize the importance of the question. This may be a matter of antigen concentration. Neither Osmond nor I wish to insist that the immediate pre-B cell has no receptor material. The critical question is whether the tolerance-sensitive phase exists at some time during the transition from zero receptors to full complement of receptors. We agree that neonatal spleen has some "pre-B" cells. In fact, CBA spleen has many marrow-like features until 5-6 weeks of age.

ALLISON: You report the clonal abortion as irreversible? If so, how do you explain the ease with which autoantibodies against thyroglobulin can be induced by appropriate manipulations such as immunization with heterologous thyroglobulin in the absence of adjuvant?

NOSSAL: There may well be low-affinity B cells which escape tolerogenesis by clonal abortion because of low antigen

concentration. Obviously, the mechanism will have its
own dosage threshold, and this may well be much lower
for T than for B cells. The main point we wish to make
is that the tolerization concentration may be grossly
higher for mature than for maturing cells.

GERSHON: Two questions: First, you related your findings
with receptor blockade to Phil Baker's with SIII. His
work suggests suppressor T cells may play a role. Have
you looked at the effect of T cell depletion on your
phenomenon? Secondly, how long does your bone marrow
tolerance last, both in the primary response, and without immediate antigen stimulation?

NOSSAL: We have not yet worked with anti-θ-treated marrow,
though this is planned. There is a very small contamination only of our marrow with recirculating T cells.
Furthermore, the model as it currently exists does not
lend itself for studies of duration of tolerance. The
There are stem cells and other lymphoid precursors
feeding in new cells all the time, and in the absence
of antigen, these could not be tolerized. Early experiments are planned to remove these cells by ^{3}H-thymid-
ine suicide. If that works, and clonal abortion is
irreversible, the tolerance should be long-lasting.

HERZENBERG: I will present data on this tomorrow, but I
just want to point out here that we find allotype suppressor cells in bone marrow, and that these are about
ten-fold more active per T cell in suppressing than
splenic T cells.

NOSSAL: This is clearly a serious point and we shall have
to investigate it carefully.

UNANUE: How long does the inhibition of antibody secretion
by antigen last? Is it reversible? Can it be induced
by anti-Ig? Is there evidence for pinocytosis and/or
digestion of the complex?

NOSSAL: We have not yet worked out ways of reversing blockade. Schrader has some evidence of blockade by anti-Ig,
but has done much more work on antigen-antibody complexes, which block very effectively. We have no hard
evidence for pinocytosis and digestion of attached antigen by single PFC, though this could be studied by
electron-microscopic radioautography. I believe in the

likelihood, however, because when I was working with
Bussard and Mazie, I frequently observed tiny fragments
of erythrocyte debris inside PFC that had been cultured for some hours.

CINADER: Kaplan and I noticed that the early descendents of
stem cells made small plaques. Does your cultured
bone marrow make progressively larger plaques when you
transfer it after progressively larger time in culture?
Secondly, you speak of clonal abortion. Allotype suppression provides some--albeit tenuous--indications
that a cell might switch to a different product. This
could abolish a clonal product which results in the
killing of the cells of the clone. This is clearly
more amenable to experimentation than is cell death.
Do you consider this a viable question in the context
of clonal deletion?

NOSSAL: We have not noted the former phenomenon. As regards
allotype suppression switching a particular cell from
the expression of one receptor to another, I do not believe that microdrop experiments would be likely to
answer the question, for purely technical reasons. The
cells simply do not live long enough in the microdrops.

CELLULAR PARAMETERS OF THE TOLERANT STATE INDUCED TO HUMAN γ GLOBULIN IN MICE AND OF ITS MODULATION BY BACTERIAL LIPOPOLYSACCHARIDES

Jacques M. Chiller, Jacques A. Louis, Barry J. Skidmore and William O. Weigle

Scripps Clinic and Research Foundation
476 Prospect Street
La Jolla, California   92037

In the years which have passed since the publication of Burnet's concept of immunological tolerance (1), a number of experimental systems have been used in an attempt to dissect its possible mode of action. The accumulation of data directed to that issue has led to the realization that certain dilemmas may exist in such an approach, among which are: 1) whether any system of experimentally-induced unresponsiveness does, in fact, parallel that biological process of tolerance which Burnet originally postulated as part of the events in clonal selection and 2) whether various systems of experimentally-induced tolerance differ in that each reflects a particular phase of the control mechanisms involved in the immune system rather than being similar in obeying the laws of a common mechanism. The present communication will first elaborate on those issues and then describe experimental details of the cellular manifestations of a system of experimental unresponsiveness which has been studied on the basis that it may represent a prototype for the phenomenon of self tolerance (2).

The theoretical genesis for the concept of clonal elimination stems from the necessity to provide a means for the biological basis of self-non-self discrimination (1). If the immune system can be viewed as a functional network of finely attuned regulatory mechanisms (3) which suppresses rather than eliminates the potential for detrimental reactions, then the necessity for clonal deletion as the pathway by which self fails to be recognized may not be a biological prerequisite. Nevertheless, an attraction still exists for the evolutionary selection of a recognition system which can respond either positively or negatively depending on the conditions of interactions between cells and antigens. In this regard an ontogenetic basis for self tolerance could be viewed as occurring at a stage in the course of lymphoid cell differentiation when a negative response is the only consequence which can result from a specific interaction between

lymphocyte and antigen. Viewed from the standpoint of a
signal hypothesis (4), it may be that the development or
expression of an antigen recognition receptor (signal 1)
precedes the development or expression of a structure also
needed for specific lymphocyte stimulation (signal 2). A
variation of the same theme may involve a temporal lag between the differentiation of specific antigen receptors and
expression of those genetic capacities in the form of
putative histocompatible structures which have been claimed
to be requirements for T cell activation by macrophages (5)
as well as for B cell activation by T lymphocytes (6). Thus,
the sequential differentiation of lymphocytes during ontogeny could provide for the establishment of self tolerance
on the basis of functional clonal elimination in that the
process could occur at a stage during the life of a lymphocyte when a negative event is the only possible sequela of
the interaction between specific lymphocyte and antigen.
Within this framework, it would appear that many experimental models of tolerance are not such that would be designed
to operate within these temporal restrictions.

In addition, systems of experimental tolerance may not
share pathways of identity. Experimentally-induced immunological tolerance is defined as the state of specific immune
refractoriness to an antigen which results from previous
exposure to that antigen. Beneath that empirical umbrella,
a myriad of experimental systems have been used to study the
phenomenon of tolerance, and the resulting observations have
been viewed within the framework of divergent, seemingly
conflicting, mechanisms. In part, the interpretative discrepancies have resulted from the attempt to channelize each
observation into a single, unifying mechanism of tolerance,
namely, that of functional clonal deletion. It is becoming
more apparent, however, that this reductionist approach may
not be appropriate inasmuch as the multitude of phenomenology ascribed as experimentally-induced tolerance most probably reflects various states of immune regulation operational within the complexities of the immune system. For
example, the conclusion that different mechanisms may be
involved in establishing an apparently similar state of unresponsiveness is implicit in the following sets of experiments. Appropriate doses of soluble bovine serum albumin
(BSA) can induce a state of specific tolerance in either
neonatal or adult rabbits (7). However, markedly different
cellular events characterize the induction phase of unresponsiveness in each instance (8). Unresponsiveness to BSA
in neonates is established without detectable production of

antibody, as evaluated by the absence in lymphoid tissues of antibody-forming cells specific to BSA. Contrariwise, the establishment of unresponsiveness in adult rabbits to the identical antigen is characterized by a transient phase of antibody formation to BSA. Therefore, although both states of tolerance appear identical when operationally defined as specific unresponsiveness to a subsequent immunologic challenge, a more accurate characterization may be that they are similar operational end products of biologically different processes.

The system of tolerance whose cellular parameters will now be considered in detail is based on the observations originally described by Dresser (9) whereby heterologous γ-globulins can be made highly tolerogenic if they are treated in a way so as to render them monomeric in solution. Specifically, adult A/J mice can be made tolerant to purified human IgG (HGG) if the antigen preparation used is rendered aggregate free by ultracentrifugation. Such deaggregated HGG (DHGG) will induce a total, specific and protracted state of unresponsiveness to subsequent immunogenic challenges with aggregated HGG (AHGG). The data seen in Table I exemplifies this situation. Mice, injected 71 days previously with 2.5 mg DHGG, fail to respond to a highly immunogenic regimen of two sequential challenges of AHGG. The unresponsive state is highly specific in that such animals respond to a non cross-reactive globulin, turkey γ-globulin (TGG) in a manner quantitatively identical to that observed in normal mice. Furthermore, this specific unresponsiveness to AHGG is observed even in tolerogen-treated mice which are subsequently challenged with both AHGG and TGG. Three additional features are germane to the description of this tolerant state. First, the induction of unresponsiveness occurs without detectable antibody formation to HGG. Second, once tolerance has been established it can be sustained when transferred adoptively into irradiated syngeneic recipients. And third, the response to AHGG which is ablated is that which is measured in the form of plaque-forming cells (PFC) which are mainly, if not exclusively, amplified (indirect) PFC and more specifically, those secreting the γ class of murine immunoglobulin.

CELLULAR PARAMETERS OF A TOLERANT STATE IN MICE TO HUMAN γ GLOBULIN

The demonstration that the antibody response obtained following the injection of immunogen (AHGG) required T cell

375

helper function was followed by the observation that mice treated with tolerogen (DHGG) could be shown to have specifically unresponsive T cells and B cells (10). In addition, each specific cell population displayed unique temporal kinetic patterns of tolerance induction, maintenance and termination (11). A synopsis of those data is given in Table II. It can be seen that in vivo T cells(thymocytes or splenic T cells) become unresponsive within a short period of time following tolerogen administration.

TABLE I

SPECIFICITY OF A TOLERANT STATE INDUCED WITH
DEAGGREGATED HGG (DHGG)

Group		Treatment (day)[a]		Response (PFC/Spleen)[b]	
	0	71	82	to HGG	to TGG
A	Sal	AHGG	AHGG	84,275	NT[c]
B	DHGG	"	"	1,725	NT
C	"	Al TGG	Al TGG	NT	62,400
D	Sal	"	"	NT	54,500
E	DHGG	AHGG + Al TGG	AHGG + Al TGG	3,350	71,300
F	Sal	"	"	86,000	62,400

[a]A/J male mice (6-8 weeks of age) were injected i.p. on day 0 with either 2.5 mg deaggregated HGG (DHGG) or saline. On day 71, groups A and B were challenged with an i.v. injection of 400 µg aggregated HGG (AHGG); groups C and D with 200 µg alum precipitated turkey gamma globulin (Al TGG); and groups E and F with both AHGG and Al TGG. On day 82, respective groups received either 200µg AHGG i.p., 200 µg AI TGG i.p. or both of the antigens.

[b]Indirect PFC specific either to HGG or TGG were assayed 4 days after the last antigenic challenge.

[c]Not tested.

TABLE II

TEMPORAL PATTERN OF IMMUNOLOGIC TOLERANCE TO HGG IN A/J MICE [a]

Site	Days of	
	Induction	Maintenance
Thymus	< 1	120 - 135
Bone Marrow	8 - 15	40 - 50
Spleen: T Cells	< 1	100 - 150
B Cells	2 - 4	50 - 60
Whole Animal	< 1	130 - 150

[a]Based on accumulated data using A/J male mice which received a tolerogenic dose of 2.5 mg deaggregated HGG.

This tolerant state is maintained for a prolonged period (> 100 days) before it spontaneously wanes. In contrast, B cells (bone marrow lymphocytes or splenic B cells) require a longer time period before they become irreversibly unresponsive and the tolerant state in those cells is maintained for a much shorter period of time (< 60 days). The whole animal displays a kinetic pattern of unresponsiveness which is essentially superimposable for that seen with T cells suggesting that in vivo, the maintenance of unresponsiveness to a T cell dependent antigen necessitates only a cellular lesion in specific T cells. In addition, these cellular dynamics demonstrate that the "phenotype" of tolerance observed after a single injection of tolerogen may be characterized cellularly as the sequential expression of various phases whose "cellular genotypes" can be either tolerant T cells and non tolerant B cells or tolerant T cells and tolerant B cells.

The time lag between the induction of tolerance in T cells and B cells could be interpreted as the dependence on T cells for B cell tolerance induction (12). However, that possibility is not supported by the results obtained from the experiments seen in Table III. Adult, thymectomized, lethally irradiated and bone marrow reconstituted (ATxBM) mice

377

were injected with either saline, AHGG or DHGG, and 15 days thereafter specific immunocompetence of their spleen cells was assayed by transferring those cells into HGG primed, lethally irradiated syngeneic recipients. It can be seen that whereas cells obtained from donor mice treated with saline or immunogen responded to AHGG following the adoptive transfer, those cells obtained from donor mice treated with tolerogen did not. The necessity for prior priming of recipient mice with AHGG can be seen by the lack of a response in irradiated, non primed recipients of ATxBM spleen cells. Therefore, within the limits of the technical value provided by ATxBM mice, it appears that the induction to tolerance in B cells can occur without the required participation of a normal complement of T cells. This conclusion is in agreement with that reached by others who have made similar findings for the induction of tolerance in B cells to T dependent antigens in a more stringent T cell depleted in vivo environment provided by congenitally athymic (nu/nu) mice (13, 14).

Although the previous observations indirectly obviate the necessity for the involvement of suppressor T cells in the establishment of B cell tolerance to HGG, they do not address themselves to the possibility that the induction and/ or maintenance of tolerance of specific helper T cells in this system requires a T cell suppressor population (15). In order to directly evaluate the possibility that this state of unresponsiveness is maintained by a positive influence rather than via a negative effect, two types of cell transfer experiments were performed. In the first case, normal and/or tolerant spleen cells were adoptively transferred into lethally irradiated syngeneic recipients and their response to AHGG was subsequently assessed. It can be seen from the data in Table IV that although adoptively transferred tolerant spleen cells remained unresponsive to ensuing immunogenic challenges, they did not suppress the ability of adoptively transferred normal spleen cells to respond to AHGG. It should be noted that these experiments include the assessment for positive unresponsiveness of spleen cells obtained from mice at various times following their treatment with tolerogen, namely, 3, 17 and 35 days post injection.

The second method by which the possibility of positive unresponsiveness within this system was evaluated was to adoptively transfer normal or tolerant cells (spleen or thymus) into normal syngeneic recipients and then assess the response of such animals to subsequent challenge of AHGG given either at the time of transfer or 4 days thereafter.

The delay of the initial immunogenic challenge was included as part of the protocol in order to allow time for the expression of a potential suppressor activity. It can be seen from the data in Table V that neither thymocytes nor spleen cells obtained from mice treated with tolerogen 67 days previously reduce the capacity of recipients of such cells to respond to HGG. Furthermore, even delaying the initial time of challenge with AHGG did not reveal any suppressive effect of tolerant cells on the response of the recipient mice. Experiments not included here which have also tested the suppressor capacity of lymphoid cells obtained from mice 7 days post tolerogen yielded similar negative effects.

TABLE III

EFFECT OF TOLEROGEN OR IMMUNOGEN ON THE ABILITY OF SPLEEN CELLS FROM AT x BM MICE TO SUPPORT ANTIBODY FORMATION IN PRIMED, IRRADIATED RECIPIENTS

Treatment		Response
ATxBM Donors[a] (day-15)	X-ray Recipients[b] (day-5)	Indirect PFC/Spleen ($\pm$SE)
Saline	10μg AHGG	1,845 (478)
AHGG	"	2,356 (682)
DHGG	"	122 (72)
Saline	None	84 (23)

[a]A/J male mice were thymectomized at 7 weeks of age and at 12 weeks were irradiated (1000 r) and reconstituted with 30×10^6 anti-θ + complement treated syngeneic bone marrow cells. Five weeks thereafter, the animals were injected with saline, 2.5 mg deaggregated HGG (DHGG) or 400 μg aggregated HGG (AHGG). Fifteen days after this treatment, 50×10^6 spleen cells from each designated donor group were transferred into appropriately treated recipients.

[b]A/J male mice were injected i.v. with 10μg AHGG and 5 days thereafter were lethally irradiated (1000 r). At that time, they were injected with designated donor spleen cells and challenged with 400μg AHGG. All mice were rechallenged on day 10 with 400μg AHGG.

[c]Indirect plaque-forming cells determined 5 days after the second challenge with HGG. (SE) = standard error of the mean.

TABLE IV

FAILURE OF TOLERANT CELLS TO SUPPRESS NORMAL CELLS IN AN ADOPTIVE TRANSFER SYSTEM

Spleen Cells Injected		Response[b]
No. x 10^{-6}	Donor Source[a]	PFC/Spleen
100	Norm.	20,800
100	3d Tol.	600
100	3d Tol. + Norm.	21,000
80	Norm.	13,800
80	17d Tol.	0
80	17d Tol. + Norm.	14,100
80	Norm.	48,100
80	35d Tol.	200
80	35d Tol. + Norm.	66,500

[a]Spleen cell suspensions obtained from either normal A/J male mice (Norm.) or from mice injected with a tolerogenic dose of 2.5 mg deaggregated HGG 3 days (3d Tol.), 17 days (17d Tol.) or 35 days (35d Tol.) previously. The designated numbers and combinations of cells were injected i.v. into irradiated (1000 r) syngeneic recipients which were challenged on the day of transfer and 10 days later with aggregated HGG (AHGG).

[b]Indirect plaque-forming cells specific to HGG assayed 5 days after the second injection of AHGG.

TABLE V

INABILITY TO CONFER TOLERANCE BY ADOPTIVE TRANSFER OF TOLERANT SPLEEN OR THYMUS CELLS INTO NORMAL MICE

Cells transferred[a]	Time of Initial Challenge[b] (Day)	Response Indirect PFC/Spleen[c] ($\pm$ SE)	
N Spleen	0	48,657	(12,816)
T Spleen	0	68,565	(13,230)
N Spleen	4	34,700	(6,228)
T Spleen	4	60,284	(19,358)
N Thymus	0	52,321	(8,188)
T Thymus	0	45,974	(10,658)
N Thymus	4	42,803	(5,904)
T Thymus	4	70,108	(6,131)
Normal donor		43,666	(3,177)
Tolerant donor		167	(71)

[a]Spleen or thymus cells were obtained from either normal mice or mice injected with tolerogen (2.5 mg deaggregated HGG) 67 days previously. Normal (N) or tolerant (T) cell suspensions were injected into normal syngeneic A/J recipients at a dose of 100×10^6 or 50×10^6 viable spleen or thymus cells respectively.

[b]On the day of transfer or 4 days later, recipient mice were injected with 400 µg aggregated HGG (AHGG). 10 days after the initial challenge, mice were rechallenged with 200 µg AHGG.

[c]Indirect plaque-forming cells determined 5 days after the second challenge with AHGG. (SE) = standard error of the mean.

On the basis of these negative observations, it is difficult to rule out the existence of a state of positive unresponsiveness within this system of immunological tolerance. However, the fact that, in contrast to the relative ease by others of obtaining adoptively transferred positive unresponsiveness (16,17, 18), the failure to obtain similar observations in this system and in a tolerant state induced in rats to the antigen sheep Ig (19) may imply a difference in the mechanism responsible for these various states of tolerance. Since there is an inherent danger in over-interpreting negative findings, the reserved conclusion which can be reached is that, insofar as it has been sought, there is at present no evidence to support the idea that the state of tolerance obtained in mice with monomeric HGG is induced or maintained by a cell mediated positive suppression mechanism. One should include the caveat that more sophisticated methodology may in fact alter such a conclusion. For example, it has been recently reported (20) that the removal of putative suppressor T cells on columns of histamine-bound Sepharose beads (21) allows the expression of the immune potential otherwise suppressed in tolerant spleen cells. Experiments are now in progress to determine whether this or other approaches yield similar results in the system of tolerance presently described.

THE EFFECT OF LIPOPOLYSACCHARIDE ON THE TOLERANT STATE INDUCED TO HGG

The observation originally made by Claman (22) that mice given bacterial lipopolysaccharide (LPS) after a normally tolerogenic dose of bovine γ-globulin do not become tolerant has been repeated using DHGG (23) and extended quantitatively to reveal that such mice not only fail to become tolerant to HGG but in fact respond anamnestically to a subsequent challenge of AHGG (24). Furthermore, that structural moiety of LPS which is necessary to induce B cell mitogenesis, namely, Lipid A (25,26,27,28), is also that portion of LPS which can modulate the induction of tolerance to a state of immunity (29). This correlation is also observed under conditions in which LPS is not mitogenic for B cells. For example, as originally described by Sultzer and Nilsson (30), spleen cells from C3H/HeJ mice do not show ^{3}H thymidine incorporation following exposure to LPS. This can be seen from the data presented in Table VI which demonstrate that in contrast to LPS-induced mitogenesis observed in either A/J or C3H/St spleen cell cultures, cells obtained from C3H/HeJ spleens are refractive to the effect of LPS but not to the effect of Con A. A similar conclusion is also valid for a wide range of LPS concentrations tested (31). In this particular strain of mice, LPS is also incapable of altering the normal induction process of tolerance. This is shown in Table VII. A dose of LPS which in conjunction with tolerogen produces immunity in the A/J strain has no effect in altering the induction of tolerance in C3H/HeJ mice. This observation is not due to a difference in the ability of the two strains to respond to the antigen HGG since the data demonstrate that both strains respond equally well to AHGG.

TABLE VI

STRAIN DIFFERENCES IN THE RESPONSIVENESS OF SPLEEN CELLS TO LPS-INDUCED MITOGENESIS[a]

| Day of Assay | CPM/Culture $(E-C)$[b] | | | | | |
| | A/J | | C3H/St | | C3H/HeJ | |
	LPS	Con A	LPS	Con A	LPS	Con A
1	---	---	4,200	3,100	0	3,200
2	4,600	47,300	16,800	28,500	0	26,600
3	3,500	97,600	9,700	37,300	0	67,500
4	---	---	2,000	88,700	0	99,900

[a]The culture methods used are based on those developed by Mishell and Dutton. Spleen cell cultures were prepared containing 2×10^6 viable cells in 1 ml of medium supplemented with 5% FCS. Duplicate cultures were incubated in the presence of either saline, 10µg E. coli K235 LPS or 5µg Con A, and at daily intervals the stimulation of DNA synthesis was assessed by a 4 hour pulse with ^{3}H-TdR (1µCi/ml, 5Ci/mmole). Cells were then harvested, washed, precipitated with 5% TCA, and the precipitates collected onto Millipore filters. Radioactive measurements were made after overnight accommodation of samples in Aquasol scintillation fluid. A/J and C3H/HeJ mice were purchased from Jackson Laboratories, Bar Harbor, Maine and C3H/St mice were purchased from L.Strong Laboratories, Del Mar, California.

[b]Net counts per minute represent the counts obtained in the mitogen supplemented cultures minus the counts obtained in the saline supplemented cultures.

TABLE VII

EFFECT OF LPS ON THE INDUCTION OF TOLERANCE TO HGG IN C3H/HeJ AND A/J MICE

Group	Treatment[a]	Response [indirect PFC/Spleen (+SE)][b] C3H/HeJ	A/J
A	Saline	8,075 (2,811)	8,958 (3,114)
B	DHGG + Saline	632 (522)	291 (179)
C	DHGG + LPS	15 (15)	21,308 (7,878)

[a]A/J or CeH/HeJ male mice were injected on day 0 with either saline, saline and 2.5 mg deaggregated HGG (DHGG) or 2.5 mg DHGG and 3 hours later with 50 µg of E.coli K235 LPS. Fifteen days after this initial treatment, all mice were challenged with 100µg aggregated HGG (AHGG) given i.v.

[b]Indirect plaque-forming cells specific to HGG enumerated at the peak of the response following the challenge injection, day 6 for groups A and B, day 4 for group C. (SE) = standard error of the mean.

In view of the positive correlation which exists between the capacity of LPS to act as a B cell mitogen on one hand and to alter the induction of tolerance on the other, it is tempting to postulate that the cellular mode of action of LPS on tolerance is confined to specific B cells only. There is at present a conflict over the exact requirements of T cells and/or macrophages for those immunologically-related functions attributed to LPS. For example, although there is evidence that LPS can act directly on B cells to stimulate both cellular replication and IgM synthesis (32), more recent data would suggest that LPS-induced mitogenesis requires both T cells and macrophages (33). The adjuvant effect of LPS on antibody formation has also been regarded as potentiating specific T cell helper function possibly due to an increase in the interaction between macrophages and T cells resulting in specific T cell proliferation (34,35,36). The direct activation of macrophage by LPS (37,38) is another biological effect whose role is difficult to evaluate inasmuch as both inductive (39) and suppressive (40) functions

have been implicated for this cell type in immunological reactions. Critical to understanding the action of LPS on tolerance induction is the question of whether the effect of
LPS on HGG tolerance can occur in spite of T cell tolerance.
Although it has been previously reported that mice making
specific antibody to HGG as the result of the dual treatment
with DHGG and LPS have tolerant thymocytes (24), the scope of
peripheral T cell unresponsiveness in this system would appear more germane to the question.

An indirect approach to that problem has now been undertaken by utilizing the observation that the antigens HGG and
equine γ-globulin (EGG) display cross tolerance, yet do not
show cross immunity (41). This phenomenon was experimentally
shown to be explainable by the fact that EGG and HGG share
antigenic recognition by T cells but not by B cells. By contrast, HGG and turkey globulin (TGG) do not cross-react in
A/J mice insofar as either tolerance or antibody formation.
It follows, therefore, that if mice, immune to HGG as the
result of the dual treatment with a tolerogenic preparation
of HGG and LPS, display specific T cell tolerance, then such
mice should be unresponsive to a subsequent challenge with
the equally T dependent antigen EGG because these globulins
cross-react at the T cell level. The prediction was tested
using the protocol seen in Table VIII. Groups of mice were
injected on day 0 with either deaggregated HGG, deaggregated
HGG + LPS, saline or LPS. All groups were challenged with
EGG on day 26, with EGG and HGG on day 36 and on day 41
spleens from individual animals were assayed for PFC specific
for either equine or human globulin. The results from this
experiment conform with with the prediction. That is, tolerogen-treated mice are in fact hyporesponsive to EGG when
compared to the response in those animals initially treated
only with saline or with LPS. To test the specificity of
such a phenomenon, an identical protocol was used to determine the effect on the response to the T cell non cross reactive globulin TGG. As before, groups of mice were injected
on day 0 with either deaggregated HGG and LPS, deaggregated
HGG, saline or LPS. All groups were challenged with TGG on
day 26, with TGG and HGG on day 36 and on day 41 spleens
from individual mice were assayed for plaque-forming cells
specific for either turkey or human globulin. The results
of this experiment are shown in Table IX and reveal that the
effect was indeed specific in that regardless of subsequent
treatment with LPS, mice initially injected with deaggregated
HGG responded to turkey globulin as well as those groups not
initially treated with the tolerogen.

TABLE VIII

PRIMING TO HGG WITH TOLEROGEN (DHGG) AND LPS FAILS TO AFFECT UNRESPONSIVENESS INDUCED TO EGG, A "T" CELL CROSS-REACTIVE ANTIGEN

Treament			PFC/Spleen Specific to (±SE)[b]	
Day 0	Day 26	Day 36	EGG	HGG
DHGG + LPS	EGG	EGG + HGG	711 (135)	16,453 (9,610)
DHGG	"	"	1,272 (195)	0
Saline	"	"	5,551 (1,221)	4,508 (1,520)
LPS	"	"	5,131 (251)	6,622 (518)

[a]A/J male mice were injected on day 0 with either 2.5 mg deaggregated HGG (DHGG) and 50 µg LPS, 2.5 mg DHGG alone, saline or 50 µg LPS. All the mice received an i.p. injection of 400 µg alum-precipitated equine γ globulin (EGG) on day 26, and 400 µg EGG i.p. and 400 µg aggregated HGG (AHGG) iv on day 36.

[b]Indirect plaque-forming cells specific either to EGG or HGG were assayed 4 days after the last antigenic challenge. (SE) = standard error of the mean.

Albeit indirect, this evidence suggests that mice immunized as the result of injecting LPS after tolerogen are specifically rendered tolerant at the level of T cells. A priori, these data would support the concept that the effect of LPS on the induction of tolerance is one whose cellular mode of action does not require a normal complement of specific T cell helper function. They do not however, eliminate the possibility that LPS and antigen may amplify a residual population of non tolerant specific T cells. An alternative to the requirement of antigen specific T cell help may be a non specifically stimulated T cell activity (? via LPS activated macrophages), a macrophage activity either directly stimulated or stimulated by LPS activated T cells, or even T cell activity specifically recognizing LPS bound on B cells. Whatever mechanism may be operational, it is painfully obvious that more precisely defined cellular parameters than those on hand will be necessary to understand either the phenomenon of tolerance heretofore detailed or its modulation by LPS.

TABLE IX

PRIMING TO HGG WITH TOLEROGEN (DHGG) AND LPS DOES NOT INFLUENCE RESPONSIVENESS TO TGG, A "T" CELL NON CROSS-REACTIVE ANTIGEN

Treatment[a]			PFC/Spleen Specific to (±SE)[b]	
Day 0	Day 26	Day 36	TGG	HGG
DHGG + LPS	TGG	HGG + TGG	4,205 (440)	6,900 (1,749)
DHGG	"	"	4,293 (439)	99 (67)
Saline	"	"	6,925 (845)	1,500 (307)
LPS	"	"	5,112 (392)	1,454 (195)

[a]A/J male mice were injected on day 0 with either 2.5 mg deaggregated HGG (DHGG) and 50 µg LPS, 2.5 mg DHGG alone, saline or 50 µg LPS. All of the animals received an i.p. injection of 400 µg alum-precipitated turkey γ globulin (TGG) on day 26 and 400 µg TGG i.p. and 400 µg aggregated HGG (AHGG) iv on day 36.

[b]Indirect plaque-forming cells specific either to EGG or HGG were assayed 4 days after the last antigenic challenge. (SE) = standard error of the mean.

ACKNOWLEDGMENTS

    We thank Ms. Emma Lum, Lee Cunningham and Linda Lewis for their excellent technical assistance, and Ms. Linda Norwood for her invaluable contributions in typing and editing this manuscript.

FOOTNOTES TO THE TITLE PAGE

    This is Publication Number 849 from Experimental Pathology, Scripps Clinic and Research Foundation, La Jolla, California. The work was supported by the U.S. Public Health Service Grant AI-07007, American Cancer Grant #IM-42D and

Atomic Energy Commission Contract AT (14-3)-410.

Dr. Chiller is supported by a Dernham Fellowship (No. D-202) of the California Division of the American Cancer Society.

Dr. Louis is supported by a Dernham Fellowship (No. D-209) of the California Division of the American Cancer Society.

Dr. Skidmore is supported by U.S. Public Health Service Training Grant AI-00453.

Dr. Weigle is supported by U.S. Public Health Research Career Award 5-K6-GM-06936.

REFERENCES

1. Burnet, F.M., The Clonal Selection Theory of Acquired Immunity. Cambridge University Press, Cambridge, 1959.

2. Weigle, W.O., Clin. Exp. Immunol. 9:437, 1971.

3. Jerne, N.K., Ann. Immunol. (Inst. Pasteur). 125C:373, 1974.

4. Bretscher, P. and Cohn, M., Science. 169:1042, 1970.

5. Rosenthal, A.S. and Shevach, E.M., J. Exp. Med. 138:1194, 1973.

6. Katz, D.H., Hamaoka, T., Dorf, M.E. and Benacerraf, B., Proc. Nat. Acad. Sci. (USA). 70:2624, 1973.

7. Weigle, W.O., Adv. Immunol. 16:61, 1973.

8. Chiller, J.M., Romball, C.G. and Weigle, W.O., Cell. Immunol. 8:28, 1973.

9. Dresser, D.W., Immunology. 5:378, 1962.

10. Chiller, J.M., Habicht, G.S. and Weigle, W.O., Proc. Nat. Acad. Sci. (USA). 65:551, 1970.

11. Chiller, J.M., Habicht, G.S. and Weigle, W.O., Science. 171:813, 1971.

12. Gershon, R.K. and Kondo, K., Immunology. 18:723, 1970.

13. Mitchell, G.F., Lafleur, L. and Andersson, K., Scand. J. Immunol. 3:39, 1974.

14. Schrader, J.W., J. Exp. Med. 139:1303, 1974.

15. Zembala, M. and Asherson, G.L., Nature. 244:227, 1973.

16. Weber, G. and Kolsch, E., Eur. J. Immunol. 3:767, 1973.

17. Droege, W., Eur. J. Immunol. 3:804, 1973.

18. Miller, J.F.A.P., Ann. Immunol. (Inst. Pasteur). 125C: 213, 1974.

19. Scott, D.W., this symposium.

20. Segal, S., Weinstein, Y., Melmon, K.L. and McDevitt,H.O., Fed. Proc. 33:723, 1974.

21. Shearer, G.M., Melmon, K.L., Weinstein, Y. and Sela, M., J. Exp. Med. 136:1302, 1972.

22. Claman, H.N., J. Immunol. 91:833, 1963.

23. Golub, E.S. and Weigle, W.O., J. Immunol. 98:1241, 1967.

24. Louis, J.A., Chiller, J.M. and Weigle, W.O., J. Exp. Med. 138:1481, 1973.

25. Andersson, J., Melchers, F., Galanos, C. and Luderitz, O., J. Exp. Med. 137:943, 1973.

26. Peavy, D.L., Shands, J.W., Adler, W.H. and Smith, R.T., J. Immunol. 111:352, 1973.

27. Rosenstreich, D.L., Nowotny, A., Chused, T. and Mergenbagen, S.E., Inf. and Immun. 8:406, 1973.

28. Chiller, J.M., Skidmore, B.J., Morrison, D.C. and Weigle, W.O., Proc. Nat. Acad. Sci. (U.S.A.). 70:2129, 1973.

29. Chiller, J.M., Louis, J.A., Skidmore, B.J. and
    Weigle, W.O., In The Immune System, edited by E. Sercarz
    and A. Williamson, Academic Press, 1974.

30. Sultzer, B.M. and Nilsson, B.S., Nature New Biol. 240:
    198, 1972.

31. Skidmore, B.J., Chiller, J.M., Morrison, D.C. and
    Weigle, W.O., Fed. Proc. 33:600, 1974.

32. Andersson, J., Sjöberg, O. and Möller, G., Transpl.
    Rev. 11:131, 1972.

33. Kagnoff, M.F., Billings, P. and Cohn, M., J. Exp. Med.
    139:407, 1974.

34. Allison, A.C. and Davies, A.J.S., Nature. 223:330,
    1971.

35. Hamaoka, T. and Katz, D.H., J. Immunol. 111:1554, 1973.

36. Armerding, D. and Katz, D.H., J. Exp. Med. 139:24,
    1974.

37. Alexander, P. and Evans, R., Nature New Biol. 232:76,
    1971.

38. Gery, I. and Waksman, B.H., J. Exp. Med. 136:143, 1972.

39. Schrader, J.W., J. Exp. Med. 138:1466, 1973.

40. Yoshinaga, M., Yoshinaga, A. and Waksman, B.H., J. Exp.
    Med. 136:956, 1972.

41. Ruben, T.J., Chiller, J.M. and Weigle, W.O., J. Immunol.
    111:805, 1973.

DISCUSSION FOLLOWING JACOUES CHILLER

KATZ: I only want to point out that there are a large number
of observations now that indicate the effects of LPS on
T cell functions, the most recent of which are those of
Dick Smith's colleagues in vitro that perhaps he will
comment on later. In view of these observations, I
think that it is possible to consider the LPS effects
on tolerance induction that Jacques has presented on the
following lines: 1) LPS may be increasing residual
helper T cell function in tolerogen-treated mice to
manifest sufficient helper activity to give a response,
and 2) LPS may be decreasing suppressor cell activity
if this may exist at all in this system.

CHILLER: The reason that we feel that LPS is not magnifying
residual specific T helper activity is that we are unable to observe a concomitant response to a T cell
cross-reacting antigen. There are, however, other
variations on the same theme. For example, T cell
activity may be directed toward LPS bound on B cells or
to antigen(s) modified by LPS. Insofar as LPS decreasing suppressor activity, the possibility certainly
exists if, in fact, the state of tolerance which we
have described is maintained by suppressor cells.

SMITH: The conclusion that T cells are not involved in the
LPS "rescue" effect (135 day tolerant animals + AHGG +
LPS) is a bit hazardous, for reasons we have come to
appreciate from our own work (Forbes, J.T., Kakao, Y.,
Smith, R.T., Fed. Proc., submitted to Science, 1974.)
We find that "pure" population of thymus competent cells
(low density, low θ, high H-2) can be triggered by LPS
to proliferation by concomitant T cell activation.
This effect is shown with very low even submitogenic
concentrations of Con A or alloantigens (not PHA,
curiously). This suggests that the antigen in your
tolerant animals could be encountering small numbers of
competent T cells (anti-HGG) which in turn could trigger
the LPS responses you describe. Moreover, it suggests
that the cell population responsive to LPS may not be
that stimulated to secrete anti-HGG in large numbers.

CHILLER: I agree that we have not formally excluded the
possibility you suggest.

G. MÖLLER: It is important to distinguish between two experimental situations. 1) Effect of LPS alone and
2) Effect of LPS plus antigen. The latter we call
synergy. In the first situation it is clearly shown
that LPS directly activates B cells in the absence of T
cells and macrophages. LPS does not activate T cells.
The synergy between LPS and antigen requires macrophages
and also T cells. The evidence suggests that it is the
T dependent antigen that activates T cells and that the
phenomenon is due to synergy between LPS and B mitogens
released from antigen-activated macrophages and T cells.

E. MÖLLER: Do you have any information to substantiate the
notion that LPS affects those exact cells which would
become tolerant?

CHILLER: We have not done qualitative experiments which
measure the spectrum of antibody-forming cells in terms
of their affinity to the specific antigen, if that is
what the question implies. On a quantitative basis,
however, the response obtained by the combination of
tolerogen and LPS is about what one obtains with immunogen alone.

SCOTT: We have some LPS data which agrees with both your
data, Jacques and with David Katz's data. We used a
hapten-carrier model in which tolerance to the carrier
prevents an immune response to TNP on such a carrier.
Rats were "tolerized" to sheep Ig, given LPS 3-6 hours
later and then challenged either one day or five days
later with TNP-sheep Ig in adjuvant; the anti-TNP response is measured six days later. In summary, as shown
in Fig. 1, we cannot prevent carrier (T cell) tolerance
with a one-day interval between tolerogen and challenge.
In contrast, with a five-day interval, we get a significant reversal in two out of four experiments. This
could reflect an expansion of helper T cells by LPS and
tolerogen but also could be due to the effect of anti-
carrier antibody acting to "help" (since there is anti-
sheep Ig in some of these animals). In contrast to
these studies on T cell tolerance, hapten-specific
tolerance induced by TNP-Rat Ig (in the Borel model) is
readily reversed by LPS with only a one-day interval in
the protocol.

INTERVAL BETWEEN TOLEROGEN (± LPS) AND CHALLENGE

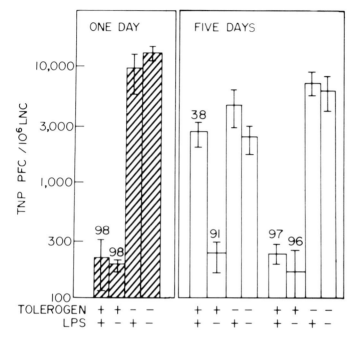

Figure 1. Effect of the interval between tolerogen and challenge on the ability of LPS to prevent carrier (T cell) tolerance. Each experiment in this figure has been done twice with identical results. Number above columns = % unresponsiveness.

GERSHON: When you make B mice tolerant with HGG and fail to break the tolerance by adding thymocytes, how do you rule out remaining tolerogen making the added thymocytes tolerant?

CHILLER: First, let me clarify that the B cells are adoptively transferred to a primed irradiated recipient so that we are not adding an exogenous source of thymocytes to the system. To rule out tolerogen carryover in this protocol, we can show that mixtures of normal and tolerogen-treated ATxBM spleen cells do, in fact, respond.

FELDMANN: There is an interesting difference in the results concerning the findings of suppressor T cells in the HGG system. Tony Basten, Roger Taylor, Huchet and myself, who have found evidence of T cell suppression, have used the CBA strain while you have used A/J. It thus seems possible that T cell suppression may be under genetic control, and thus it would be of interest when you repeat your experiments on T suppressor cells to HGG to have CBA controls.

CHILLER: I agree that this should and will be done.

BASTEN: I should like to comment on the apparent discrepancies between Dr. Chiller's data which have failed to show suppression with HGG and ours. First, we were not examining an HGG Ig_1 response per se but a polyvalent IgG anti-DNP response in a hapten-carrier collaborative system. Secondly, the target for suppression was an HGG-primed spleen cell population which could behave differently from normal cells in an interaction. Thirdly, the suppressor effect was present for only a short period of time from approximately three to fifteen days. Thus, spleen cells transferred 67 days after tolerance induction would not be expected to suppress. Finally, tolerance could only be demonstrated by injecting at least 10^9 cells (10^8 cells being ineffective). I would hope that interchange in protocols may well resolve these issues.

CHILLER: The differences in the two spleens may, in fact, account for the differences in the conclusions. What is most germane, however, is whether the tolerant state we have described is, in fact, maintained by a population of specific suppressor cells. If this were to be so, then I would expect that to be the case even 67 days after tolerance induction since such treated animals are, in fact, specifically unresponsive. With regard to the dose of cells transferred, we have not yet gone up to higher numbers than 10^8 spleen or thymus cells. Finally, let me say that I concur with Dr. Basten that this issue is certainly resolvable by an exchange of materials and protocols and that it will indeed be done.

MITCHELL: An additional difference between the Basten system and the Chiller system (to those mentioned by Feldmann and Basten) is that the latter one is looking at an IgG_1 response to HGG versus a presumably mixed allotype response to DNP.

G. MÖLLER: I would like to reiterate the point I tried to make earlier. In synergy experiments (LPS plus antigen) helper cells (T cells and macrophages) are needed. Therefore, synergy will be weaker in nude mice. It is a mistake to conclude that this is due to an effect of LPS on T cells: it is antigen that requires T cells in this synergy.

CHILLER: In this vein I should add that we have not yet been capable of converting tolerance to immunity with LPS in nude mice. However, this may be also interpretable as reflecting the paucity of B cells which can form γ_1 antibody to HGG in such mice.

EFFECT OF ANTIGEN STRUCTURE ON THE INDUCTION
OF TOLERANCE IN T CELLS

Marc Feldmann, Sirkka Kontiainen and Marvin B. Rittenberg

Imperial Cancer Research Fund Tumor Immunology Unit
Department of Zoology
University College, London

INTRODUCTION

Whereas B cell tolerance has been extensively studied in vitro, there are fewer studies of T cell tolerance in vitro. Having developed an assay for the induction of T helper cells in vitro (1), it, thus, became possible to compare the induction of tolerance in primed and unprimed T cells in vitro, with that of B cells, using antigenic molecules of different physical structure.

METHODS

Basically, the Marbrook/Diener culture system was used as described previously (2, 3). Antigens, details of culture and assay techniques, have all been published elsewhere (4, 5). For use as donors of primed spleens, CBA mice were injected i.p. with 100 µg of dinitrophenylated fowl gamma globulin (DNP-FγG) emulsified in complete Freund's adjuvant with 20 µg dinitrophenylated polymeric flagellin (DNP-POL) in saline or with KLH adsorbed on bentonite.

RESULTS

The presence of antibody-forming cell assays for fowl gamma globulin (FγG) and flagellin and of thymus-independent antigens bearing these determinants makes it possible to compare the induction of tolerance in FγG (or flagellin) reactive helper cells and antibody-forming cell precursors. Basically, primed spleen cell suspensions were incubated with protein, then washed and challenged with the hapten protein to measure the helper response, and the thymus-independent antigen to measure the B cell response against the protein.

Table I shows results of this kind using DNP-FγG-primed mice, incubated with deaggregated FγG or FγG linked to POL via an antibody bond and then challenged with 0.1 µg/ml DNP-FγG and 0.1 µg/ml FγG-POL. Responses to DNP reflect

helper cell function, to FγG, B cell function. Only the
FγG-POL induced B cell tolerance under the conditions
studied, whereas both induced T cell tolerance, indicating
that both soluble and aggregated ("polymeric") antigens
induce T cell tolerance, whereas the latter is more efficient for B cells.

TABLE I

CAPACITY OF DIFFERENT FORMS OF FγG TO INDUCE TOLERANCE

TOLERANCE INDUCTION (μg/ml)		CHALLENGE		RESPONSE	
				Anti-DNP	Anti-FγG
NIL		DNP-FγG and FγG-POL		1022	1410
Soluble FγG	100	"	"	110	1367
"	10	"	"	263	1130
"	1	"	"	415	1095
FγG-POL	100	"	"	310	225
"	10	"	"	115	672
"	1	"	"	165	1810

Spleen cells from mice primed to DNP-FγG were incubated
over night (14 hours) at 37^{0}, washed and challenged with
1 μg/ml DNP-FγG and FγG-POL. Suppression of anti-DNP response reflects T cell tolerance. Suppression of anti-FγG
response reflects B cell tolerance. The FγG-POL used for
challenge was not the same as used for tolerance induction.
The immunogen contained less FγG and did not induce tolerance.

A similar experiment of this type is shown in Table II
using mice primed to DNP-POL. Incubation with polymeric
flagellin (POL) or monomeric flagellin (MON) abrogated the
response to the thymus-dependent antigen DNP-MON, indicating
tolerance of T helper cells, whereas only POL induced tolerance in B cells. These results indicated that both primed
T and B cells may become tolerant after in vitro incubation
with tolerogens. To look at tolerance induction in unprimed

T cells, various sources of unprimed T cells were incubated
with keyhole limpet hemocyanin (KLH) prior to challenge with
an immunogenic concentration of KLH (and helper cell induction). The results in Table III are plotted as the % of an
optimal response (cells incubated with chicken gamma globulin, CGG) remaining after KLH pre-treatment, using the
optimal number of cultured helper cells in vitro (tested over
range 10^5 to 10^6). A hierarchy of sensitivity to tolerance
induction was found with unprimed spleen and cortisone-
resistant thymus (CRT) the most sensitive, with lymph node
cells (LN) next and primed spleen the most resistant to tolerance induction. This closely parallels the variation in
antigen dose which stimulates T helper cells of various organ
sources (6).

Complexes of antibody and antigen have been reported to
induce a state of partial tolerance, termed "antibody-
mediated tolerance". Most of the published work in this
field has dealt with B cell tolerance. Table IV indicates
that complexes of KLH and purified anti-KLH induced partial
tolerance in T helper cells to KLH. For comparison the
degree of tolerance in T helper cells to 10 μg KLH is shown.

TABLE II

COMPARISON OF T AND B CELL TOLERANCE TO FLAGELLIN
IN CELLS PRIMED TO DNP-POL

TOLERANCE INDUCTION (μg/ml)	CHALLENGE		RESPONSE	
			Anti-DNP	Anti-flagellin
NIL	DNP-POL		2680	862
	DNP-MON,	POL	1812	1172
MON 10	"	"	260	945
1	"	"	495	1200
10^{-1}	"	"	1410	1024
POL 10	"	"	202	433
1	"	"	430	1160
10^{-1}	"	"	1562	920

Spleen cells from DNP-POL-primed mice were incubated for 4
hours with POL or MON, washed and challenged with DNP-POL
10^{-1} μg/ml, DNP-MON 1 μg/ml or POL 10^{-2} μg/ml. IgM response
was measured at day 4.

TABLE III

SENSITIVITY OF T CELL POPULATIONS TO TOLERANCE INDUCTION

CELLS CULTURED	INDUCTION (μg/ml KLH)	CHALLENGE (μg/ml KLH)	RESPONSE %
Spleen	10	10^{-2}	18
"	1	"	60
CRT	10	10^{-1}	12
"	1	"	56
LN	100	1	10
"	10	"	16
"	1	"	92
Primed spleen	100	10^{-2}	11
"	10	"	38

Cells were incubated for 4 hours at 37°, washed and then cultured for 4 days to induce KLH-reactive "helper cells". Graded numbers of these cells were cultured with TNP-KLH and a source of B cells normal spleen for a further 4 days. Results are expressed as a percentage of response of KLH helper cells which had been incubated with CGG instead of KLH for the first 4 hours.

TABLE IV

ANTIBODY-MEDIATED TOLERANCE IN CORTISONE-RESISTANT THYMOCYTES

INDUCTION	CHALLENGE (μg/ml)	RESPONSE %
NIL	10^{-1} KLH	100
10 μg KLH 37°	"	12
4°	"	16
1 μg KLH + 1 μg anti-KLH	"	18
1 μg FγG + 1 μg anti-KLH	"	97

CRT were incubated for 4 hours prior to washing and then challenged with 10^{-1} μg/ml KLH. After 4 days helper cells were harvested and added with TNP-KLH to a B cell source.

DISCUSSION

The results presented above indicate that tolerance may be induced in T cells in vitro just as reported previously for B cells (4, 7, 8). The results obtained so far do not permit any detailed conclusions about T cell tolerance, in general, but point out certain aspects.

First, there are marked variations in the ease of in vitro T cell tolerance induction, depending on the organ source and whether the mice had been primed. The correlation between this T cell heterogeneity in ease of tolerance induction with other T cell sub-populations (T_1, T_2, etc.) is not yet known.

Secondly, "monomeric" antigens such as deaggregated FγG or MON induced tolerance in primed T cells but not primed B cells, suggesting that while a polymeric nature is of importance for B cell tolerance in vitro (4, 7, 8, 9) as in vivo (10), it is not for T cells in vitro (see above) just as it is not in vivo (11).

Thirdly, antigen-antibody complexes can induce T cell tolerance (antibody-mediated tolerance) in much the same way as these complexes can induce B cell tolerance in vitro (12, 13).

As yet, no attempts have been made to test the reversibility of T cell tolerance induction and the role, if any, of suppressor T cells in T cell tolerance is not known.

SUMMARY

Induction of tolerance in T and B cells in vitro was compared. Unlike B cells, T cells were rendered tolerant by non-polymeric antigens such as monomeric flagellin and de-aggregated gamma globulin. T cells were rendered tolerant by keyhole limpet hemocyanin and by antigen-antibody complexes containing hemocyanin. T cells taken from various organs of unprimed mice, or from the spleens of primed mice, could also be rendered tolerant but with varying concentrations of antigen.

ACKNOWLEDGMENTS

This work was supported by USPHS grants AM13173 and CA12355.

The present address of Sirkka Kontianinen is at the Department of Bacteriology and Serology, University of Helsinki, Finland, and the present address of Marvin B. Rittenberg is at the Division of Immunology and Allergy, University of Oregon Medical School, Portland, Oregon, U.S.

REFERENCES

1. Kontianinen, S. and Feldmann, M., Nat. New Biology. 245:285, 1973.

2. Marbrook, J., Lancet. 2:1279, 1967.

3. Diener, E. and Armstrong, W.D., Lancet. 2:1281, 1967.

4. Feldmann, M., J. Exp. Med. 135:735, 1972.

5. Feldmann, M., Greaves, M.F., Parker, D.C. and Rittenberg, M.B., Eur. J. Immunol. In press, 1974.

6. Kontianinen, M. and Feldmann, M., Eur. J. Immunol. In press, 1974.

7. Diener, E. and Armstrong, W.D., J. Exp. Med. 129:591, 1969.

8. Feldmann, M., Nat. New Biology. 231:21, 1971.

9. Feldmann, M., Cont. Topics Molecular Immunology. In press, 1974.

10. Howard, J.G. and Mitchison, N.A., Prog. Allergy. In press, 1974.

11. Weigle, W.O., Adv. Immunol. 16:1, 1973.

12. Feldmann, M. and Diener, E., J. Exp. Med. 131:247, 1970.

13. Diener, E. and Feldmann, M., Transplant. Rev. 8:76, 1972.

INDICATIONS OF ACTIVE SUPPRESSION IN MOUSE
CARRIERS OF LYMPHOCYTIC CHORIOMENINGITIS VIRUS

Rolf Zinkernagel and Peter Doherty
(Communicated by G.L. Ada)

Department of Microbiology
The John Curtin School of Medical Research
Canberra A.C.T., Australia

In Nature, mouse carriers of lymphocytic choriomeningitis (LCM) virus are infected in utero and circulate high titres of virus throughout life (1). A similar state of persistent tolerant infection (2) is readily induced experimentally by injecting neonates with large doses of LCM virus. The possible analogy between the LCM carrier state and self tolerance was first discussed by Burnet and Fenner (3) when proposing the concept of immunological tolerance. This model is, however, of more than historical interest to immunologists. The recent development of a sensitive in vitro ^{51}Cr release assay for thymus-derived lymphocytes (T cells) sensitized to LCM virus (4-6) has made feasible direct examination of tolerance mechanisms in the T cell compartment.

THE CYTOTOXIC ASSAY

Monolayers of C3H mouse L929 Fibroblasts (L cells) are grown in flat-bottomed hemagglutination trays, infected with a high multiplicity of LCM virus and labelled with ^{51}Cr. These target cells, together with control uninfected L cells, are overlaid with the lymphoid cell population to be tested at a ratio of 30:1, and %^{51}Cr release is measured 16 hours later (6). Cell-mediated lysis is a function of specifically sensitized thymus-derived lymphocytes, being completely eliminated by prior incubation of immune spleen cells with anti-Θ ascitic fluid and complement (4, 5). Culture supernates have no specific activity, either in the presence or absence, of normal spleen cells. Cytotoxic capacity is in no way diminished by prior incubation with anti-Ig serum and complement or by addition or deletion of macrophages (7).

The experimental usefulness of this assay is greatly enhanced by the fact that cytotoxic activity is restricted by the H-2 gene complex (7, 8). Specific lysis of LCM-infected L cells occurs only when targets and T cells share at least one set of H-2 antigenic specificities (H-2^k).

Also, reciprocal restriction of cell-mediated lysis between BALB/c (H-2^d) and CBA/H (H-2^k) mice has been demonstrated using LCM-infected peritoneal macrophages as target cells.

STATUS OF ANTIGEN REACTIVE CELLS IN CARRIER MICE

There is good evidence against clonal deletion of B cells in LCM carrier mice. Much of the virus in carrier serum is complexed with Ig (9), indicating that antibody-forming cell function is intact. Adoptive immunization of carriers with syngeneic immune spleen cells from actively infected mice results in formation of very high titres of specific antibody, the levels being considerably greater than those recognized in any other host-LCM virus combination (1, 10). This may be interpreted as representing provision of specific T cell help to primed B cells in the carrier recipient.

The status of T cells in LCM carrier mice is, however, less clear. Total numbers of lymphocytes bearing the ⊖ allo-antigen are apparently equivalent to those found in normal mice (11), but there is disagreement in the literature as to whether any of these T cells are reactive for LCM-viral antigen (11-13). Spleen preparations from LCM-carrier mice have, in our hands, shown no evidence of specific T cell activity (Table I). The question remains whether clonal deletion or active suppression of T cells is central to persistent tolerant infection of mice with LCM virus.

ALLOGENEIC ABROGATION OF T CELL TOLERANCE

Tolerance of rats to sheep erythrocytes can be transiently broken by inoculation with allogeneic normal lymphocytes (14, 15). We have used this phenomenon to investigate the T cell status of mouse carriers of viscerotropic (WE3) LCM virus. Mice from a CBA/H (H-2^k) carrier colony were injected intravenously (i.v.) at various intervals with 5.0 x 10^7 spleen cells from syngeneic or allogeneic normal mice. These carrier recipients were all killed on the same day, and spleen preparations (16) were assayed together for cytotoxic T cell activity. Two separate experiments are shown in Fig. 1. In both cases injection of allogeneic spleen cells resulted in generation of high levels of cell-mediated lysis. Maximal release of ^{51}Cr was observed at 11 days after inoculation, but later intervals have not yet been examined.

TABLE I

ABSENCE OF SIGNIFICANT CYTOTOXIC ACTIVITY IN SPLEEN PREPARATIONS FROM CBA/H CARRIER MICE

Experiment[a]	Cell Population	Carrier Age (days)	$\%^{51}$Cr Release from L cells	
			Infected	Normal
1	Carrier	56	22.9 + 0.7	22.3 + 2.0
	Normal		23.0 + 1.1	20.0 + 1.4
	LCM Immune[b]		90.1 + 1.0	21.0 + 1.9
2	Carrier	42	28.0 + 2.2	25.4 + 1.0
	Normal		28.4 + 0.4	23.5 + 0.6
	LCM Immune		87.2 + 1.8	22.8 + 0.6
3	Carrier	10	16.9 + 1.4	18.7 + 2.9
		15	19.3 + 2.1	16.4 + 1.6
		19	18.9 + 1.0	18.1 + 2.0
		24	18.0 + 0.4	16.3 + 0.6
		42	20.3 + 1.1	17.6 + 0.5
	Normal		20.3 + 0.5	17.3 + 1.7
	LCM Immune		75.2 + 1.7	19.3 + 2.0

[a] Results for 1 and 2 are the positive and negative controls for experiments shown in Fig. 1.

[b] Injected intracerebrally with 300 LD_{50} of WE3 LCM virus 7 days previously.

The sensitized T cells may be considered to be of carrier, not donor, origin for two reasons. Firstly, lysis of normal targets, which presumably reflects activity of transferred T cells specific for host alloantigens, had returned to background levels by day 11 (Expt. 2, Fig. 1). Apparently, these donor lymphocytes had been eliminated before maximal cytotoxicity for LCM-infected monolayers. Secondly, lysis of LCM-infected L cells occurs only when targets and T cells share at least one set of H-2 antigenic specificities (8). Lymphocytes from LCM immune BALB/c x C57BL/F1 ($H-2^{b/d}$) mice do not induce specific release of ^{51}Cr from LCM-infected L cells ($H-2^k$). Furthermore, when spleen preparations from syngeneic or allogeneic LCM-immune mice were inoculated into CBA/H carriers, the syngeneic T cells went on to generate high levels of cytotoxic activity by day 9 (Table II). However, in carriers injected with an allogeneic immune population, specific effector activity was observed only on day 6, presumably due to the allogeneic abrogation effect.

At present, our understanding of the conditions governing allogeneic abrogation of T cell tolerance in LCM is very incomplete. Two further attempts to induce cytotoxic activity in carrier mice at 9 and 11 days after transfer of allogeneic normal cells failed completely. Also, we have no explanation as to why, in the first experiment (Fig. 1, Table II), allogeneic normal spleen cells were much more effective than an allogeneic immune population. The phenomenon is, however, almost certainly valid. Generation of cytotoxic T cells is associated with considerable reduction of virus titres in the spleens of the carrier recipients (Table III). Elimination of LCM virus from tissues of acutely-infected mice has been shown, in cell transfer experiments, to be largely a function of sensitized thymus-derived lymphocytes (17).

EVIDENCE FOR ACTIVE SUPPRESSION

The above results support the concept that allogeneic confrontation derepresses or removes from suppression functional T cell activity (14, 18, 19). By analogy with other experimental systems, the fact that the responsiveness of normal syngeneic cells is apparently depressed in the carrier environment, whereas transferred syngeneic immune cells generate further cytotoxic capacity, is also in accord with the idea that suppressor T cells may be active in the LCM-carrier state (15). Experiments to establish the presence of suppressors are, however, at a preliminary stage.

TABLE II

CYTOTOXIC ACTIVITY OF CBA/H CARRIER SPLEEN CELLS FOLLOWING ADOPTIVE IMMUNIZATION WITH 5.0 x 10^7 SYNGENEIC OR ALLOGENEIC IMMUNE SPLEEN CELLS[a]

Cells Transferred	Days after transfer	%51 Cr release from L cells	
		Infected	Normal
CBA/H	3	33.5 + 1.8	21.1 + 1.0
	6	22.7 + 0.9	18.5 + 1.6
	9	67.1 + 2.8	23.7 + 1.5
	12	40.5 + 1.7	20.8 + 2.2
BALB/c x C57BL/F1	3	27.1 + 1.4	20.9 + 1.1
	6	41.2 + 1.1	22.1 + 0.8
	9	24.7 + 1.1	19.8 + 0.8

[a]This experiment was done at the same time as Expt. 1 in Fig. 1. Donors were dosed 7 days previously with 300 LD_{50} of WE3 LCM virus.

TABLE III

VIRUS TITRES IN SPLEENS OF CBA/H CARRIER MICE INJECTED WITH ALLOGENEIC NORMAL SPLEEN CELLS AT VARIOUS INTERVALS

Days after inoculation	Virus Titre[a]
5	3.8
7	4.0
9	1.6
11	0.4
No cells	4.2

[a] $\log_{10}$ Ic LD_{50} per 10^6 nucleated spleen cells, assayed in WEHI mice which are uniformly susceptible to LCM.

This is Expt. 2 from Fig. 1.

Normal CBA/H mice were adoptively immunized with syngeneic carrier lymphoid cell populations and challenged with virus 24 hours later. The response of mice dosed with carrier spleen and mesenteric lymph node preparations was greatly suppressed (Table IV). Mice given carrier thymocytes also generated much lower levels of cytotoxic activity. Suppression by thymocytes has also been described for other tolerance models (20, 21).

This effect may reflect activity of suppressor T cells. However, there are several other quite feasible alternative explanations. Carrier spleen preparations contain very high concentrations of infectious virus (Table III). Injection of large doses of LCM virus causes considerable depression of the cytotoxic T cell response (2, 5). Also, the transferred spleen and lymph node cells would presumably contain many antibody-forming cells (9).

TABLE IV

CYTOTOXIC ACTIVITY OF SPLEEN PREPARATIONS FROM NORMAL CBA/H MICE DOSED 8 DAYS PREVIOUSLY WITH 5.0×10^7 SYNGENEIC CELLS FOLLOWED BY 3,000 LD_{50} OF WE3 LCM VIRUS I.V. 24 HOURS LATER

Experiment	Cell Inoculum	Virus at 24 hrs	%51Cr release from L cells	
			Infected	Normal
1	Carrier spleen	-	23.0 ± 2.0	20.8 ± 1.8
	Carrier spleen	+	26.5 ± 1.9	20.9 ± 1.5
	Normal spleen	-	21.8 ± 1.5	19.4 ± 1.3
	Normal spleen	+	84.5 ± 2.7	20.1 ± 0.4
	No cells	-	21.8 ± 0.8	19.3 ± 1.8
2	Carrier spleen	+	30.2 ± 1.7	25.3 ± 2.5
	Carrier MLN	+	31.2 ± 1.6	27.0 ± 2.0
	Carrier thymus	+	36.3 ± 1.5	25.6 ± 1.2
	Normal spleen	+	82.6 ± 3.2	28.6 ± 1.7
	No cells	-	29.8 ± 0.9	24.0 ± 1.7

CONCLUSIONS

Thymus-derived lymphocytes specific for LCM virus cannot normally be demonstrated in spleen preparations from LCM-carrier mice. However, following inoculation with allogeneic but not syngeneic normal spleen cells, high levels of cytotoxic T cell activity may be generated in the carrier recipients. These sensitized T cells almost certainly originate from a suppressed population in the carrier. Adoptive transfer of carrier spleen and lymph node cells to normal syngeneic mice results in considerable depression of host responsiveness, but the nature of this suppressor mechanism has not yet been analyzed.

ACKNOWLEDGMENTS

We wish to thank Mr. Tony Duffy for help with the LCM-carrier colony and Miss Gail Essery for capable technical assistance.

REFERENCES

1. Lehmann-Grube, F., Virol. Mongr. 10:1, 1971.

2. Hotchin, J., Virol. Mongr. 3:2, 1971.

3. Burnet, F.M. and Fenner, F., The Production of Antibodies, 2nd edition, Macmillan, Melbourne, 1949.

4. Zinkernagel, R.M. and Doherty, P.C., J. Exp. Med. 138:1266, 1973.

5. Doherty, P.C., Zinkernagel, R.M. and Ramshaw, I.A., J. Immunol. 112:1548, 1974.

6. Zinkernagel, R.M. and Doherty, P.C., Scand. J. Immunol. In press.

7. Doherty, P.C. and Zinkernagel, R.M., Transplant. Rev. Volume 19, in press.

8. Zinkernagel, R.M. and Doherty, P.C., Nature (London). In press.

9. Oldstone, M.B.A. and Dixon, F.J., J. Exp. Med. 129: 483, 1969.

10. Volkert, M., Hannover Larsen, J. and Pfau, C., Acta Path. Microbiol. Scand. 61:268, 1964.

11. Oldstone, M.B.A., Lymphocytic Choriomeningitis and Other Arenaviruses, edited by F. Lehmann-Grube, Springer-Verlag, Berlin, p. 185.

12. Cole, G.A., Prendergast, R.A. and Henney, C.S., Lymphocytic Choriomeningitis and Other Arenaviruses, edited by F. Lehmann-Grube, Springer-Verlag, Berlin, p, 207.

13. Marker, O. and Volkert, M., _Lymphocytic Choriomeningitis and Other Arenaviruses_, edited by F. Lehmann-Grube, Springer-Verlag, Berlin, p. 207.

14. McCullagh, P., _J. Exp. Med._ 132:916, 1970.

15. McCullagh, P., _Transplant. Rev._ 12:180, 1972.

16. Blanden, R.V. and Langman, R.E., _Scand. J. Immunol._ 1:379, 1972.

17. Mims, C.A. and Blanden, R.V., _Infect. Immunity._ 6:695, 1972.

18. Katz, D.H., _Transplant. Rev._ 12:141, 1972.

19. McCullagh, P., Aust. _J. Exp. Biol. Med. Sci._ 51:773, 1973.

20. Gershon, R.K., Cohen, P., Hencin, R. and Liebhaber, S.A., _J. Immunol._ 108:586, 1972.

21. Ha, T.-Y., Waksman, B.H. and Treffers, H.P., _J. Exp. Med._ 139:13, 1974.

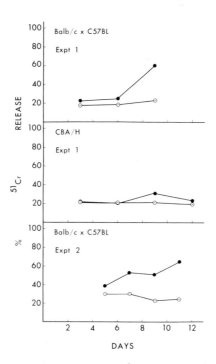

Fig. 1. Carrier CBA/H mice (6-10 weeks) were injected
i.v. with 5.0 x 10^7 CBA/H or BALB/c x C57BL/Fl spleen cells
and were all killed and assayed on the same day. Carrier
spleen preparations were overlaid (30:1) on ^{51}Cr-labelled
LCM-infected (o) or normal (O) L cells. ^{51}Cr release was
measured 16 hours later and expressed as mean $\pm$ SEM.

INTERACTIONS BETWEEN T CELLS WHICH RESULT IN SUPPRESSION OF T CELL FUNCTIONS

Richard K. Gershon

Department of Pathology
Yale University School of Medicine
New Haven, Connecticut 06510

INTRODUCTION

When properly stimulated, T cells are known to be able to produce or cause to be produced factors which can specifically suppress the immune response (1). In some instances this suppression only affects the response against the antigen which originally activated the T cells. In other instances the suppression produced has little antigen specificity. The relationship between the specific and nonspecific effects is not clear at present.

It is now well known that interactions between cell populations of T cells play an important role in determining the immune response (2). In this paper I would like to discuss interactions between sub-populations of T cells which have immunosuppressive consequences. In particular, I would like to focus on the interactions between spleen-seeking and lymph node-seeking thymic T cells.

SUPPRESSIVE INTERACTIONS BETWEEN T CELLS

We have studied interactions between thymic T cell populations in the following manner. We inoculate parental thymocytes into lethally (850 R) irradiated F1 mice. We then measure the amount of DNA the inoculated thymocytes synthesize by pulsing the recipient mice with the thymidine analog 5-iodo-2-deoxyuridine-labelled with I^{125}. This substance is incorporated into the DNA of synthesizing cells, and all IUDR not intimately associated with DNA is excreted from the animal within 12 to 24 hours (3). Thus, 24 hours after the inoculation of isotope, we kill test mice and harvest their lymphoid tissues. The gamma emissions are counted in a gamma counter, and the % of the inoculated isotope is determined. We have found that in the first five days after lethal irradiation almost no uptake of this isotope occurs (3). Further, inoculation of recipient mice with syngeneic thymocytes, without the addition of exogenous antigen, does not significantly increase host DNA synthesis

Analysis of the dose response kinetics of parental thymocytes inoculated into lethally irradiated mice, by the
techniques described above, have strongly suggested that
there are suppressive interactions between the inoculated
cells (4). Thus, doubling the dose of inoculated thymocyte
doubles the number of cells localizing in recipient's lymphoid tissue but does not nearly double the amount of DNA
the inoculated cells synthesize. Interestingly, after a
latent period of 1 to 3 days, the cells undergo a period of
rapid increase in DNA synthesis. This increase usually
peaks on day 4 and is followed by a sharp fall in DNA synthetic activity. The time the cells seem to be shutting
themselves off coincides with the time of peak antigenic competition, suggesting perhaps T cells are elaborating immunosuppressive factors which render them temporarily incapable
of responding both to the antigen which stimulated them and
to other antigens.

SUPPRESSIVE EFFECTS OF SPLEEN-SEEKING T CELLS

A. Effects on DNA synthesis.

In the experiments to be described, we determined what
effect interactions between the cells which localize in the
spleen and those which localize in the lymph nodes might
have (5). To do this, we lethally irradiated recipient
mice, inoculated them with parental thymocytes and at intervals thereafter removed the spleen (and the cells which had
localized in it) by splenectomy. We did concomitant experiments with Chromium 51-labelled cells to determine what effect the splenectomy had on the localization of the inoculated cells. Removal of the spleen three hours after cell
inoculation and at any interval thereafter did not affect
the subsequent localization of cells in the lymph nodes. It
did, however, under some circumstances lead to a marked augmentation of the DNA-synthetic response in the lymph nodes
(Fig. 1). Splenectomy at 3 hours produced the greatest augmentation. The augmentation produced by splenectomy at 24
or 48 hours was significantly less, and splenectomy at 72
hours failed to produce a significant increase.

One of the striking features of this experiment was the
fact that in order to produce maximum effects, splenectomy
had to be performed very early. However, the effects of
splenectomy were not seen until 4 or 5 days later. The significance of this observation and its relation to similar
observations by other workers is discussed in detail in the
accompanying paper (this volume).

These results indirectly support the notion that the response of the cells in the recipient's spleen was suppressing the response of the cells in the lymph nodes. Direct evidence to support this point was obtained by retrieving the inoculated cells from the spleens removed at 3 hours and reinoculating them into other lethally irradiated mice along with normal thymocytes. The results of such an experiment are presented in Fig. 2. As before, splenectomy 3 hours after the inoculation of cells led to an increase in the lymph node response of primary recipient mice. Reinoculation of the cells harvested from their spleens produced a marked depression of the response of normal thymocytes in other mice.

B. Effects on antibody production.

Based on these observations, Wu and Lance did similar experiments, but instead of using DNA synthesis as their assay, they determined the plaque-forming response in the lymph nodes of mice immunized in the foot pads with sheep red blood cells (6). They inoculated lethally irradiated mice with syngeneic spleen and three hours later performed splenectomies. Shortly thereafter, they injected sheep red blood cells subcutaneously into the foot pads. They found an increased number of plaques in the lymph nodes of the splenectomized recipients compared to controls. Interestingly, when they performed the same experiment using lymph node cells, in lieu of spleen cells they found that splenectomy failed to produce an increase.

These results suggested to them that there might be a splenic T cell which acted to suppress the response of the cells in the lymph nodes. To test this notion, they inoculated lethally irradiated mice with a combination of syngeneic lymph node cells and large numbers of syngeneic thymocytes. The addition of syngeneic thymocytes was suppressive of the plaque-forming response in the lymph nodes in mice with intact spleens but not in splenectomized recipients. Thus, these experiments support the notion that a spleen-localizing T cell can suppress the response of lymph node cells.

DIFFERENCES BETWEEN SPLEEN AND LYMPH NODE CELLS

We have confirmed the finding of Wu and Lance that splenectomy of recipients of spleen cells but not of lymph node cells increases the response to antigen of the cells which localize in the recipient's lymph node. The results in Fig. 3 show that splenectomy of the recipients of parental spleen cells produces a significant increase in the response of the cells which localize in the lymph node. It has no such effect on the lymph node localizing cells of an inoculum of parental lymph node cells. These experiments suggest that the cell which regulates the lymph node response is present in the thymus and the spleen but not in the lymph node. It does not appear that the splenic microenvironment per se causes the cells to produce their suppressive effects.

EFFECTS OF CYTOTOXIC DRUGS

During the course of these experiments, we noted that the sham-splenectomized animals also often made an augmented lymph node response (5). The sham splenectomy, however, never increased the response in the spleen nor did it cause augmented traffic of cells to the lymph nodes. We tested the possibility that the sham splenectomy was producing its effects releasing endogenous cortisone with the following protocol: We inoculated lethally irradiated mice with thymocytes, spleen cells or lymph node cells and at intervals thereafter inoculated the recipient mice with 1 milligram of cortisone acetate.

We found that cortisone, injected three hours after the cells were inoculated, often led to a marked increase in the lymph node response of the parental thymocytes. Similar to splenectomy, waiting until 24 or 48 hours after cells were inoculated to inject the cortisone, either reduced its effect or actually decreased the lymph node response. The cortisone never augmented the response of the thymocytes which localized in the recipient's spleens nor did it augment lymph node localization of the inoculated cells. In contrast to splenectomy, cortisone injection could augment the lymph node response of both spleen and lymph node cells (Fig. 3). These results are compatible with the notion put forth above that suppressor T cells are activated very early in the response to antigen. Their activation can render them susceptible to cytotoxic drugs such as cortisone. We have reproduced the effects of cortisone by using other cytotoxic drugs, most notably cyclohexamide (to be published). They also suggest that spleen-seeking T cells may be especially important in the interactions which lead to activation of the suppressor populations but are clearly not absolutely required.

RELATION TO TOLERANCE

The relation of these effects to the induction of tolerance is unknown. However, it has been shown by Claman and Bronsky that the inclusion of actinomycin-D, with a tolerance-inducing dose of bovine gamma globulin (BGG), changes the BGG from a tolerogen to an immunogen (7). In addition, Brent has presented preliminary evidence suggesting that prior splenectomy increases the resistance of mice to tolerance induction (8). Further work is required to relate these intriguing findings to the ones we have presented above.

ACKNOWLEDGMENTS

This work was supported by research grants CA08593 and AI 10497 as well as by a Research Career Development Award number CA10,316 from the National Institutes of Health.

REFERENCES

1. Gershon, R.K., Contemporary Topics In Immunobiology. 3:1, 1974.

2. Asofsky, R., Cantor, H. and Tigelaar, R.E., In Progress in Immunology, edited by B. Amos, Academic Press, New York, p. 369, 1971.

3. Gershon, R.K. and Hencin, R., J. Immunol. 107:1723, 1971.

4. Gershon, R.K. and Liebhaber, S.A., J. Exp. Med. 136: 112, 1972.

5. Gershon, R.K., Lance, E.M. and Kondo, K., J. Immunol. 112:546, 1974.

6. Wu, C.Y. and Lance, E.M., Cell. Immunol. In press.

7. Claman, H.N. and Bronsky, E.A., J. Immunol. 95:718, 1965.

8. Brent, L., In Immunological Tolerance to Tissue Antigens, edited by N.W. Nisbet and M.W. Elves, Orthopaedic Hospital, Oswestry, England, p. 49, 1971.

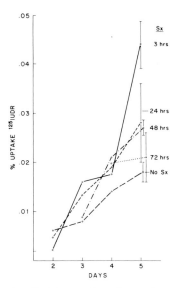

Fig. 1. Effect of time of splenectomy on the DNA-synthetic response of parental thymocytes in the lymph nodes of lethally irradiated Fl mice. The thymocytes were inoculated at 0 hour.

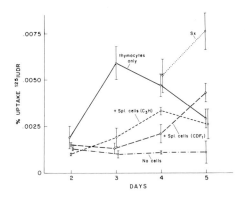

Fig. 2. Effect of inoculating parental (C3H) thymocytes recovered from the spleens of lethally irradiated parental or Fl mice together with non-spleen-passaged parental thymocytes on the DNA-synthetic response of the cells in the lymph nodes of lethally irradiated Fl mice. Spleens were harvested 3 hours after thymocyte inoculation. Also presented is the DNA synthetic response of the parental thymocytes in the lymph nodes of the Fl spleen cell donors (Sx).

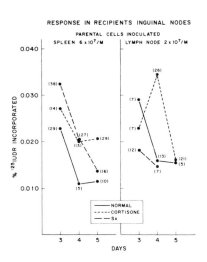

RESPONSE IN RECIPIENTS INGUINAL NODES

Fig. 3. The DNA-synthetic response of parental spleen and lymph node cells in the inguinal lymph nodes of lethally irradiated F1 mice. Three hours after the parental cells were inoculated, some recipient mice were inoculated with 1 mg of cortisone and others were splenectomized. Each determination is the mean of 3 test mice and the numbers in parentheses are the coefficients of variation. (Parental thymocytes and their cortisone-resistant fraction, both react in a fashion similar to the spleen cells and, therefore, quite different from the lymph node cells; that is to say, both splenectomy and cortisone treatment at 3 hours post inoculation can increase their response.)

GENERAL DISCUSSION - SESSION IV

MECHANISMS OF T CELL TOLERANCE

William Weigle, Chairman

WEIGLE: I would like to open the discussion by asking Gus
Nossal if he could explain the discrepancy between his
results showing a rapid induction to tolerance in vitro
with small amounts of DNP-HGG in bone marrow cells and
Jacques Chiller's results in vivo showing a delay in
the induction of tolerance to HGG which requires large
amounts of the tolerogen.

NOSSAL: We have been very puzzled by your marrow B cell
kinetics as the studies with Osmond have shown a very
rapid cell renewal in marrow small lymphocytes. This
suggests that any event which takes two to three weeks
must be addressing itself to some sub-population. Maybe the exigencies of your read-out system which involves addition of T cells and two antigen injections,
focuses particular empnasis on the most mature elements
of marrow. In that case, perhaps the last residuum of
these non-tolerizable cells must leave the marrow before
you read it as tolerance in marrow.

WEIGLE: It is not unrealistic to assume that in contact
with natural antigen that two or more exposures are involved. In response to Gus' comment that different
populations of bone marrow cells are present, I suggest
that the latent period in Chiller's experiments may be
the result of a population of cells that is slowly replaced in bone marrow. It may be that this population
is antigen-driven to maturity and only when mature can
tolerance be induced. It seems that there may be a
difference in the mechanism at play in the in vivo induction of tolerance to HGG and the in vitro induction
of tolerance to DNP-HGG.

CHILLER: The two systems differ in that Nossal is using in
vitro dissociated bone marrow cultures and we are looking at kinetics in the marrow of the intact animal.
That the two may show differences may not be surprising
and not really reflect mechanism differences at the
cellular level.

G. MÖLLER: Dr. Nossal should actually be happy that it

takes longer to induce tolerance in B cells in adult
mice. The mature B cells should, according to Nossal's
(and originally Lederberg's) idea be much more difficult to tolerize and actually may not become tolerant.
Therefore, they must first be chased out before the
animals express tolerance.

MITCHELL: The point against Göran Möller's comment on the
time required for B cell tolerance in immature versus
mature T cells is that Chiller has shown that the time
required for B cell tolerance induction in spleen is
less than that for bone marrow B cells.

Also, I have been trying to relate Unanue's comment this morning on the effect of ligand in the medium
on the re-expression of Ig on cells with the observation of Nossal that tolerance is induced in bone marrow cells by antigen in vitro. Can Nossal discount an
inhibition of re-expression of Ig in reactive B cells
(which have been stripped as a result of antigen binding) accounting for the apparent tolerance induction
in bone marrow B cells?

LESKOWITZ: I am directing this question to Nossal. Would
your model allow any prediction on differences in persistence of tolerance if tolerance is due to either a
"clonal abortion" mechanism?

NOSSAL: I would predict that the kinetics of tolerance loss
would be identical to the kinetics of new lymphocyte
formation from precursor cells, provided that one can
ensure total absence of antigen. Of course, operationally this is very difficult to achieve.

LESKOWITZ: I have obtained data which are similar to those
Marc Feldmann has reported. They involve tolerance
induction to the azobenzene arsonate group (ABA) towards which both T and B cells respond. When monovalent ABA conjugates are given (ABA-tyr), only T cells
are tolerized, and when polyvalent conjugates are
given (ABA-poly-L-tyr), both T and B cells are tolerized. Did you suggest that different mechanisms may be
involved for T and B cell tolerance, since my results
could favor this too?

FELDMANN: I'm glad to hear that monovalent ABA induces tolerance in T cells, but not B cells, as my statements

were in complete agreement. Deaggregated gamma globulin only induced tolerance in T cells;only if FγG is
complexed to POL was B cell tolerance found.

KATZ: I would like to draw attention to the fact that the
cell surface events involved in tolerance induction in
T cells must be quite different from the surface events
occurring in tolerization of B cells. Now we heard
earlier from Emil Unanue that the surface events following binding of DNP-D-GL to specific B cells are
quite unique as compared to metabolizable molecules.
Nevertheless, in attempts to tolerize T cell responses
elicited by DNCB skin painting in guinea pigs, Baruj
and I have been unable to tolerize DNP-reactive T cells
with this molecule (J. Immunology. 112:1158, 1974).
Moreover, in a perhaps more clearly defined T cell determinant recognition system; namely, sensitivity to
ABA-tyrosine, recent studies in my laboratory by Wes
Bullock and ourselves have been similarly unsuccessful
in inducing T cell tolerance with ABA-D-GL. In fact,
and to our surprise, the ABA-D-GL was immunogenic for
ABA-specific T cells. The point here is that these
contrasting findings with B and T cells must be telling
us something relevant about differences either in tolerance-inducing signals and/or cell surface binding
characteristics between these two cells.

LESKOWITZ: I agree, but ABA conjugates of d-polymers in my
hands are neither tolerogenic nor immunogenic.

HUMPHREY: Perhaps the explanation offered by David Katz that
skin sensitivity is not abrogated by DNP-D-GL treatment
is explicable as he suggested by the fact that specificity in the skin reaction is not for DNP but for DNP
conjugated with unidentified skin elements. A clearer
answer might be obtained by using arsonylbenzene azo-
tyrosine derivatives since the determinant for skin
reactivity is the ABA tyrosine. I have made ABA-SIII
for testing this point in guinea pigs, but the experiment has not been done.

KATZ: I agree with John Humphrey entirely. It was perhaps
not sufficiently clear, but as I mentioned a few mo-
ments ago, Wes Bullock and ourselves have been studying
ABA sensitivity in guinea pigs in attempts to circumvent the DNCB skin painting specificity problems and
have found that ABA-D-GL is ineffective in inducing T

cell tolerance in ABA skin sensitivity. Moreover, this molecule is immunogenic in the sense of inducing as well as eliciting ABA-specific skin sensitivity reactions. John Humphrey's idea of using ABA-SIII is·an excellent one--indeed, I believe Graham Mitchell has preliminary evidence to the effect of showing that ABA-SIII does not induce tolerance in ABA-specific T cells.

MITCHELL: We have heard that tolerance with respect to de-layed-type hypersensitivity is difficult to induce with ABA-SIII, DNP-D-GL, etc., yet Feldmann can achieve quite easily helper T cell tolerance in vitro. Does this in any way suggest a difference in the ease of tolerance induction in these two T cell functions?

KATZ: I would think that such findings do indeed suggest different thresholds of tolerance induction in T cells mediating, respectively, delayed sensitivity and helper functions. Strong confirmation of this has recently come out in experiments performed by John Silver, a senior medical student in Baruj's laboratory, in which they compared the effective dose of deaggregated BGG necessary to induce tolerance in helper cell function versus delayed hypersensitivity in guinea pigs, using the model of supplemental carrier immunization described by us five years ago (J. Exp. Med. 131:261, 1970). What Silver and Benacerraf have shown is that whereas helper cell activity can be abrogated by very low doses (10 μg) of deaggregated BGG, delayed sensitivity is not affected unless 100-fold higher doses are employed. Of course, such differences could very well reflect the activity (stimulated by low doses of deaggregated BGG) of BGG-specific suppressor cells acting to inhibit helper cell function while having no effect on delayed sensitivity reactions. Nonetheless, the threshold of sensitivity of these two T cell functions to inactivat-ing mechanisms can be readily distinguished under these circumstances.

TAYLOR: Regarding the question of valency, there is some evidence for a generalization that T cells respond (by immunity or tolerance) to monomeric or monovalent anti-gens, while in the absence of T cell help, B cells can only respond to multivalent antigens. I want to ask if Dr. Nossal has given us an exception to this in the tolerance induced by $DNP_{0.9}BGG$ in bone marrow because if this is true, it should be possible to induce toler-

424

ance in these early B cells with the hapten alone, just as T cells can be tolerized with ABA-tyrosine. However, in order to preserve this generalization, I would like to suggest either that there is something special about BGG (and other immunoglobulins) as tolerogens, perhaps in that they provide extra bonding through the Fc region; or that this kind of tolerance induction was really thymus-dependent.

NOSSAL: I do not want to say too much about the tolerization of T cells by monomeric antigens as the results we have on the subject are too preliminary. We have some results that could suggest difficulty of tolerizing mature T cells quickly and which are not inconsistent with a "clonal abortion" approach. I believe here it will be necessary before citing results that are deemed publishable to do an extensive "base" titration in which the numbers of T and B cells are widely varied with respect to each other. Also, we have models which suggest that kill day is an important variable. It seems likely to me that for both T and B cells there will be subpopulations with different characteristics of tolerizability.

SMITH: I want to make two points. First, several presentations have been concerned with the characteristics of subpopulations of cells selected in Fl hybrids at intervals after injection of parental cells. We have examined that question carefully and found that the selected population after injection of immunocompetent parental thymus cells (prepared on BSA gradients) into irradiated Fl hybrids has the following characteristics: 1) Low susceptibility to cytotoxic effects of anti-θ plus GPC; 2) High anti-H-2 susceptibility; 3) Absence of PHA response; 4) Retention of some Con A response; 5) Low or absent Ig; 6) De novo susceptibility to stimulation by LPS; and 7) Three to five-fold increase in alloantigen response. These characteristics are those of cells responding to in vitro MLC. The only surprise is that PHA responses are gone, and despite absence of detectable B cells, LPS responses are detected--in fact, very strong. This seems quite analogous to the in vitro synergy of alloantigen and LPS we described in an earlier session. These data describe a subpopulation quite different from the average peripheral T cells but very much like those of thymus competent cells. Clearly different generalizations on T cell functions must be made when the T cell source used in tolerance or suppressor effects are from this or from the usual peripheral lymph node or spleen source.

The second point concerns the opposite model--the possible effect of F1 cells on parent--as raised by the very nice work of Britton. Bill Adler and I found in studies first reported in 1968 that F1 cells proliferated in MLC when presented with mitomycin-treated parental target spleen cells. Since this was on the surface incompatible with graft vs. host and graft data, we therefore accepted a large burden of proof to establish that the observation did not have a trivial or irrelevant mechanism. Bryan Gebhardt has essentially resolved most of the alternative possibilities by showing that the F1 is the proliferating cell, that blastogenic factor of parental cell origin is not involved by any assay we can devise. The most compelling observation has been that the responding F1 cells are clonal with respect to each parent--that, activation of an MLC toward one parent--followed by suicide with BUDR and light, leaves a subpopulation responding to the other parent at the same time abrogating that to the first parent and vice versa. These data (Gebhardt, B., Nahao, Y. and Smith, R., Federation Proceedings, 1974) have been derived in multiple strain combinations including congenics differing only for genes of the MHC locus. This suggests that whatever the initiating stimulus or the receptor bearing structure responsible for recognition of parent, that the stimulating structure is determined by or linked to the H-2 locus. It seems possible that an in vivo expression of such recognition might be considered in interpreting Britton's data and perhaps involving F1 resistance to parental tumors.

PAUL: In the study which you mention, the question of recognition of the "responding" F1 cells by the mitomycin-blocked parental "target" cell is critical. Indeed, Harrison and I and several others have shown that this explains at least some instances of F1-parent mixed lymphocyte reactions. In this regard have you demonstrated that responsiveness of the F1 is independent of T lymphocytes in the parental target cell populations.

SMITH: We haven't determined that critically, but one would still have the difficulty of explaining the clonal character of the phenomenon.

BASTEN: I should like to ask Dr. Benacerraf or Dr. McDevitt whether there is any evidence that suppressor effects could be H-2 linked.

GERSHON: We have looked into a number of strains. The only possible linkage is with H-2^p, but further work is required to make this a firm conclusion.

MCDEVITT: In dealing with immune response differences between CBA/H and CBA/J, it is necessary to consider the effect of an M-locus (MLC locus, Festenstein, H. Transpl. Proc., 1973) difference between these two strains which may be associated with an Ir gene effect. In addition, these two strains may have developed differences in the major histocompatibility complex as well.

    If Dr. Basten is asking whether anyone has studied the genetics of T cell suppression, the answer is no, not yet.

ACTIVITY OF SUPPRESSOR CELLS AS A MECHANISM OF TOLERANCE

BYRON H. WAKSMAN, CHAIRMAN

ACTIVITY OF SUPPRESSOR CELLS AS A MECHANISM OF TOLERANCE

INTRODUCTION

Byron H. Waksman

Department of Microbiology
Yale Medical School
New Haven, Connecticut 06510

The concepts of "suppressor cells" introduced by Gershon in 1969 (1, 2) has given rise to a great deal of new research activity (reviewed in 3, 4). Suppressor cells have been shown to play a role or are suspected of playing a role in immunologic states (Table I) which include essentially all the immunologic regulatory mechanisms recognized today. It would be difficult to exaggerate their probable importance if suppressor cells should prove to be responsible for tolerance or non-reactivity to self-antigens and aberrations in their function responsible for autoimmunization. If they are also concerned with some part of the unresponsiveness to tumors usually attributed to "enhancing" antibody or antigen-antibody complexes, their significance would be still greater. We shall hear evidence at this meeting that these assumptions are at least in part correct.

Recent work has focussed on the development of suitable in vitro models in which to study suppressor cell activity (Table II) and has permitted the definitive demonstration in some instances that they are T cells (1, 2, 5, 6, 7) which may act by way of diffusible mediators (8, 9, 10). Suppression then exhibits points of similarity to cell cooperation. A systematic study of suppressor cells in any in vivo or in vitro model must address itself to some of the questions which I have assembled in Table III. Though we all believe in the economy of nature, it would be unwise a priori to assume that answers to these questions will prove the same in all systems examined. Recent studies provide a few indications of the complexities yet to come.

TABLE I

CELLULAR SUPPRESSOR PHENOMENA IN VIVO

Failure of response in "low-responder" mice
Regulation of T-independent response (e.g. to SIII)
Regulation of IgE response

Tolerance (to SRBC, contact allergens, autoantigens)
Chronic allotype suppression, idiotype suppression

Antigenic competition, preemption
Suppression during systemic GVH
"Enhancement" by humoral antibody?

Feedback-inhibition factor in delayed sensitivity

TABLE II

SUPPRESSOR PHENOMENA IN VITRO

Mitogen-induced suppression of antibody formation
Mitogen-induced suppression of proliferation
Suppression by allogeneic stimulation
Suppression by specific soluble antigens

Enhanced suppression after adult thymectomy,
hydrocortisone

Role of weakly adherent cells, histamine receptor cells

Role of macrophages

TABLE III
SUPPRESSOR T CELLS (STC)

1. Classes of suppressor experiment

   a. Short-term
   b. Long-term
   c. Modulation of response of other cells to antigen
      or mitogen (specificity of suppression)

2. What are suppressor T-cells (STC)?

   a. Organ localization of STC
   b. Proof that STC are T cells
   c. Relation of STC to maturation of T cells
   d. Physical separation of STC

3. Nature of stimulus to STC, leading to suppression

   a. Antigen
   b. Mitogen
   c. Mediators produced by target cells

4. Cell functions required for STC action

   a. DNA, RNA, protein synthesis
   b Mediators of suppressor effect

5. Types of target system

   a. T cells stimulated by antigen, mitogen
   b. B cells   "   "   "   "

6. Cell function which is target of STC

   a. DNA synthesis, mitosis
   b. RNA synthesis, blast transformation
   c. Protein synthesis, antibody release, lymphokine re-
      lease

7. Agents affecting STC function

   a. Age, stress
   b. adjuvants
   c. Immunosuppressants

8. STC in immunologically unusual strains of mice

   (NZB, SJL, SWAN, BALB/c)

The cells in a number of studies have been either thymocytes (5,6,11) or spleen-seeking T-lymphocytes (12). They may be short-lived (13) proliferating (14) cells comparable to the T subpopulation which has now come to be spoken of as post-thymic (15) or T_1 (16). That suppressor cells are distinct from other T cells and can be isolated is, of course, unproven, but this possibility is under investigation in several laboratories. They are weakly adherent to glass wool (4) and appear to possess histamine receptors (17) like those characteristic of immune "killer" T cells (18). It has frequently proved difficult to disentangle their contribution from that of macrophages which are also adherent cells (19,20), and it is not unlikely that they will prove to be macrophage-dependent or to express themselves by stimulating an appropriate type of macrophage activity.

Reports of suppressor B cells in, e.g. the response to virally induced tumors (21), may be concerned with cells which act by producing enhancing antibody. The mind boggles at the possibility that macrophages and helper T cells must cooperate with antigen, may act in turn to stimulate suppressor T cells, which then, in concert with macrophages, produce a suppressor effect. This is a compl ballet which it will be our duty and our pleasure to unravel.

The target of the suppressor effect, in adequately studied cases, appears to be cell proliferation or, more specifically, DNA synthesis (22,23) although inhibition of other types of macromolecular synthesis is by no means ruled out. One thinks immediately of lymphokines which depress cell proliferation, notably "proliferation-inhibitory factor", "cloning-inhibition factor" and the "inhibitor of DNA synthesis" (see 24). Yet suppressive molecules which resemble antibody (9) or which possess immunologic specificity but differ from immunoglobulin in other respects (25) have also been incriminated. The most interesting factors are those described as "chalones" (26,27,28) which have been extracted from normal lymphoid tissue. "Chalone" is an old term that finds a convenient application here describing a molecule which inhibits proliferation of cells similar to those which produced it.

Of no less importance than the nature of the suppressor cell, its mediator(s) and its target is the type of

stimulus which elicits suppressor cell activity. Folch and
I have suggested elsewhere (23) that there are three quite
different classes of suppressor model:

a) Short-term experiments measured in days (less than
a week). Here the observed suppression may be nonspecific
as in competition of antigens (2,29,30) and acute graft-
vs-host disease (31) or specific as in preemption (32) and
its target may be a T cell or a B cell response (29). In
these cases the activation of unprimed cells exposed to
antigen several days earlier appears to result in the suppressor effect. In the interesting case of regulation
in the rat IgE response to DNP-conjugates of Ascaris protein investigated by Tada and his coworkers (6), the T cell
response to the carrier suppresses the B cell response to
the hapten. While the two stimuli are simultaneous, the
T cell effect comes into play after several days (33) and
this pattern may well apply to most cases of competition
involving multiple antigens given simultaneously (34).

b) Long-term experiments measured in days, weeks, or
months in which priming with antigen results in later responses to the same antigen. Here one would include experiments on tolerance (35,36), including tolerance to
autoantigens (37,38) and possibly chronic allotype suppression (39). Available evidence suggests that the
suppressor effect in these cases results from the response
of specific T cell clones, amplified by priming and activated by re-exposure to the same antigen.

c) Single stimulus experiments. The remarkable fact
has been brought out by Baker and his colleagues (22) that
the response to the thymus-independent antigen pneumococcal
polysaccharide elicits regulation by T cells which apparently do not react to the antigen itself but to the responding B cells. This mechanism is mimicked in the system
involving stimulation of B cells in vitro by lipopolysaccharide endotoxin acting as a mitogen in that the response is
damped down by T cells not directly responsive to the
mitogen (40). Similarly, the response of T cells to
specific alloantigen elicits regulation by other T cells not
stimulated by the antigen but rather by the responding cell
themselves (5). Single stimulus experiments appear to fit
better the designation "regulatory mechanism" than conventional short or long-term experiments. They may find
their explanation in the recently demonstrated fact that

recognition of antigen by T lymphocytes   suffices to stimulate (perhaps by release of mediators) adjacent lymphocytes
which do not themselves participate in the recognition
event (41).

REFERENCES

1. Gershon, R.K. and Kondo, K., Immunology. 18:721, 1970.

2. Gershon, R.K. and Kondo, K., J. Immunol. 106:1524,
    1971.

3. Gershon, R.K., Contemp. Topics in Immunobiol. 3:1,
    1971.

4. Folch, H. and Waksman, B.H., Cell. Immunol. 9:12, 1973.

5. Gershon, R.K. Cohen, P., Hencin, R. and Liebhaber, S.A.,
    J. Immunol. 108:586, 1972.

6. Okumura, K. and Tade, T.,   J. Immunol. 107:1682, 1971.

7. Rich, R.R. and Pierce, C.W., J. Exp. Med. 137:649,
    1973.

8. Kantor, F.S., Hall, C.B. and Lipsmeyer, E.A., In
    Cellular Interactions in the Immune Response,edited by
    S. Cohen, G. Cudkowicz and R.T. McCluskey, S. Karger,
    Basal, p. 213, 1971.

9. Feldmann, M., In Lymphocyte Recognition and Effector
    Mechanisms, edited by K. Lindahl-Kiessling and D. Osoba,
    Acad. Press, New York/London, p. 605, 1974.

10. Rich, R.R. and Pierce, C.W., J. Immunol. 112:1360,
    1974.

11. Ha, T.Y. and Waksman, B.H., J. Immunol. 110:1290, 1973.

12. Gershon, R.K., Lance, E.M. and Kondo, K., J. Immunol.
    112;546, 1974.

13. Kappler, J.W., Hunter, P.C., Jacobs, D. and Lord, E.,
    J. Immunol. In press.

14. Moorhead, J.W. and Claman, H.N., J. Immunol. 112:333, 1974.

15. Stutman, O., Yunis, E.J. and Good, R.A., J. Exp. Med. 132:583, 601, 1970.

16. Raff, M.C. and Cantor, H., In Progress in Immunology, edited by B. Amos, Acad. Press, New York/London, p. 83, 1971.

17. Shearer, G.M., Melmon, K.L., Weinstein, Y. and Sels, M., J. Exp. Med. 136:1302, 1972.

18. Plaut, M., Lichtenstein, L.M., Gillespie, E. and Henney, C.S., J. Immunol. 111:389, 1973.

19. Sjöberg, O., Clin. Exp. Immunol. 12:365, 1972.

20. Scott, M.T., Cell. Immunol. 5:469, 1972.

21. Corczynski, R.M., J. Immunol. In press.

22. Baker, P.J., Stashak, P.W., Amsbaugh, D.F. and Prescott, B., J. Immunol. 112:404, 1974.

23. Folch, H. and Waksman, B.H., J. Immunol. In press, 1974.

24. David, J.R. and David, R.A., Progr. Allergy. 16:300, 1972.

25. Tada, T., Okumura, K. and Taniguchi, M., J. Immunol. 111:952, 1973.

26. Houck, J.C., Irausquin, H. and Leikin, S., Science. 173: 1139, 1971.

27. Florentin, I., Kiger, N. and Mathé, G., Eur. J. Immunol. 3:624, 1973.

28. Garcia-Giralt, E. and Macieira-Coelho, A., In Lymphocyte Recognition and Effector Mechanisms. edited by K. Lindahl-Kiessling and D. Osoba, Acad. Press, New York/London, p. 457, 1974.

29. Möller, G., J. Immunol. 106:1566, 1971.

30. Eidinger, D. and Pross, H., Scand. J. Immunol. 1:193, 1972.

31. Blaese, R.M., Martinez, C. and Good, R.A., J. Exp. Med. 119:211, 1964.

32. O'Toole, C.M. and Davies, A.J.S., Nature. 230:187, 1971.

33. Okumura, K., Tada, T. and Ochiai, T. Submitted.

34. Taussig, M.J., Curr. Topics Micro. Immunol. 60:125, 1973.

35. Gershon, R.K. and Kondo, K., Immunology. 21:903, 1971.

36. Asherson, G.L., Zembala, M. and Barnes, R.M.R., Clin. Exp. Immunol. 9:111, 1971.

37. Allison, A.C., Denman, A.M. and Barnes, R.D., Lancet. 2:135, 1971.

38. Monier, J.C., Controle par le Thymus et les Cellules T, des Phénomènes d'Auto-Immunisation et de Compétition Antigénique, Ediprim, Lyon, 1972.

39. Herzenberg, L.A., Chan, E.L., Ravitch, M.M., Riblet, R.J. and Herzenberg, L.A., J. Exp. Med. 137:1311, 1973.

40. Yoshinaga, M., Yoshinaga, A. and Waksman, B.H., J. Exp. Med. 136:956, 1972.

41. Harrison, M.R. and Paul, W.E., J. Exp. Med. 138:1602, 1973.

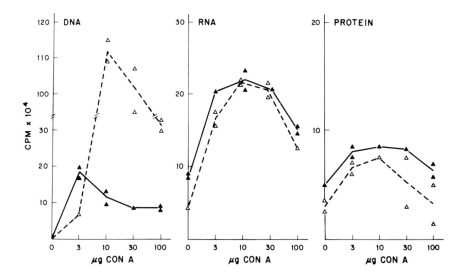

Fig. 1. Dose-response curves obtained with normal adult rat spleen cells (▲) and with nonadherent cells (passed through glass wool) (△), each cultured at 2×10^6/ml with concanavalin A. There is marked suppression of DNA synthesis (^{3}H-thymidine uptake at 48-72 hours) in the whole cell culture and no evidence of suppression of early RNA or protein synthesis (^{3}H-uridine and ^{3}H-leucine uptake at 0-24 hours). From ref. 23.

LACK OF ACTIVITY OF CONTRA-SUPPRESSOR T CELLS AS A MECHANISM OF TOLERANCE

Richard K. Gershon

Department of Pathology
Yale University School of Medicine
New Haven, Connecticut 06510

In 1967 we were engaged in a search for a suppressor cell which played an active role in shutting off the immune response. The stimulus for the search was some observations we had made on the behavior of an unusual hamster tumor, originally described in 1960 by Dr. H.S.N. Greene (1). Dr. Greene had noted that tumor-bearing animals were resistant to rechallenge with cells of the same tumor and rarely developed metastases. However, shortly after tumor resection the animals became susceptible to rechallenge and many, subsequently, developed widespread disseminated metastases.

We had noted that the resistance to reinoculation was mediated by a strong cell-mediated immune response which at its height could reject greater than 10,000 times more tumor cells than were required to produce tumors in normal hamsters (2). In spite of this strong response, the primary tumor continued to grow until the death of the animal although, as noted by Dr. Greene, metastases hardly ever appeared. Immunosuppressive treatments such as the administration of ALS caused the primary tumor to grow faster and led to metastatic dissemination (3). Resection of the primary tumor early after the original inoculation led within 24 hours to a very sharp fall in the specific immune capacity to reject the tumor (4). Adoptive transfer of cells harvested from animals 24-96 hours after tumor resection was able to supress the immune response in syngeneic recipients (5-7). We felt that the excision must have activated a class of suppressor cells as it was inconceivable that the immunity could disappear so rapidly without an active suppressive event taking place. The idea that suppression was due to the production of enhancing antibody seemed unlikely to us; again, because of the rapidity of the changes and also because we could not envision a mechanism by which the tumor could lead to such a rapid production of antibody without postulating, in addition a regulatory cell which controlled the antibody production.

Being thus sensitized to the notion of suppressor cells, we were particularly impressed with those experiments which showed that cytotoxic drugs could lead to augmented immune responses (8) and could even prevent the induction of tolerance (9). Thus, when Davies et al published their paper, "The Failure of Thymus-Derived Lymphocytes to Make Antibody" in 1967 (10), we were taken with the notion that our suppressor cell might lie within this lymphocyte population. When we went to work in the laboratory of Tony Davies late in that year, we soon became disabused of that notion. It was very clear from his data that the thymus-derived lymphocytes were acting as helper cells. Perhaps if Davies et al had given their paper a different title indicating in it that thymus-derived lymphocytes performed a helper function, the notion that they were also suppressor cells might never have occurred to us. In spite of the fact that as we learned more about T cells, we considered it less likely that they would be suppressor cells, we decided to pursue the notion anyway. Thus, we designed some experiments to see what possible role thymus-derived lymphocytes might play in the induction of immunological tolerance.

Thymus dependence of tolerance to sheep red blood cells (11).

Since we knew that bone marrow-derived lymphocytes were incapable of making antibody to sheep cells in the absence of thymus-derived lymphocytes, we decided to see if, when presented with large amounts of antigen in the absence of helper cells, the bone marrow-derived or B cells would then become tolerant. We performed a series of experiments, the general protocol of which is outlined in Fig. 1. Apparently, this figure has been found by many people to be excessively complex and difficult to follow. To those that find it so, please ignore it. It is presented only to illustrate the scope of the experiments done and the specificity controls performed. The results I will present below are a simplified version of the results presented in our original paper (11). In essence, the experiments were quite simple. Mice were deprived of their T cell complement by thymectomy, lethal irradiation and bone marrow grafting. We have subsequently learned that this procedure reduces their T cell complement by about 90% (unpublished observations). Some of the deprived mice were reconstituted with 15×10^6 syngeneic thymocytes, a number known to produce a modest reconstitution of the immune response in mice deprived of thymocytes by the above method. Both groups of mice, the deprived and the reconstituted, were started immediately on a 30 day course of inoculations of large numbers of sheep cells in an attempt to produce tolerance. The 30 day course was chosen because of parallel experiments we were doing in mice with thymus grafts which will be explained and expanded on below. At the end of the tolerance inducing regimen, we discarded mice which made antibody during the course of tolerance induction. The remaining mice were then split into two groups. One group got an additional inoculum of normal thymocytes (15×10^6), while the other received no further cells. The thymocytes were added to see if the tolerance-inducing regimen had rendered the animal's own cells unable to cooperate with normal thymocytes.

The results of one such experiment are presented in Figs. 2-4. <u>Figure 2 shows the effect of the antigen pre-treatment in thymus-deprived mice.</u> Mice which received no thymocytes and were not pre-treated with antigen made a small but significant immune response on day 7 which disappeared by day 15. Pre-treatment with antigen abolished this small response. The addition of 15 million thymocytes to control mice produced a significant increase in the immune response on day 7. The response of the thymocyte-reconstituted animals pre-treated with antigen was markedly suppressed on day 7; the added thymocytes did not increase the response significantly. By day 15, however, the response in these mice reached control levels. In fact, it reached control levels on day 10 (data not presented). This suppression of the early (day 7) response with return to normal on day 10 was seen in all four experiments done using this protocol. It is also worth emphasizing that the results presented are the total antibody response. The mercapto-ethanol resistant antibodies were never affected by the pre-treatment with antigen.

We interpreted these results at that time and have not changed our minds since to indicate that there are two classes of B cells. One of these can react with sheep red blood cells in the absence of thymus help: a) to make small amounts of mercapto-ethanol-sensitive antibody when properly immunized and b) to become tolerant without thymus help when treated with excess antigen. There exists also a second class of B cells which can be neither activated nor rendered tolerant without T cell help. We have subsequently developed this notion of two classes of B cells somewhat further, and readers who are interested in the subject are referred to Ref. 12 in which the subject is treated in greater detail and other supporting evidence is discussed.

The results presented in Fig. 3 stand in marked contrast to the results obtained by pre-treating thymus-deprived mice. Pre-treatment of animals which had been given 15 x 10^6 thymocytes at the time the pre-treatment schedule was started rendered these animals refractory to the helping activity of added normal thymocytes at day 15 as well as day 7. Of some importance in this experiment is the increased antibody made on day 7 by the control animals given a second inoculation of thymocytes compared to those that were not. The significant increase in the immune response produced by the second injection of thymocytes shows that the reason the thymocytes could not help the pre-treated animals was not due to the preemption of space by the first injection of thymocytes; there was room for the newly added cells to function. The fact that they could not function in pre-treated mice could not be explained by the notion that residual antigen made them tolerant as they functioned quite well in the mice that were pre-treated with the same amount of antigen in the absence of thymocytes.

The difference in the subsequent immune response produced by the presence of thymocytes during the tolerance-inducing regimen is shown in Fig. 4 where the results of the two types of pre-treated mice are compared.

These results clearly indicate that the thymocytes and the excess sheep red blood cell antigen were acting in concert to: a) either shut off the host B cells or b) create a milieu in which the added normal thymocyte was being made tolerant, or both. Subsequent experiments have established that the second of the three listed possibilities was the correct one. This was shown by two lines of evidence; one showing the infectious nature of the tolerance-inducing stimuli (13), and the other showing the presence of reactive B cells capable of making anti-sheep cell antibody when properly stimulated (14).

The infectious nature of T cell dependent tolerance (13). Spleen cells from mice made tolerant in the presence of T cells were able to specifically suppress the anti-sheep red blood cell response of immuno-competent syngeneic recipient mice after adoptive transfer. Adoptive transfer of spleen cells of mice given the same tolerance-inducing regimen of sheep red blood cells in the absence of thymocytes had no effect on the anti-sheep red blood cell response. These results suggest that T cells can produce a specific suppressor factor when confronted with the large amounts of sheep cells which we tentatively named IgY. The reasons we rejected the notion that it was a T-dependent B cell that was producing the suppression on adoptive transfer were considered in detail (13).

TABLE I

EFFECT OF ANTI-THETA TREATMENT ON INFECTIOUS TOLERANCE

Treatment of cells	Antibody titer of* all mice	Number of responding mice	Antibody Titer	
			Responding mice	Non-responding mice
anti-θ + GPC	3.2 + 2.7	7/12	5.3 + 1.5	.4 + 4
GPC only	<0	1/12	4	$\overline{1}$

*Mean of $\log_2$+ S.D.

One experiment on infectious tolerance which has not heretofore been published is presented above in Table I. Treatment of the tolerant cells with anti-theta serum and guinea pig complement abrogated the suppression in 7 of 12 recipient mice. However, 5 of the 12 mice had a very suppressed response which were not much greater than the response of 11 of the 12 mice inoculated with cells incubated only in the guinea pig complement. The reason why the anti-theta serum acted in such a fashion is obscure. The experiment gives the impression that suppression may be close or akin to an all or none phenomenon produced by a very small number of cells. Therefore, when the cell number is reduced by killing with anti-theta serum, the probability that there will be a sufficient number to have an effect on secondary transfer is markedly reduced. Whatever the explanation for these results, it seems fairly clear that theta-positive T cells are in some way responsible for the infectious tolerance.

This experiment, however, does not carry us much further than the original experiments. It only shows that the pheno-

menon is thymus-dependent, which we knew because it did not
occur unless T cells were added during the tolerance-inducing
regimen. It does not directly answer the question of whether
the suppression is being mediated by a thymus-dependent B
cell. In fact, no experiment which is assayed by antibody
titration can answer that question. As long as B cells are
present in an animal, it is always limnally possible that
they are the real suppressor cells. Thus, our more recent
experiments on T cell suppression have been done in B cell-
deprived mice in which we measured the effect of T cells on
other T cells. With this new system we have been able to
show T cell suppression of T cell effects (12) in many instances. We have not yet, however, been able to show antigen specificity in these types of experiments and, thus, it
is still possible that the mechanisms of the two phenomena
are different.

Absence of tolerant B cells in tolerant mice (14).
The above experiment showed that it was possible, indeed likely, that the T cells which were added to the animals made tolerant in the presence of T cells, were being
specifically shut off. The following experiments make it
seem unlikely that a major portion of the B cells in the
tolerant animals were themselves tolerant. In the experiments reported above, we added normal thymocytes to the tolerant animals and immunized them with sheep cells. In some
experiments we did specificity controls in which we added
normal thymocytes and immunized the recipients with horse
cells. Surprisingly, this procedure substantially boosted
the tolerant animal's anti-sheep red blood cell response
(Fig. 5, left hand panel). Although the animals made significant amounts of anti-horse red blood cell antibody, the
results reported in Fig. 5 concern only the specific anti-
sheep cell response. Multiple absorptions with horse red
blood cells failed to diminish this titer whereas one absorption completely removed all the antibodies which could
agglutinate horse cells.

These experiments showed that there were at least two
requirements for the production of anti-sheep red blood cell
antibodies in the sheep red blood cell tolerant mice. One
is that normal thymocytes had to be added to the animals
and the other is that these thymocytes had to be stimulated
with an antigen other than sheep cells. These results are
very reminiscent of those reported by McCullagh (15). He
showed that normal thoracic duct lymphocytes injected into
syngeneic rats could not overcome a state of sheep cell

446

tolerance. He further showed that within three days, the injected cells themselves became tolerant. If, however, the added thoracic duct cells were either allogeneic to the host or the host was allogeneic to the cells, they could then abrogate the tolerance. These findings are a little different from those reported by Katz et al in their studies on the allogeneic effect (16). Those authors could demonstrate a boosting of the antibody response only when the B cell was allogeneic to the T cell. McCullagh found he could overcome tolerance even when the T cell did not recognize the B cell as foreign, as long as some form of histoincompatibility was present.

Rendering cells immune (refractory) to infectious tolerance.

Putting McCullagh's and our experiments together, I offer the following explanation. A tolerance-inducing factor (IgY) present in our tolerant animals rendered the normal thymocytes tolerant to sheep red blood cells. The addition of more sheep red blood cells did not overcome the tolerogenic effect. If, however, the normal thymocytes were stimulated with horse red blood cells, they released a nonspecific factor, perhaps similar to the "thymus-replacing" factor of Schimpl and Wecker (17) which prevented the added thymocytes from becoming tolerant to the sheep red blood cells. Failing to become tolerant, the thymocytes were able to react with residual antigen left from the tolerance-inducing regimen and cause the B cell, which had not been rendered tolerant, to make anti-sheep red blood cell antibody. The fact that the horse red blood cells failed to boost the sheep cell response unless normal thymocytes were added indicates quite strongly that the product made after stimulating T cells with the horse cells does not break a state of existing tolerance in the T cells but merely renders them refractory to tolerance-inducing stimuli made by other T cells. It is important to re-emphasize that the residual sheep cell antigen was not responsible for rendering the added thymocytes tolerant, as those cells behaved quite normally in animals given equal amounts of sheep cells but which had been deprived of T cells before the sheep red cells were injected.

The importance of the role played by the residual sheep red blood cells in the production of the response is emphasized by two experiments. One is presented in the right hand panel in Fig. 5. Adding sheep cells to the horse cell inoculum can increase the anti-sheep cell response, although adding sheep cells without horse red blood cells produces no antibody response at all. In addition, we have shown in other experiments that adding horse cells and fresh thymocytes to the cells of the tolerant animals which were removed from that animal and put into another syngeneic host fails to elicit a sheep cell response. Thus, removal from the antigen depot renders the sheep cell antibody-stimulating effect of horse red blood cells inoperative. The results in Fig. 6 (which are the same as those in Fig. 2 except that the effect of adding horse cells on the sheep cell response is added to the figure) show that the addition of the horse cells was unable to help the thymus-independent B cell response which had been rendered tolerant in the absence of T cells. This was true whether or not additional normal thymocytes were added; the recipient animals made a reasonable response to the horse cells. These observations further support the contention put forth above.

Tolerance as the avoidance of concomitant immunity.

At this point I would like to generalize a bit based on the results reported above and on the recent work of Mark Feldmann (18). I suggest that under normal conditions of stimulation with antigen, T cells put out both specific helper and specific suppressor substances. It is well known that they also put out non-specific helper and suppressor factors. The precise role for the non-specific factors has not yet been clearly delineated. It would seem that a major role of the non-specific helper substance is to render target cells refractory to specific tolerance-inducing signals. Thus, one might think that tolerance induction is the main specific T cell signal which can either be rendered ineffective or turned into an immunogenic signal by the non-specific T cell released or T cell-dependent (macrophage?) factors. It seems that immunization leads under most normal circumstances to a conflict between tolerance-inducing and immunity-inducing signals. The key to producing tolerance is the avoidance of concomitant immunity. Thus, a particular antigen might act as a good tolerogen because it fails to stimulate non-specific activating substances which prevent the induction of tolerance. A particularly good candidate for this type of tolerogen would be deaggregated bovine gamma globulin (BGG). We have noted in studies on the effect of immunization on spleen cell responses to PHA in vitro, that immunization with deaggregated BGG can produce non-specific suppressor effects and gives no indication of producing antagonizing augmentative effects (19). On the other hand, the aggregated form of the antigen produces much greater suppressor effects but also produces antagonizing booster affects.

It may also be that certain defined antigens fail to produce antibody responses in the cells of mice with certain histocompatibility antigens (20) because they interact with the non-responder T cells in a fashion that fails to produce an anti-tolerance stimulating factor. It is known, with at least one of these antigens, that T cells recognize the antigen but that the recognition event leads to tolerance rather than immunity (21). Suppressor T cells have been implicated as a causative agent in this tolerance induction (22). We have shown that this antigen produces much less antigenic competition in non-responder then in responder mice (unpublished), again, suggesting that more negative stimuli are produced by immunogenic forms of the antigen but that tolerogenesis occurs when interfering positive factors are absent or depressed.

A recent observation by Rich and Pierce lends further credence to this notion (23). They have found a soluble immune response suppressor in the supernatant of Con A-activated T cells. This substance can profoundly suppress the five day plaque-forming response in Mishell-Dutton cultures if added to the antigen stimulated spleen cell cultures at initiation. They are much less effective when added at 24 hours after initiation and are without effect when added 48 or more hours after initiation. Thus, it seems within 48 hours of initiation the cells become refractory to the suppressor factor. It would be interesting to know whether pre-stimulation of the cultures with horse cells would make them refractory to the addition of suppressive factors and sheep cells at 48 hours.

Other examples which show the necessity for the suppressor factor to act very early in the immune response, in order for it to be effective, can be found in our experiments on removal of spleen-seeking T cells form lethally irradiated Fl mice inoculated with parental T cells (24). We found that if the spleen-seeking fraction of the parental inoculum was removed three hours after the initiation of the immune response, the response of the lymph node seeking fraction was markedly augmented. Removal of the spleen-seeking fraction at 24 or 48 hours after initiation reduced the effectiveness of the maneuver and after 72 hours abrogated it entirely. This was true even though the increased DNA synthetic activity was not seen until 120 hours after cell inoculation.

Baker has found that in order for ALS to augment the immune response to pneumococcal polysaccharide, it must be added at 0 hours (25). If he waits until 24 hours after initiation to treat the mice with ALS, it is much less efficacious and by 48 hours it is without effect.

Thus, there is beginning to appear a body of evidence suggesting that suppressor factors act very early in the immune response. We suggest that their inability to suppress the response when added later stems from a refractoriness induced in the target cells by the production of non-specific activating factors. This may be why neonatal tolerance is often difficult to break by the adoptive transfer of normal cells and easily broken by the adoptive transfer of immune cells (26).

Additional evidence supporting the above hypothesis can be gleaned from an analysis of data on the effect of adding different numbers of T cells to mice prior to attempts at inducing tolerance. We have pooled the data from 10 separate experiments and present them in Fig. 7. Mice treated in the absence of T cells, essentially, make no antibody. 100% of normal mice treated in the same way make antibodies, the titers of which are distributed between 6 and 8 ($\log_2$) tubes. Treatment of thymus-deprived mice, reconstituted with 15×10^6 thymocytes, yields two populations; one of which can be considered tolerant. Their antibody titer is between $\overline{1}$ and 1. Another population of these mice is immune with their titers distributed in a fashion very similar to those of the normal mice. There is very little difference in the absolute titers of the two groups of mice. When the number of thymocytes the mice are reconstituted with is raised to 60×10^6, these same two populations remain. However, the percent of mice in the tolerant population is significantly reduced and that in the immune population is significantly augmented. These results clearly demonstrate that the more T cells there are (and probably the more that are stimulated), the more difficult it becomes to avoid concomitant immunization and, therefore, the production of tolerance. The implication is that when extra T cells are present and being stimulated with the sheep cells, they are preventing the other T cells from becoming tolerant. The conclusion is based on the assumption that the extra T cells are not preventing tolerance by diluting the amount of antigen at the cellular level. I think this is a reasonable assumption. Thus, one might say when excess numbers of T cells are stimulated by whatever means (adjuvants, addition of extra T cells, aggregation of antigen, etc.) they produce factors which render other cells unresponsive to tolerogenic stimuli.

Other observations which are explainable or at least compatible with this theory include the known rapid loss of susceptibility of newborn mice with age (26). As mature T cells develop, they may cancel out the tolerogenic stimuli. (It is also possible that the T cells of newborn mice are especially rich in suppressor activity as Mosier's recent work (personal communication) indicates. The two notions are not mutually exclusive.)

The recent demonstration that endotoxin turns a tolerogenic form of human gamma globulin (HGG) into an immunogen (27) can also be explained by excess T cell activity cancelling out tolerogenic stimuli. Although endotoxin is a potent B cell mitogen (28), it also acts to potentiate T cell activity (29, 30). Thus, while endotoxin is without mitogenic activity on normal T cell populations, it markedly augments the mitotic response of antigen-stimulated T cells.

An interpretive summary of the results presented up to now is as follows. The B cell population of adult CBA mice can be divided into two sub-populations. One of these reacts with sheep red blood cells to form mercaptoethanol-sensitive antibodies in the absence of significant numbers of T cells. This population can be rendered tolerant by pre-treatment with antigen. The tolerance so produced cannot be broken by adding T cells to the tolerant mice. Another population of B cells which includes most of the cells responsible for the production of mercaptoethanol-resistant antibodies require T cell help to make their product. These cells cannot be rendered tolerant by overwhelming them with antigen in the absence of T cells. T cells can, when stimulated with large amounts of antigen, release or cause to be released factors which render other T cells specifically incapable of functionally responding to the antigen which activated them. (We have no evidence that this factor also acts on B cells.) When larger numbers of T cells are stimulated, they release or cause to be released, factors which render other T cells refractory to the specific immunosuppressive effects of the above-mentioned factor.

These results imply that ostensible tolerance need not require the deletion of a clone of responsive cells. Rather

unresponsive or suppressed cells may exist in an unresponsive mouse. A number of laboratories have presented evidence that such may be the case. I would like to present
here some evidence from our laboratory which bears on the
subject.

The existence of immune cells in operationally tolerant mice.

We have utilized the so-called split Claman approach to
study the effect of different antigen doses on T cell education (31, 32). In these experiments we lethally irradiated recipient mice, re-populated them with syngeneic thymocytes and immunized them with different doses of sheep red
blood cells. We measured the amount of DNA synthesized by
the injected thymocytes by determining the amount of the
thymidine analog 5-iodo-2-deoxyuridine (labelled with I^{125})
the stimulated T cells incorporated (33). We have found
that the more antigen used for stimulation of the thymocytes,
the more DNA they synthesize (33, 34). We have tested the
immunological capacities of the immunized cells by retrieving them from the spleens of the primary recipients and re-
transferring them to thymus-deprived indicator mice (34).
We have found that a dose of 0.2 cc of a 1% sheep red blood
cell suspension (in the presence of the adjuvant pertussis)
is the optimal immunizing dose (34). Increasing the amount
of antigen decreases the ability of the harvested T cells
to augment the response of thymus-deprived mice. In fact,
immunizing T cells with 0.2 cc of a packed sheep red blood
cell suspension leads to a total absence of helper cell
activity, even though considerable amounts of DNA is synthesized by the cells during the immunization procedure.

We have previously shown that DNA synthesis leads to
the generation of long-term memory cells (35). Thus, we
tested the possibility that the excess antigen was producing
long-term memory cells which were being made tolerant or
being actively suppressed directly or indirectly by the excess antigen. We harvested the spleen cells of lethally
irradiated, thymocyte reconstituted, sheep red blood cells
immunized mice a week after the start of the immunization
procedure. We transferred the recovered splenic T cells to
indicator mice which had been thymus-deprived one month previously. We immunized the indicator mice on the day of
transfer three weeks later and three weeks after that. The
results of one such experiment are presented in Fig. 8. It
can be seen that thymocytes immunized with a large dose of
sheep red blood cells, although devoid of any demonstrable

helper activity on the day of transfer into thymus-deprived recipients, became quite efficacious with time at boosting the anti-sheep red blood cell response. The thymocytes immunized with the 1% suspension were efficient right after transfer and lost activity with time. It is unlikely that a transfer of antigen along with the splenic T cells of the immunized mice acted to immunize small numbers of non-tolerant T cells in the secondary recipients. Thymocytes immunized with packed sheep cells plus pertussis were much better than thymocytes immunized with packed sheep cells alone at boosting the anti-sheep red blood cell response late after transfer (though neither was effective initially). If any antigen was transferred with the educated T cells, it should have been transferred equally in both groups.

The acquisition of significant helper activity with time rules out such explanations as non-specific cytotoxicity, "exhaustive differentiation" or cell migration for the lack of such activity earlier. Since the magnitude of the initial DNA synthetic response made by the thymocytes correlated with their late helper activity, the DNA synthesis was probably not immunologically irrelevant. It would seem more likely that the DNA synthesis was involved, at least in part, in the generation of memory cells. The reason these memory cells could not express their full potential for at least six weeks is not clear. The correlation between the rise in their activity and the fall in helper activity of the cells immunized with the low dose of sheep red blood cells is intriguing. The possibility that a short-lived suppressor cell was responsible for the lack of earlier helper activity deserves consideration. Simpson and Cantor have noted a correlation between the presence of suppressor activity and the presence of cytotoxic T cells, which also appeared to be short-lived cells (personal communication). We are presently exploring this notion.

Although not totally relevant to the discussion at hand, the appearance of highly active helper cells in the absence of significant amounts of DNA synthesis after immunization with the 1% suspension of sheep red blood cells deserves a comment. Byfield and Sercarz have also noted the appearance of short-lived memory cells in the absence of detectable DNA synthesis (36) as have we in other situations (21). Transference of receptors from T cell to T cell comes to mind as a possible mechanism for the generation of such helper activity. We are planning to experimentally test this concept.

The experiments reported above also bear on the notion that avoidance of concomitant immunization is an important factor in tolerance induction. Immunization of thymocyte-reconstituted B mice with a packed sheep red blood cell suspension and pertussis will almost always cause the production of antibody. As we have shown above, such immunization of T cells in mice lacking B cells produces tolerance in the T cells. We suggest that the way concomitant immunization was avoided in this situation was that the T cell-dependent helping factors which might have been made during tolerance induction were wasted as there were no B cells for them to act upon. Thus, concomitant immunization was avoided. Perhaps this is how some cytotoxic agents, particularly those with a predilection for killing B cells, can produce tolerance to sheep red blood cells. By killing the B cells which may be helped by the helping T cell factors, they prevent those cells from becoming immunized. Thus, the avoidance of concomitant immunization takes place and the tolerance-producing effects predominate.

Thymus dependence of recovery from tolerance.
The mice used in the studies on the thymus dependence of tolerance reported above (Figs. 1-4) were followed for several months, being occasionally reimmunized. None of these mice had a source of new T cells after the initial experiments were completed. Thus, they were all thymus-deprived and some were reconstituted with 15×10^6 thymocytes prior to the start of tolerance induction. Half of the mice made tolerant in the presence of thymocytes and half that were made tolerant in the absence of thymocytes were reconstituted with an additional 15×10^6 thymocytes after tolerance induction. The precise anti-sheep red blood cell titers present in these mice 15 days after immunization with sheep red blood cells are presented in Figs. 2-4.

In the data presented in Table II, we have arbitrarily chosen the presence of an antibody titer greater than four as an indication of the absence of tolerance, as all control mice had titers greater than that after a second immunization. Mice which never received T cells never made antibody titers greater than four. On the other hand, those animals made tolerant in the absence of T cells but then given an inoculation of normal thymocytes showed no evidence of residual tolerance in the secondary response.

TABLE II

NUMBER OF MICE WITH ANTIBODY TITERS GREATER THAN 4

Treatment		Day of Test				
Before Tolerance Induction	After Tolerance Induction	15(1)*	50(2)	76(3)	83(4)	113(5)
+T**	+T	0/15	10/15	15/15	15/15	15/15
	-T	0/20	5/20	5/20	13/20	20/20
-T	+T	2/10	9/10	10/10	10/10	10/10
	-T	0/20	0/20	0/20	0/20	0/20

*Indicates number of immunizations with SRBC after termination of tolerance-inducing regimen.

**+T means 15 x 10^6 thymocytes were inoculated into thymectomized, lethally irradiated bone marrow reconstituted mice.

In the case of mice made tolerant in the <u>presence of T cells and then inoculated with normal thymocytes</u>, there was significant recovery from tolerance (see Fig. 3 for the level of tolerance in the primary response) in the secondary response and total recovery by the time of the tertiary response. These results indicate that the tolerance induced in the added thymocytes was quite short-lived (the infectious tolerance produced on adoptive transfer is equally short-lived) (37). Of particular interest and importance in the context of existence of tolerant cells are the results seen in the mice that were made <u>tolerant in the presence of T cells and then given no further T cells</u>. Some of these mice had recovered from tolerance in the secondary response, more in the quaternary response and by the quinternary response they were all making significant amounts of anti-sheep red blood cell antibody. Thus, tolerance produced in the thymocyte population by the large amounts of sheep red blood cells was longer lived than was the infectious tolerance. Nonetheless, these T cells eventually regained the capacity to cooperate with the B cells in the production of anti-sheep cell antibody.

These experiments suggest but do not prove that there were tolerant T cells present. It is possible that there very small numbers of non-tolerant T cells which eventually proliferated so that sufficient numbers were present to perform a cooperative response. The experiments reported below with chromosomally-marked T cells indicate that the latter situation does not occur. The difference in longevity of tolerance induced by suppressor T cells versus that produced directly by antigen can be explained either by an added direct contribution of the antigen or by the fact that the tolerant cells may have been exposed to more suppressor material during tolerance induction.

T cell tolerance in chromosomally-marked cell populations.
There is one other set of experiments that we did while working in the laboratory of Tony Davies that have previously been reported only in part (12, 38), but which bear on the question of whether or not tolerant cells exist, which I would like to present. In these experiments we gave standardly-prepared B mice an histocompatible thymus graft that contained chromosomally (T6)-marked cells (39). Over the course of the next 30 days, we gave these mice large doses of sheep red blood cells. We used the 30 day period because we knew that 30 days after transplant the mitotic cells in the thymus graft switch from T6 to host type and that from this time on there is no longer seeding of T6 thymocytes to peripheral tissues (39). At the termination of the pretreatment schedule, we removed the thymus grafts of half the mice and these animals had no further source of any T cells. At intervals thereafter we immunized the mice with sheep cells or with horse cells and measured the mitotic response of the T6 cells as well as the antibody response made by the mice. Some of the mice were immunized directly and some had their spleen cells transferred to lethally irradiated syngeneic recipients.

Sheep red blood cell pre-treatment severely depressed both the T6 mitotic response and the antibody response to sheep cells. The specificity of this suppression of T6 mitosis was poor as has previously been noted (40) in that the mitotic response to horse red blood cells was also diminished although not as severely as the specific suppression. The mitotic response to a totally unrelated antigen, oxzazolone, was normal. The antibody response to the horse red blood cells, however, was not significantly affected by the pretreatment. With time the anti-sheep red blood cell antibody response recovered and actually acquired secondary response type characteristics, as it was predominantly IgG in both mice with or without intact thymus grafts. The findings of a hyper-immune state when tolerance wanes has previously been noted, but the question of whether the memory was acquired before or after tolerance induction could not be decided (41). In this case, however, the nature of the T6 mitotic response after the waning of tolerance gave some added clues as no source of T6 cells was present after the period of tolerance induction. However, one group of mice--those with intact thymus grafts--had a source of new T cells without T6 chromosomes. The mitotic response of cells transferred from both groups of mice to lethally irradiated recipients 11-12 weeks after the termination of tolerance induction is given in Table III. In mice with intact thymus grafts, 65% of the cells in mitosis were of the T6 genotype three days after stimulation with SRBC and only 40% were T6 in mice stimulated with horse red blood cells. The mitotic response of their peripheral blood cells cultures with PHA was 49%. In mice whose thymus grafts were removed at the termination of the tolerance induction, the T6 response was about 90% in both groups as was the response of their peripheral blood cells to PHA. Since the cells which respond mitotically to PHA are essentially all T cells (42), these results suggest that the peripheral T cell pool had been diluted about 50% in mice with intact thymus grafts. However, the T6 cells responded preferentially to the non-T6 cells when stimulated with SRBC indicating a form of memory. As noted above, we have previously shown that memory is reflected in T cell mitosis. These memory cells were probably formed during the tolerance induction. If the memory was generated by antigen remaining after the termination of tolerance induction, it should have affected the non-T6 cells coming from the thymus, and we should not have seen a preferential T6 effect after stimulation with sheep cells.

TABLE III

PERCENTAGE OF CELLS IN MITOSIS WITH T_6 CHROMOSOMES THREE DAYS AFTER STIMULATION WITH VARIOUS MATERIALS

	Experimental Group	
Mitotic Stimulus	Thymus Graft Excised	Thymus Graft Intact
SRBC	91	65
HRBC	86	40
PHA	87	49

Thus, these studies support the notion that memory cells can be functionally depressed without deletion of a cell clone. Further experiments are required, however, to answer the important question of whether the waning is due to the loss of a cell which is actively suppressing the response or to a waning of a suppressor meterial produced during the tolerance induction.

SUMMARY

We have shown that B cells of adult CBA mice are made up of at least two sub-populations. One of these is thymus independent in that it responds to sheep red blood cells without much T cell help and in addition can become tolerant to sheep cells without T cell help. After it is made tolerant to SRBC, T cell help does not break its unresponsive state. A second population fails to react to sheep cells without T cell help, either to become immune or tolerant. Induction of tolerance in the first population does not detectably alter the response of the second, indicating the two cells may come from separate lines.

In addition, we showed that sheep red blood cell stimulated T cells can make, or cause to be made, factors which render other T cells specifically unresponsive to sheep cells. Whether this factor(s) also acts on B cells is not clear. If it does, it does so at much higher thresholds. Antigen-stimulated T cells can also make, or cause to be made, factors which render other T cells refractory to, or at least increase the threshold requirements for, the suppressive signal. The latter factor has less antigen specificity than the former.

We have also presented several models which indicate that suppressed immune T cells may exist in operationally tolerant mice. These cells have longer lives than the suppressing agents.

From these data we have put forth a theory in which we suggest that immunization of T cells usually causes them to make specific suppressor factors. When they also make sufficient amounts of the non-specific activating factor, immunity results. When they fail to do this, a state akin to immunological tolerance results. Factors which favor the latter situation include antigen solubilization and reduction in numbers of mature T cells, either by experimental maneuvers or by stimulating an immature immune system. Intrinsic adjuvanticity (such as antigen aggregation) or extrinsic adjuvants are factors which favor the former.

ACKNOWLEDGMENTS

Figure 1 and the data in Figs. 2-4 are reprinted from Reference 11 with the kind permission of Blackwell Scientific Publications, Oxford, England. Figure 8 is reprinted from Reference 34 with the kind permission of the Macmillan Journals Limited, London, England.

REFERENCES

1. Greene, H.S.N. and Harvey, E.K., Cancer Res. 20:1094, 1960.

2. Gershon, R.K., Carter, R.L. and Kondo, K., Nature. 213: 674, 1967.

3. Gershon, R.K. and Carter, R.L., Nature. 226:368, 1970.

4. Gershon, R.K., Carter, R.L. and Kondo, K., Science. 159:646, 1968.

5. Gershon, R.K. and Carter, R.L., J. Nat. Cancer Inst. 43:533, 1969.

6. Gershon, R.K. and Kondo, K., J. Nat. Cancer Inst. 43: 545, 1969.

7. Gershon, R.K. and Kondo, K., J. Nat. Cancer Inst. 43: 1169, 1971.

8. Chanmougan, D. and Schwartz, R.S., J. Exp. Med. 124: 363, 1966.

9. Claman, H.N. and Bronsky, E.A., J. Immunol. 95:718, 1965.

10. Davies, A.J.S., Leuchars, E., Wallis, V. and Koller, P.C., Transplantation. 5:222, 1967.

11. Gershon, R.K. and Kondo, K., Immunology. 18:723, 1970.

12. Gershon, R.K., Contemporary Topics in Immunobiology. 3:1, 1974.

13. Gershon, R.K. and Kondo, K., Immunology. 21:903, 1971.

14. Gershon, R.K. and Kondo, K., Science. 175:996, 1972.

15. McCullagh, P.J., J. Exp. Med. 132:916, 1970.

16. Katz, D.H., Paul, W.E., Goidl, E.A. and Benacerraf, B., J. Exp. Med. 133:169, 1971.

17. Schimpl, A. and Wecker, E., Nat. New Biol. 237:15, 1972.

18. Feldmann, M., Nat. New Biol. 242:84, 1973.

19. Gershon, R.K., Gery, I. and Waksman, B.H., J. Immunol. 112:215, 1974.

20. Benacerraf, B. and McDevitt, H.O., Science. 175:273, 1972.

21. Gershon, R.K., Maurer, P.H. and Merryman, C.F., Proc. Nat. Acad. Sci. 70:250, 1973.

22. Kapp, J., Pierce, C. and Benacerraf, B., Fed. Proc. (abs.). 33:773, 1974.

23. Rich, R.R. and Pierce, C.W., J. Immunol. 112:1360, 1974.

24. Gershon, R.K., Lance, E.M. and Kondo, K., J. Immunol. 112:546, 1974.

25. Baker, P.J., Stashak, P.W., Amsbaugh, D.F. and Prescott, B., J. Immunol. 112:404, 1974.

26. Billingham, R.E., Brent, L. and Medawar, P.B., Phil. Trans. Roy. Soc. 239:357, 1956.

27. Louis, J.A., Chiller, J.M. and Weigle, W.O., J. Exp. Med. 138:1481, 1974.

28. Gery, I., Kruger, J. and Spiesel, S.Z., J. Immunol. 108:1088, 1972.

29. Armerding, D. and Katz, D.H., J. Exp. Med. 139:24, 1974.

30. Ohrbach-Arbouys, S. and Gershon, R.K., J. Immunol. Submitted.

31. Miller, J.F.A.P. and Mitchell, G.F., Transpl. Rev. 1:3, 1969.

32. Claman, H.N. and Chaperon, E.A., Transpl. Rev. 1:92, 1969.

33. Gershon, R.K. and Hencin, R., J. Immunol. 107:1723, 1971.

34. Spiesel, S.Z. and Gershon, R.K., Nat. New Biol. 238: 271, 1972.

35. Gershon, R.K., Kruger, J., Naysmith, J.D. and Waksman, B.H., Nature. 232:639, 1971.

36. Byfield, P. and Sercarz, E., J. Exp. Med. 129:897, 1969.

37. Gershon, R.K. and Kondo, K., Immunology. 23:321, 1972.

38. Gershon, R.K., Fed. Proc. (abs.) 29:626, 1970.

39. Davies, A.J.S., Transpl. Rev. 1:43, 1969.

40. Gershon, R.K., Wallis, V., Davies, A.J.S. and Leuchars, E., Nature. 218:280, 1968.

41. Dresser, D.W. and Mitchison, N.A., Adv. Immunol. 8: 129, 1968.

42. Doenhoff, M.J., Davies, A.J.S., Leuchars, E. and Wallis, V., Proc. Roy. Soc. B. 176:69, 1970.

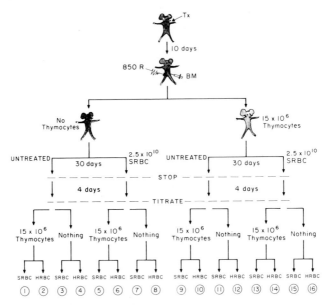

Fig. 1. Experimental protocol for demonstrating the thymus dependence of tolerance to sheep red blood cells.

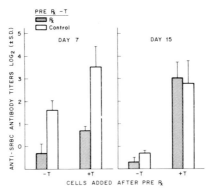

Fig. 2. The effect of pre-treating thymus-deprived recipients with large doses of sheep cells on the subsequent immune response to that antigen. Some of the pretreated mice received 15 x 10⁶ thymocytes 4 days after the cessation of the pre-treatment schedule (+T) (see text). Control mice were treated the same way as test mice except they received no antigen during the pre-treatment period. All mice were immunized with a 20% suspension of sheep red blood cells 4 days after the cessation of pre-treatment. The results presented are hemagglutination titers on day 7 and 15 after immunization.

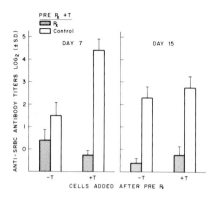

Fig. 3. The effect of pre-treating thymus-deprived
recipients reconstituted with 15 x 10⁶ thymocytes with large
doses of sheep cells on the subsequent immune response to
that antigen. Some of the pre-treated mice received 15 x
10⁶ thymocytes 4 days after the cessation of the pre-treatment schedule (+T) (see text). Control mice were treated
the same way as test mice except they received no antigen
during the pre-treatment period. All mice were immunized
with a 20% suspension of sheep red blood cells 4 days after
the cessation of pre-treatment. The results presented are
hemagglutination titers on day 7 and 15 after immunization.

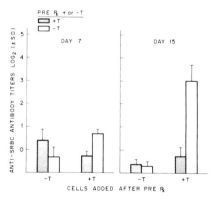

Fig. 4. Effect of the presence of 15 x 10⁶ thymocytes
during the course of pre-treatment with sheep red blood
cells on the subsequent immune response of mice immunized 4
days later with a 20% suspension of that antigen. Some of
the pre-treated mice also received 15 x 10⁶ thymocytes at
the time of immunization (+T) (see Figs. 2 and 3).

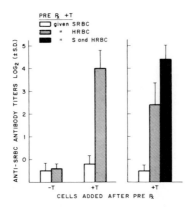

Fig. 5. Effect of horse red blood cell immunization on the anti-sheep red blood cell response of mice made tolerant to sheep red blood cells in the presence of 15 x 10⁶ thymocytes. Some of the mice were reconstituted with an additional 15 x 10⁶ thymocytes at the time of immunization (+T). The results are the anti-sheep cell titers 15 days after immunization with either sheep cells, horse cells or both and are from two separate experiments.

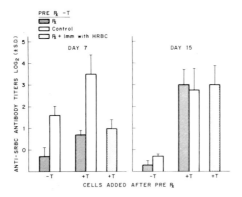

Fig. 6. Effect of horse red blood cell immunization on the anti-sheep red blood cell response of mice made tolerant to sheep red blood cells in the absence of 15 x 10⁶ thymocytes. Some of the mice were reconstituted with an additional 15 x 10⁶ thymocytes at the time of immunization (+T). The results are the anti-sheep cell titers 7 and 15 days after immunization with either sheep cells or horse cells. Control mice were not pre-treated with antigen and were immunized with sheep cells.

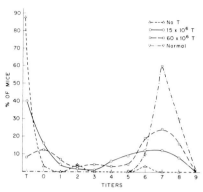

Fig. 7. The distribution of antibody titers in mice given 12-14 injections of 0.2 cc of packed sheep red blood cells over the course of 30 days. The titers were obtained 4 days after the last injection of sheep cells. Three groups of mice were thymus-deprived. One received no reconstitution with thymocytes, another was reconstituted with 15 x 10⁶ and the third with 60 x 10⁶ thymocytes. A fourth group was untreated. The results are pooled from ten separate experiments in which greater than 200 mice were studied. Each point represents the % of mice in each group with a given antibody titer. The sum of all points in each group should equal 100.

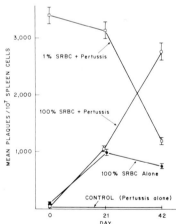

Fig. 8. Number of plaque-forming cells in the spleens of thymus-deprived radiation chimeras reconstituted with thymocytes "educated" with 0.2 ml of different concentrations of sheep red blood cells with or without the inclusion of pertussis. The mice were boosted with a 20% suspension of sheep red blood cells at different intervals after reconstitution. Each point is the geometric mean + SE of the results from five individual mice. ☐ , 1% sheep red blood cells + pertussis; ◯ , 100% sheep red blood cells + pertussis; ● , 100% sheep red blood cells alone; and ____ , control, pertussis alone.

DISCUSSION FOLLOWING RICHARD GERSHON

WAKSMAN: Several workers have described a thymus in sharks and even in cyclostomes. How does this fit with your suggestion about phylogenesis?

GERSHON: I know of no published evidence that sharks have thymuses. I think one of the reasons for the notion that T cells preceded B cells phylogenetically is historical; at one time we thought that cellular immunity was T cell-mediated and antibody-mediated immunity was B cell mediated and that the two systems were separate. Since graft rejection preceded humoral immunity in phylogenesis we assumed T cells preceded B cells. We now know that earthworms reject grafts and have no thymus, indicating that more primitive rejection mechanisms exist and rule out graft rejection as a T cell marker. My icthyologist friends have been unable to demonstrate a thymus or thymus-dependent lymphoid functions. I have reviewed the evidence on the subject recently (Contemporary Topics in Immunobiology, 3:1, 1974).

E. MÖLLER: Have you reproduced suppression in vitro, and if so, do supernatants of tolerant cells work?

GERSHON: To the first question, yes; the second, I haven't tested. Others have found T cell-dependent suppressor supernatants.

NOSSAL: Dr. Gershon could you give us a speculative intellectual framework for T cell suppressor effects? I have three competing notions in my mind. First, there could be IgT-antigen complexes directly tolerizing T and B cells (Feldmann) Secondly, there could be an excessive release of lymphokines ("super-helper"). Thirdly, there could be anti-idiotype effects (Herzenberg; Jerne). Which, if any, of these ideas do you favor?

GERSHON: None of the mechanisms you mention can be ruled out at present. My own personal feeling is that an informational event must transpire. I like the idea of an IgT suppressor which is carried to appropriate target cells by antigen and has a stop signal in its Fc moiety.

FELDMANN: Just a comment to concur with Dick. Basically a

highly subtle difference could exist between helper
IgT and suppressor IgT. The data on the mechanism of
help with IgT requires binding to macrophages. Any
change in IgT which abrogates its capacity to bind
to macrophages would swing the system wholely towards
suppression, as immunization could not occur.

GERSHON: An important point. As we have shown, non-specific
helper effects can render suppressor signals inoperative. Macrophages are clearly a source of non-specific
factors which help T cells to respond.

DRESSER: Would you go along with the suggestion that there
is only one kind of antigen generated T-cell. This
immune T-cell mediating graft rejection, delayed hypersensitivity and, in the context of the present discussion, help and suppressor activity, where the T
cell recognises a B (T) cell binding an antigen molecule. The difference between help and suppression would
lie at the level of the "target" cells reaction to a
potentially lethal attack. Do you have evidence which
would convincingly exclude this model.

GERSHON: There is really very little hard information which
bears directly on mechanisms, although too much help
can be ruled out as the cause of specific suppression.
Your suggestion is both feasible and clever, but as I
mentioned above, not one I personally find appealing.

MITCHELL: Dick Gershon would predict that the shark, which
he says lacks T cells should be totally refractory to
tolerance induction. Do we know anything about tolerance induction in phylogenetically early species?

GERSHON: Dick Gershon would certainly not make such a prediction! He showed clearly, or at least it seemed clear
to him, that subpopulations of B cells are easily rendered tolerant. These were the B cells he speculated
were similar to those in the shark (and the nude mouse
also). Thus, he suggests that sharks and nude mice
should be easily rendered tolerant.

BASTEN: I should like to comment on Dr. Gershon's results
with erythrocyte antigens. The site of action of the
suppressor effect appears to be a non-tolerant carrier-
reactive cell rather than the AFCP which is consistent
with our findings in a hapten-carrier collaborative

system; furthermore the results do not support supra-priming as the mechanism of suppression.

In your experiments with the sheep and horse erythro-cyte you found no evidence of cross-reactivity. How-ever, in our system where carrier-primed cells are the target for suppression, there is cross-reactive sup-pression demonstrable at the level of the T cell - the existence of cross-reactivity in a suppressor system clearly has important implications in regulation of the immune response, particularly to self antigens.

GERSHON: We did find cross-reactions in some situations (Immunology 18:723, 1970), and so know that at least some types of T cells react with both sheep and horse erythrocytes. Perhaps the difference in specificity between our results is quantitative; your suppressors seem to be more active than ours.

BENACERRAF: I would like to challenge your statements:
1) that IgG B cells cannot be tolerized in the absence of T cells.
2) Thymus-independent antigens are the only ones to stimulate restricted responses.

There is ample evidence that high affinity IgG B cells are easily tolerized in certain systems in the absence of T cells.

Also restricted clonal responses have been obtained in rabbits with pneumococcus organisms and in guinea pigs with DNP-oligo-lysine, both thymus-dependent responses.

GERSHON: May I modify those statements. The first state-ment I must restrict to erythrocyte-bound antigens. Certainly David Katz and you and your colleagues have presented evidence to the contrary using DNP-D-GL. Very little information is available using other antigens. My guess is that it will turn out that, in general, thymus-dependent B cells will be highly but not absol-utely resistant to tolerance induction in the absence of T cell help. The second statement can be modified as follows: the less T cells that participate in the response to an antigen, the more restricted is the sub-sequent antibody heterogeneity.

TAYLOR: It may well be possible to get suppression by ex-

cess helper cells. We have found a radiation-resistant
suppressor T-cell, in a system very much like that
described by Dr. Herzenberg. Presumably this could
be due to excess helper function.

THE MODE AND SITES OF ACTION OF SUPPRESSOR T CELLS IN THE ANTIGEN-INDUCED DIFFERENTIATION OF B CELLS

Tomio Tada

Department of Pathology
Chiba University School of Medicine
Chiba, Japan

With the recognition of the presence of inhibitory activity of T cells in certain types of humoral antibody responses, there have been uncovered various perplexing activities of T cells in the immune response (1-13). These are not only concerned with the T cell's suppressive effect on the magnitude of B cell response but also with the role of T cells in the induction of immunological tolerance, autoimmunity, class distribution of antibodies, allotype expression and immunological maturation. Thus, it seems to me that everybody is having to face the more sophisticated roles played by T cells in various immunological phenomena. In order to analyze the possible role of suppressor T cells in the induction and maintenance of tolerance, one has to know the mode and sites of action of suppressor T cells in the course of antibody response.

It has been recognized that the suppression by T cells is mediated by both antigen-specific and non-specific means. While both pathways may be equally important for the regulation of antibody response, I am going to deal mostly with the antigen-specific suppression by T cells, since it seems to be more pertinent for understanding some forms of immunological tolerance. I would like to discuss the mode and sites of action of suppressor T cells in antigen-induced differentiation of B cells for production of different classes of antibodies using as our models of hapten-specific antibody responses in rodents. A special emphasis is put on some selective roles of T cells on the proliferation and maturation of the B cell lineage.

Antigen-specific suppression by T cells.
We have been able to demonstrate the suppressive effect of T cells on certain T cell dependent antibody responses in rodents. In our earlier studies concerning IgE antibody response in the rat, it was found that passively transferred T cells from donors immunized with a carrier antigen can effectively suppress an ongoing hapten-specific IgE antibody

response, provided the recipient animals were immunized with the homologous hapten-carrier conjugate (12). Neither the T cells obtained from normal rats nor those primed with the hapten coupled to a different carrier showed such suppressive activity; therefore, this suppression was definitely antigen-specific. A similar antigen-specific suppression of IgM antibody response by carrier-specific T cells was also demonstrated in the mouse immunized with a hapten-carrier conjugate (13). These results suggested that a suppression of antibody response occurred through an interaction between carrier-specific T cells and hapten-specific B cells analogous to that observed in the induction of antibody response.

From these results it was predicted that if animals were preimmunized with carrier by certain means so as to produce suppressor T cells, it would be inhibitory for the antibody response upon subsequent immunization with hapten-carrier conjugate. This prediction was proved to be true in two experimental systems. In the rat preimmunization with carrier in complete Freund's adjuvant (CFA) one month before immunization with hapten-carrier conjugate completely prevented the induction of hapten-specific IgE antibody response (14). Treatment of such preimmunized animals with anti-thymocyte serum caused partial recovery of the antibody response (15). In the rabbit preimmunization with carrier protein in CFA also greatly reduced the amount of anti-hapten IgG antibody produced by subsequent immunizations with hapten-carrier conjugate, accompanied by a striking decrease of antibody affinity for the hapten (16). These features are clearly analogous to those of hapten-specific immunological tolerance, inasmuch as the production of high affinity antibody and a certain class of antibody was preferentially suppressed by carrier-preimmunization.

Time-dependent suppressive effect of T cells in the antibody response.

In order to investigate more detailed mechanisms in this antigen-specific suppression produced by carrier-primed T cells, we have devised an in vivo system of sequential IgM and IgG antibody responses in the mouse against a hapten 2,4-dinitrophenyl (DNP) coupled to Keyhole limpet hemocyanin (KLH) (17, 18). BALB/c 6J mice were immunized with a single dose of DNP-KLH (100 µg) intraperitoneally (i.p.) with 10^9 Bordetella pertussis vaccine (BPV). DNP-specific antibody response was estimated by the hemolytic plaque method of Cunningham and Szenberg using sheep erythrocytes coated with DNP_{29}-BSA by $CrCl_3$. Direct plaque-forming cells (PFC) were considered to be producing IgM antibody, and indirect PFC produced by the addition of rabbit anti-mouse IgG was considered to be the IgG producer.

By this immunization procedure BALB/c mice produced normal sequential IgM and IgG antibody responses. The peak direct PFC response occurred on day 3, amounting to about 50,000 PFC/spleen. The number of indirect PFC at this time was low and variable, but reached its maximum on day 6, amounting to 10,000 PFC/spleen. Both direct and indirect PFC responses were short lived and barely detectable on day 10 (see Fig. 1).

To test the effect of carrier-primed suppressor T cells on the above antibody response, donor BALB/c mice were immunized with two i.p. injections of 100 μg of KLH at a two-week interval. As a control, some donor animals were immunized with an unrelated antigen, bovine gamma globulin (BGG) by the same schedule. They were killed two weeks after the second immunization, their thymuses and spleens removed and cell suspensions were prepared in Eagle's minimal essential medium (MEM). These cells will be referred to as KLH-primed or BGG-primed thymocytes and spleen cells.

To see the effect of KLH-primed cells on the anti-DNP antibody response, 5×10^7 KLH-primed thymocytes or spleen cells were passively transferred into the recipient mice simultaneously with, 2 days after or 3 days after the primary immunization of the recipient, DNP-KLH and BPV. The kinetics of IgM and IgG antibody responses of the recipient were examined by enumerating direct and indirect PFC in their spleen at various times after the immunization. Figures 1a and 1b depict the pertinent results obtained in this experiment. If animals were given KLH-primed thymocytes on day 0, the peak IgM antibody response was only slightly suppressed, but this was followed by a more rapid decrease in direct PFC numbers than in the control mice that had been given BGG-primed thymocytes. On the other hand, indirect PFC response was greatly suppressed in the group given KLH-primed cells on day 0, and in some mice it was almost undetectable (Fig. 1a). An essentially similar pattern of suppression was produced by KLH-primed spleen cells: a slight suppression of peak IgM antibody response and almost negative IgG antibody response. This suppressive effect of KLH-primed spleen cells was completely eliminated by the in vitro treatment of the cells with anti-Θ and complement before the cell transfer.

473

A reverse experiment was performed by immunizing recipient animals with DNP-BGG in place of DNP-KLH, that were concurrently given KLH-primed or BGG-primed thymocytes. In this case meaningful numbers of direct and indirect PFC were obtained on day 6, both of which were suppressed by BGG-primed cells but not by KLH-primed cells.

The effect of KLH-primed cells given 2 days after the immunization of the recipient was not so different from the effect produced by cell transfer on day 0; although the KLH-primed cells produced somewhat stronger suppression in the peak IgM antibody response than when given on day 0, the effect was preferentially directed to late IgG antibody response. Here again, BGG-primed cells had no effect on the anti-DNP antibody responses of the recipients.

However, if the recipients were given KLH-primed cells on day 3, a markedly different effect was observed. As shown in Fig. 1b, the number of direct PFC, which was already at the maximal before the cell transfer, declined very rapidly following the passive transfer of KLH-primed thymocytes or spleen cells at a much greater rate than observed in the control animals given BGG-primed cells. This suppressive effect on direct PFC was already evident on day 4 only 24 hours after the transfer of KLH-primed cells and became more pronounced on day 6. By contrast, the cell transfer on day 3 produced much less suppressive effect on indirect PFC response than that induced by the same KLH-primed cells given on day 0 or 2. It is apparent that KLH-primed cells given on day 3 were effective in suppressing the pre-established IgM antibody response, resulting in an earlier termination of the response, whereas they were no longer very effective in inhibiting the IgG antibody response which was just starting at the time of cell transfer.

Such a suppressive effect of KLH-primed cells was also detected in the secondary antibody response. In this case animals were primarily immunized with DNP-KLH 4 weeks before the secondary immunization with the same antigen with or without BPV as adjuvant. On both immunization regimens, animals produced good secondary antibody response which was characterized by increases in both maximal direct and indirect PFC in their spleen as observed 3 days after the secondary challenge. If 5×10^7 KLH-primed thymocytes or spleen cells were given simultaneously with the secondary immunization, the numbers of both direct and indirect DNP-specific

PFC moderately decreased. Whereas the control animals produced 236,000 direct and 128,000 indirect PFC on day 3, the animals given KLH-primed thymocytes produced 115,000 direct and 21,000 indirect PFC on day 3. The statistical analysis indicated that P value for the difference in direct PFC was <0.05, but that for indirect PFC was <0.001. Therefore, it was concluded that the effect of suppressor T cells in the secondary antibody response was more profound in IgG than in IgM antibody response.

Specificity of T cell-mediated suppression.

The above results indicate that T cells primed with a carrier antigen can suppress the hapten-specific IgM and IgG antibody responses if recipient animals are immunized with the hapten coupled to the homologous carrier. However, this does not necessarily mean that direct interaction between hapten-specific B cells and carrier-specific T cells is essential for the observed suppression of antibody response. Such suppression could be induced by a non-specific factor elaborated by T cells via interaction with an unrelated antigen.

In order to investigate this possibility, animals were given either KLH-primed cells or BGG-primed cells, and then subsequently immunized with the mixture of DNP-BGG and uncoupled KLH or with the mixture of DNP-KLH and uncoupled BGG. If the interaction between the uncoupled carrier and corresponding T cells elaborate non-specific factors that suppress anti-DNP antibody response, it should be predictable that the hapten-specific PFC is suppressed by the concurrent injection of uncoupled heterologous carrier and corresponding T cells.

As a control for this experiment, normal mice were immunized with the mixture of DNP-KLH and BGG or DNP-BGG and KLH. DNP-specific PFC response in these groups immunized with two antigens was slightly lower than that induced by a single hapten-carrier conjugate, probably due to the result of antigenic competition. However, even if such animals were concomitantly given the cells primed with the second carrier on which immunizing hapten was not coupled, no significant suppression of anti-DNP PFC responses was observed; animals given KLH-primed cells produced comparable numbers of direct and indirect PFC to those of the control upon immunization with DNP-BGG and KLH. Similarly, no suppression was detectable in animals given BGG-primed cells upon subsequent immunization with DNP-KLH and uncoupled BGG. Thus, it is suggested that in order to elicit effective suppression,

the hapten must be present on the same carrier by which suppressor T cells were primed.

These results indicate that the suppression of B cell
response by T cells is definitely antigen-specific, and that
the suppressive effect of T cells on IgM and IgG antibody
responses differs primarily according to the time point at
which suppressor T cells were administered to the recipient
animals. The latter differential effect of T cells on IgM
and IgG antibody responses may be interpreted in terms of
the inherently different susceptibility of B cells to the
suppressive influence of T cells. At first glance the insensitivity of early IgM antibody response as compared to
the late IgG and IgM antibody responses seems to have some
bearing on its relative independency of the T cell function,
whereas the latter two responses are known to be strongly
T cell dependent. Thus, it is probable that the T cell dependent process in antibody response is more susceptible to the
regulatory influence of T cells.

Susceptibility of B cells to suppressive influence of T
cells.
Keeping the above observation in mind, the present results appear to fit the recent concept of differentiating
events occurring in B cells following antigenic stimulation.
It has been recognized that B cells having μ chain determinants on their surface are the precursors of both IgM and IgG-
forming cells (19-21). Such virgin B cells, termed $B\mu$ cells,
would differentiate either directly into IgM-forming cells
or into the cells having both μ and γ chains on their surface
($B\mu\gamma$ cells) that consequently become $B\gamma$ cells, the precursors
of IgG-forming cells. The former, the direct process of
maturing into IgM-forming cells may be largely T cell independent, while the latter, the process of becoming $B\gamma$ cells
may be T cell dependent. If we assume that the inert sensitivity of B cells to the suppressive influence of T cells is
related to such a T cell dependency of B cells, we would be
able to guess the sites of action of suppressor T cells.
Suppressor T cells given on day 0 or 2 were unable to suppress
the direct process from $B\mu$ cells to IgM-forming cells, while
being able to prevent the indirect processes from converting
into $B\mu\gamma$ and $B\mu$ cells, which perhaps take place in the early
stage of immunization. This would naturally result in the
preferential suppression of both IgG and late IgM antibody
responses. However, after the critical time of day 3, suppressor T cells preferentially inhibited the T cell dependent
part of the IgM antibody response, resulting in the rapid

termination of the antibody formation, while being unable to effectively inhibit the IgG antibody formation, probably due to the relative insensitivity of the late maturation process from Bγ cells to IgG-forming cells. The hypothetical scheme for the site of action of suppressor T cells in the differentiation process of B cells is presented in Fig. 2.

Such interpretations may also be possible for the secondary antibody response. The secondary antibody response is characterized by a quick response of greater magnitude which reflects the presence of a pool of memory B cells. Since the degree of suppression in the secondary antibody response was much less than that in the primary antibody response, a considerable part of the memory B cells may be present in a state insensitive to the suppressive influence of T cells. However, the stronger suppression of IgG antibody response than that of IgM antibody response suggests that a sufficiently overt number of memory B cells for IgG antibody response is present in a sensitive state to the suppressor T cells, which is most likely to be the Bμ memory cell. Such Bμ memory cells would either directly mature into IgM-forming cells in a T cell independent pathway or indirectly differentiate into IgG-forming cells under the influence of T cells, and this latter process may have been suppressed by primed T cells.

The observed disparity in the sensitivity between IgM and IgG antibody responses seems to accord with the widely observed preponderant effect of neonatal thymectomy on IgG rather than IgM antibody response (22-24), and to the preferential suppression of IgG antibody response caused by infection of tolerance by T cells (10, 25). It may also be related to the shift of IgM to IgG response by preimmunization with a carrier as was observed by Miller et al (26). In any event, the results now point to the selective role of T cells in the regulation of class distribution of antibodies and to the sequence of antibody formation.

Effect of suppressor T cells on antibody affinity.
Another important factor for understanding the possible role of suppressor T cells in the induction of immunological tolerance is the apparently very rigid specificity of both T and B cells for the corresponding determinants of the immunizing antigen. This strict specificity suggests that suppressor T cells somehow interfered with the processes of selection and emergence of B cells by a given antigen, resulting in the suppression of certain T cell dependent

477

populations of B cell lineage. Since anti-hapten antibodies are known to be heterogeneous with respect to their affinity for hapten, we studied what subpopulations of B cells with respect to the affinity of their receptors were selectively suppressed by carrier-specific suppressor T cells.

The effect of suppressor T cells on the avidity of antibody produced in the primary antibody response was studied by the passive administration of 5×10^7 KLH-primed thymocytes or spleen cells into recipient animals that were concomitantly immunized with 100 μg of DNP-KLH plus 10^9 pertussis vaccine. A control group of mice was not given KLH-primed cells, but was immunized by the same schedule. The relative avidity of the antibody produced by PFC was determined by the inhibition of plaque formation in the presence of 10^{-4} to 10^{-8} M ε-DNP-L-lysine (27). The percent inhibition by a given concentration of the free hapten was calculated in comparison with the number of PFC obtained without free hapten. The molar concentration of ε-DNP-L-lysine resulting in 50% reduction in the number of PFC (I_{50}) was considered to represent the variables of average avidity of the antibody produced by PFC.

In the primary antibody response the concentrations of ε-DNP-L-lysine required for 50% inhibition of both direct and indirect PFC in the KLH-primed cell recipients were much higher than those required in the control group. Since the PFC producing high avidity antibody are inhibited from lysing DNP-coupled SRBC by low concentrations of free hapten, the higher values in I_{50} in the suppressed groups indicate that suppressor T cells caused a decrease in the average avidity of anti-DNP antibodies produced by PFC.

The same decrease in avidity was observed in the secondary antibody response. In this experiment an adoptive secondary response was utilized in order to exclude the possible influence of remaining serum antibodies produced by the primary immunization. Recipient 600 R irradiated mice were reconstituted with 5×10^7 spleen cells obtained from syngeneic mice immunized one month before with 100 μg of DNP-BGG in CFA. They were further given a cell transfer of 5×10^7 KLH-primed thymocytes or spleen cells. A control group of irradiated mice was only repopulated with DNP-BGG-primed spleen cells. Within a hour after the cell transfer, all mice were immunized with 100 μg of DNP-KLH together with 10^9 pertussis vaccine to elicit an adoptive anti-DNP secondary antibody response. The numbers and average avidities of PFC

were examined on day 7 at a time when animals were producing
the highest numbers of both direct and indirect PFC.

As can be expected, the average avidities of both direct
and indirect PFC in the control animals were higher than
those in the primary antibody response, indicating that the
antibody response had matured both in IgM and IgG classes.
KLH-primed thymocytes and spleen cells produced a moderate
suppression in both direct and indirect PFC responses. The
I_{50} values of the suppressed groups were considerably higher
than those of the control unsuppressed group, indicating
that the average avidity of PFC decreased by the administration of suppressor T cells. The average avidities of the
suppressed group was no more than those of normal primary
antibody response, which indicates that suppressor T cells
caused a definite arrest of antibody maturation. The examination of antibody affinity (K_0) of pooled antiserum also
disclosed that association constants in groups given KLH-
primed T cells were much lower than those of the control
which paralleled the decrease in the avidity of PFC.

In order to learn the distribution of PFC among subpopulations of B cells with respect to their avidity, the absolute frequency of PFC detected in the presence of series of
hapten concentrations was determined, and the difference in
the number of plaques inhibited by any two ligand concentrations was calculated. It was found that direct PFC on day 3
in the control group were distributed among a wide range of
avidities, reflecting the high degree of heterogeneity of
responding B cells at this early stage. However, it was
clearly seen that the frequency of PFC in the suppressed
group that had been given KLH-primed thymocytes on day 0
tended to distribute in low avidity subgroups, indicating
that the cells producing high avidity antibody had been
preferentially suppressed. Hence, the decrease in the average avidity of PFC in suppressed groups is considered to be
due to the selective loss of PFC with high avidity and the
relatively stable level of low avidity PFC.

The effect of suppressor T cells on the avidity distribution of PFC in the adoptive secondary antibody response was
essentially similar to that observed in the primary antibody
response. While the distribution profiles of both direct
and indirect PFC in the control group showed a definite
"shift" toward the high avidity subgroups, those in the suppressed were nearly the same as in the primary antibody response. A significant difference in the frequency of PFC in

absolute terms between suppressed and unsuppressed groups was observed among high avidity subgroups: the absolute numbers of PFC among high avidity subgroups are significantly lower in the suppressed group than in the control unsuppressed group, indicating that the suppressor T cells preferentially affected the cells which had been destined to produce high avidity antibody. Since the affinity of antibody produced by a single antibody-forming cell is assumed to be identical or closely related to that of receptors of precursor B cells, the decrease in the avidity of antibody produced by PFC should result from selective suppression of B cell populations possessing high affinity receptors for antigen. The correlation between the changes in average avidity of PFC and the association constant of serum antibody (K_0) in the adoptive secondary antibody response also support this concept.

Selective roles of T cells in the antibody response.
These observations seem to be consistent with the previous finding that IgM antibody response was more severely suppressed than T cells given simultaneously with primary and secondary immunizations, inasmuch as IgG antibody generally possesses a higher affinity for hapten than does IgM antibody. It has been pointed out that T cell independent IgM antibody formation, in general, does not mature even after repeated immunization (28, 29). Thus, it is of interest to find that the IgM as well as IgG antibody response in the present system does mature and this maturation has been inhibited by suppressor T cells. These results suggest that the maturation of antibody response is dependent on the function of T cells and that such a T cell dependent process is strongly affected by suppressor T cells. As the specificity of this T cell-mediated suppression has been firmly established, it seems probable that carrier-primed T cells exert selective pressure on the precursor population of hapten-specific antibody-forming cells with respect to both the class and affinity of antibodies to be produced by the latter cell type.

Although it is not known at the present time how such selective pressure is exerted by suppressor T cells, the findings undoubtedly have some bearing on the induction and maintenance of some forms of immunological tolerance. The preferential suppression of high affinity antibody as well as the antigen-dependent arrest of differentiation of antibody-forming cell precursors are quite analogous to the fea-

tures of immunological tolerance. I feel that it is extremely important to interpret these conflicting effects of
T cells in the light of the concept of cell selection by
antigen (30). It is widely held that selection of precursor
B cells to differentiate and to synthesize antibody is primarily dependent on the effective concentration of antigen
in the micro-environment of B cells, and thus, B cells with
high affinity for antigen are more easily selected to proliferate and to expand their progeny.

However, Gershon and Paul (31) have presented evidence
using the adoptive cell transfer system that the affinity as
well as the amount of antibody depends on the nature of the
carrier molecule and on the number of T cells possessed by
the immunized animal. They postulated that T cells may function by increasing the rate of antigen-stimulated proliferation of B cells, and thus leading to more rapid changes in
the population of B cells upon which selective pressure by
antigen is being exerted. Therefore, the changes in the
affinity in their experiments are largely explained by the
increase in the rate of proliferation of B cells in the presence of adequate numbers of T cells.

On the other hand, we have reported that affinity of
produced antibody in the rabbit is influenced by the carrier-
specific T cells (16). We found that a partial depletion
of T cells by surgical or chemical thymectomy caused a marked
enhancement of antibody formation accompanied by a striking
increase in antibody affinity. Conversely, over-stimulation
of T cells by preimmunization with the carrier caused a depressed formation of anti-hapten antibodies whose affinity
was considerably lower. We interpreted these phenomena as
the consequence of T cells' regulatory function on the selection and emergence of high affinity B cells.

Possible mechanism of T cell-mediated suppression.
To delineate these phenomena, the existence of two kinds
of antigen-specific subcellular components in the rat would
seem to lend a clue. We have recently reported the presence
of antigen-specific suppressor activity in the cell-free
extract of T cells primed with carrier antigen (32, 33). I
do not intend to get into details here, but immunochemical
and physicochemical properties of this inhibitory T cell
component are shown in Table I. This soluble component was
extractable from mechanically disrupted thymocytes and spleen
cells primed with a carrier antigen (Ascaris extract) and
exerted a strong inhibitory effect on an ongoing IgE antibody

response against DNP-Ascaris protein. This component was
absorbable by immunoadsorbents composed of Ascaris protein,
indicating that it has an affinity to the immunizing antigen.
However, the component had no immunoglobulin determinants as
was revealed by absorption with various anti-immunoglobulin
antisera (32). The activity was associated with a protein
with a molecular weight range between 35,000 and 50,000
daltons (33).

On the other hand, our more recent study (34) has proven
that the same thymocytes and spleen cell extracts contain
another carrier-specific subcellular component which exerts
a definite "helper" effect in neonatally thymectomized rats,
that otherwise cannot produce anti-hapten antibodies upon
immunization with DNP-Ascaris protein. This component was
identified in all respects as a molecule similar to the IgT
reported by Dr. Feldmann in vitro (35-38). This was evidenced
by the presence of Fab and μ chain determinants in the
absorption studies, and by the comparable molecular weight
to 7S IgG (Table I).

TABLE I

PROPERTIES OF TWO DIFFERENT T CELL COMPONENTS
IN THE REGULATION OF ANTIBODY RESPONSE

	Suppressor	Helper
Specificity	Carrier	Carrier
Ig determinants	-	Fab, μ
Determinants for ATS	+	-
Molecular weight	<100,000	>100,000 <200,000
Signal	"off"	"on"
Possible nature	Receptor (?)	IgT

From these observations we are trying to analyze the suppressive and inductive effects of T cells on various antibody responses with regards to the balance and selectivity of these two subcellular components. Some affirmative evidence for the presence of the carrier-specific inhibitory component in mice has been obtained.

Taken collectively, these findings, our tentative hypothetical scheme for the selective roles of T cells in the antigen-dependent differentiation of B cells is shown in Fig. 3, a part of which was borrowed from Dr. Mitchell's review (39). In this scheme the given antigen would select B cells depending primarily on the binding affinity of B cell receptors to antigen. Some of such selected B cells would differentiate into IgM antibody-forming cells without participation of the T cell function (T cell independent antibody formation). However, the majority of B cells that were selected by antigen do not proliferate and differentiate into antibody-forming cells without the help of T cells, even if antigen-induced capping of the receptor might have occurred. The T cells' helper component (IgT) which is specific for the carrier part of the antigen would bind to the antigen that is already present on the surface of B cells and now gives rise to an "on" signal. Therefore, it is predictable that T cells' help would preferentially be given to the cells that can capture antigen more easily, the cells having high affinity receptors. In this way the rapid increase of antibody affinity following primary and secondary immunization can be explained. This interpretation does not contradict the widely held selectional theory presented by Drs. Siskind and Benacerraf (30).

On the other hand, since the suppressor molecule found in the rat system also has the specificity and affinity for the carrier molecule, it would also affect the cells which can easily bind antigen, the high affinity cell populations. In this reverse situation the high affinity cells, which were already selected by antigen, would be preferentially given the "off" signal that ultimately lead to the functional silence of B cells (tolerance). In this way the preferential suppression of high affinity cells by specific suppressor T cells would be explained.

A major point in this scheme is that the target site for suppressor or helper T cells is placed on B cells that were already "selected" by antigen. I think it is not necessary to assume that antigen, when introduced in animals,

first reacts with T cells before B cells. Since the receptors for the antigen are already present on B cells before
immunization, the reaction between antigen and B cell receptors would take place instantly after antigen injection.
Although such B cells have to await the consequence of T
cell activation which would occur concomitantly or later,
the first step may be the direct interaction of B cells with
antigen (selection). I think it is reasonable to assume that
the fate of such selected B cells to differentiate or to stop
differentiation is determined later when the T cells' inductive or inhibitory signal becomes available.

Although it is unclear how such "on" or "off" signals
are provided by IgT or the inhibitory T cell factor, as a
working hypothesis we postulate that the inhibitory T cell
component having no immunoglobulin determinants might be a
receptor of T cells as an expression of immune response (Ir)
gene. Such a receptor may be released according to the rapid
turnover of surface proteins of T cells, but under certain
conditions it would transform into IgT with the operation of
the constant heavy chain (CH) gene and would consequently
become a helper molecule. Based on the suggestion made by
Bretscher and Cohn (40), it seems to be reasonable to assume
that rearrangement or association of the receptor molecules
on the B cell surface by T cell products may be an important
factor to determine the fate of the antigen-selected B cells
as to differentiate or to become tolerant. Keeping this
assumption in mind, the inhibitory component having a molecular weight of less than 60,000, being most likely univalent,
may not be able to rearrange the receptors to give rise to
an "on" signal in B cells. In contrast, IgT, being divalent,
would act as the hypothetical "carrier antibody" of Bretscher
and Cohn or would be able to use a convenient vehicle of
macrophage to make an "on" signal on the surface of B cells
as proposed by Feldmann and Nossal (41). Alternatively,
suppressor molecules may compete with IgT for available
antigen to delete the helper effect of the latter or somehow
inactivate the activity of helper molecule by combination
with antigen. However, until futher information is available, the nature of these antigen-specific subcellular components of T cells and the way of their interaction with B
cells remain a matter of broad speculation, and I should
stop the argument.

REFERENCES

1. Baker, P.J., Stashak, P.W., Amsbaugh, D.F., Prescott, B. and Barth, R.F., J. Immunol. 105:1581, 1970.

2. Jacobson, E.B. and Herzenberg, L.A., J. Exp. Med. 135:1151, 1971.

3. Droege, W., Nature. 234:549, 1971.

4. Allison, A.C., Denman, A.M. and Barnes, R.D., Lancet. 2:135, 1971.

5. Kerbel, R.S. and Eidinger, D., Eur. J. Immunol. 2:114, 1972.

6. Gershon, R.K., Cohen, P., Hencin, R. and Leibhaber, S.A., J. Immunol. 108:586, 1972.

7. Yoshinaga, M., Yoshinaga, A. and Waksman, B.H., J. Exp. Med. 136:956, 1972.

8. Rich, R.R. and Pierce, C.W., J. Exp. Med. 137:649, 1973.

9. Katz, D.H., Paul, W.E. and Benacerraf, B., J. Immunol. 110:107, 1973.

10. Gershon, R.K. and Kondo, K., Immunology. 18:723, 1970.

11. Ha, T.Y. and Waksman, B.H., J. Immunol. 110:1290, 1973.

12. Okumura, K. and Tada, T., J. Immunol. 107:1682, 1971.

13. Okumura, K. and Tada, T., Nature (New Biol.). 245:180, 1973.

14. Tada, T., Okumura, K. and Taniguchi, M., J. Immunol. 108:1535, 1972.

15. Okumura, K., Tada, T. and Ochiai, T., Immunology. 26:257, 1974.

16. Taniguchi, M. and Tada, T., J. Exp. Med. 139:108, 1974.

17. Tada, T. and Takemori, T., J. Exp. Med. Submitted.

18. Takemori, T. and Tada, T., J. Exp. Med. Submitted.

19. Lawton, A.R., Asofsky, R., Hylton, M.B. and Cooper, M.D., J. Exp. Med. 135:277, 1972.

20. Pierce, C.W., Solliday, S.M. and Asofsky, R., J. Exp. Med. 135:698, 1972.

21. Kishimoto, T. and Ishizaka, K., J. Immunol. 109:1163, 1972.

22. Taylor, R.E. and Wortis, H.H., Nature. 220:927, 1968.

23. Sinclair, N.R.StC. and Elliott, E.W., Immunology. 15:325, 1968.

24. Mitchell, G.F., Grumet, F.C. and McDevitt, H.O., J. Exp. Med. 135:126, 1972.

25. Gershon, R.K. and Kondo, K., Immunology. 21:901, 1971.

26. Miller, J.F.A.P., Basten, A., Sprent, J. and Cheers, C., Cell. Immunol. 2:469, 1971.

27. Davie, J.M. and Paul, W.E., J. Exp. Med. 135:660, 1972.

28. Paul, W.E., Benacerraf, B., Siskind, G.W., Goidl, E.A. and Reisfeld, R.A., J. Exp. Med. 130:77, 1969.

29. Baker, P.J., Prescott, B., Stashak, P.W. and Amsbaugh, D.F., J. Immunol. 107:719, 1971.

30. Siskind, G.W. and Benacerraf, B., Advan. Immunol. 10:1, 1969.

31. Gershon, R.K. and Paul, W.E., J. Immunol. 106:872, 1971.

32. Tada, T., Okumura, K. and Taniguchi, M., J. Immunol. 111:952, 1973.

33. Okumura, K. and Tada, T., J. Immunol. 112:783, 1974.

34. Taniguchi, M. and Tada, T., J. Immunol. Submitted.

35. Feldmann, M. and Basten, A., J. Exp. Med. 136:49, 1972.

36. Feldmann, M. and Basten, A., Nature (New Biol.). 237: 13, 1972.

37. Feldmann, M. and Basten, A., J. Exp. Med. 136:737, 1972.

38. Feldmann, M., Cone, R.E. and Marchalonis, J.J., Cell. Immunol. 9:1, 1973.

39. Mitchell, G.F. In The Lymphocyte; Structure and Function, edited by J.J. Marchalonis, Marcel Dekker, Inc., New York. In press.

40. Bretscher, P. and Cohn, M., Nature. 220:444, 1968.

41. Feldmann, M. and Nossal, G.J.V., Transplant. Rev. 13: 3, 1972.

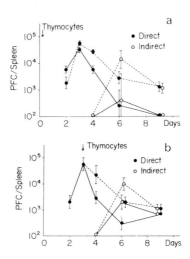

Fig. 1a and 1b. Suppressive effect of KLH-primed thymocytes on the hapten-specific PFC response in mice immunized
with DNP-KLH. The broken lines are the kinetics of PFC
response of control mice that were given BGG-primed thymocytes. Note the differential effect of suppressor T cells
on direct (closed circles) and indirect (open circles) PFC
responses primarily depending on the time of cell transfer
(arrow).

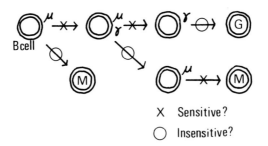

Fig. 2. Possible sites of action of suppressor T cells
in the differentiation process of B cells. The sites which
are shown to be sensitive to the suppressive influence of
T cells are apparently T cell dependent processes.

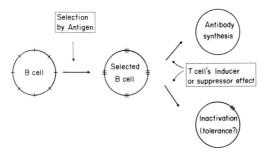

Fig. 3. A hypothetical schema for the selective roles of T cells in the antigen-induced differentiation of B cells. T cells' inductive or suppressive signals are given preferentially to the cells that have already been selected by antigen, and thus the B cells with high affinity receptors for antigen are more sensitive to the regulatory influences of T cells.

DISCUSSION FOLLOWING TOMIO TADA

WAKSMAN: I question one thing you have said, Dr. Tada. Your failure to find evidence of a diffusible mediator with a "second party" system triggered together with your test system is reminiscent of the detailed studies, more than 10 years ago, of antigenic competition by Amkraut and by Schechter. One laboratory was unable to establish competition between antigens involving two haptens on separate carriers. Yet the other investigators later showed that such competition was possible. Similarly, the first studies of cooperation implied that carrier and determinant had to be attached for cooperation to occur. Later studies achieved cooperation even when they were separate, the allogeneic effect involves such a case. I suspect that further studies will provide clear examples of this in suppression. Isn't this the basis of antigenic competition when a secondary response to one antigen suppresses the primary response to another?

TADA: I certainly agree with you that there exists non-specific suppression by antigenic competition. Although I did not mention in my presentation, the immunization with the mixture of DNP-KLH and uncoupled BGG significantly reduced the number of DNP-specific PFC, which was most likely caused by antigenic competition. However, further suppression was not produced by the passive transfer of BGG-primed T cells.

HUMPHREY: Dr. Tada, could you elaborate on how soon after immunizing with carrier you look for suppressor activity, and for how long it remains detectable?

TADA: So far, we have not looked for the time course of appearance and disappearance of suppressor T cells. We just decided to take T cells two weeks after the immunization with soluble antigen because it worked perfectly all right in the rat system.

HERZENBERG: Chuck Metzler and I have been doing some work in a very similar system to Dr. Tada's which could answer part of John's question. We have found that suppressors can be stimulated in ordinary DNP-KLH primed mice of the type we use for donors in adoptive transfer for experiments. C3H mice were primed with DNP-KLH 6 weeks prior to transfer. If these mice are boosted with aqueous

DNP-KLH or KLH three days before transfer, this IgG
anti-DNP response is suppressed. Mixture of splenic
T-cells (nylon wool) from the boosted mice with spleen
cells from 6 week-primed, unboosted donors suppresses
the normal IgG adoptive secondary response seen when
primed, unboosted donor cells are transferred alone.

GERSHON: In response to John Humphrey's question; we have
done some "parking" experiments. That is, we put suppressor T cells into B mice and studied their effects
at various subsequent intervals. We found that they
have quite a short life-span, about 3-6 weeks, very
similar to the situation with cytotoxic T cells.

I would also like to compliment Dr. Tada on his
elegant presentation. I think, however, that all his
results can be explained by T-T interactions. The B
cell functions that were lacking in the suppressor T
cell-inoculated mice were those that are most thymus-
dependent. This is the type of effect one might expect
if the active T cell component of the recipient were
reduced.

Finally, I would like to emphasize the point Dr.
Tada made, that three days after immunization the animals become refractory to suppressor effects. This
type of change with time after immunization seems to be
a generalized phenomenon in "suppressorology".

TADA: I think it is a very good point. But at the present
time, we do not have any evidence that suppressor T
cells directly knock down helper T cells. So my
tentative conclusion is that the suppression might have
been induced by the competition between helper and
suppressor molecules for the available antigen on the
"selected" B cells.

DRESSER: Can you summarize the difference between your protocol and that used by Katz and Benacerraf and their
colleagues to demonstrate a carrier or helper effect?
They look very similar, so I find it confusing that
apparently opposite results can be obtained.

TADA: The combination of T and B cells is quite the same as
that used by Drs. Katz and Benacerraf and their colleagues, since we learned it from their studies. But

491

the immunization regimen to obtain suppressor T cells is different, and also we used mostly thymocytes from primed animals. Perhaps, immunization with soluble KLH somehow caused proliferation of suppressor T cells rather than of helper T cells.

KATZ: This is an important point worth emphasizing. In our studies, we also find that soluble antigen in high doses appears to favor elicitation of suppressor cells vs. helper cells. Immunization in complete Freunds adjuvant favors precisely the reverse and alum-absorbed antigen falls somewhere in between depending on dose, timing, etc.

CLAMAN: I am somewhat worried about the use of thymocytes from mice immunized twice over a 2 week period as a source of "suppressor T cells." Such thymocytes may in fact be a "mixed bag." In the mouse, a single injection of SRBC leads, after 2-4 weeks, to the presence of in- direct PFC in the thymus. Furthermore, upon transfer to lethally irradiated mice, these "immune thymus cells" can mount an adoptive direct and indirect PFC response without added BM. Therefore, it looks as if thymus from an immunized animal may contain not only B cells but B cell precursors. Are you sure you are not transferring antibody-forming potential?

TADA: It is not likely because the suppressor effect is abrogated by the treatment with anti-θ or anti-thymo- cyte serum and complement. Therefore the observed effect was definitely caused by T cells. Furthermore, we were looking for the DNP-specific antibody response in the recipient which could not be transferred by KLH-primed thymocytes.

THE ROLE OF SUPPRESSOR T CELLS IN THE DEVELOPMENT OF LOW-DOSE PARALYSIS TO TYPE III PNEUMOCOCCAL POLYSACCARIDE

Phillip J. Baker[1], William H. Burns[2], Benjamin Prescott[3],
Philip W. Stashak[1] and Diana F. Amsbaugh[1]

Laboratory of Microbial Immunity[1]
and the Laboratory of Microbiology[3]
National Institute of Allergy and Infectious Disease and
the Laboratory of Oral Medicine[2]
National Institute of Dental Research
National Institutes of Health
Bethesda, Maryland 20014

The abbreviations used are: Ab, antibody; SSS-III, Type III pneumococcal polysaccharide; Pnc-III, formalin-treated Type III pneumococci: T cell, thymus-derived cells; B cells, bone marrow-derived precursors of Ab-forming cells; ALS, anti-mouse lymphocyte serum; ATS, anti-mouse thymocyte serum; PFC, plaque-forming cells; LDV, lactic dehydrogenase virus; i.p., intraperitoneal.

INTRODUCTION

The Ab response to SSS-III is governed by the activities of two types of T cells having opposing functions; such regulatory cells have been referred to as amplifier and suppressor T cells (1-3). The ability of ALS or ATS to increase the magnitude of the Ab response to SSS-III is due to the inactivation of suppressor T cells; these cells, in contrast to amplifier T cells, have a negative influence on the Ab response normally produced after immunization (1-3). Since suppressor T cells act primarily by limiting the extent to which clones of Ab-forming B cells proliferate in response to antigen (3), the present study was conducted to determine whether they play a role in the development of low-dose paralysis to SSS-III (4-6).

MATERIALS AND METHODS

The immunlogical properties of the SSS-III and ALS (Lot 13162) used have been described (2-4, 7-9). The SSS-III content of Pnc-III was determined by the anthrone method (10); here, SSS-III was used as a polysaccharide standard. Pooled sera from infected mice were used as the source of

LDV; the virus titer (about 10^8 ID_{50} units/ml) was determined by endpoint titration of serum lactic dehydrogenase of mice infected, 72 hours previously (11).

PFC-making Ab specific for SSS-III were detected by a modification of the technique of localized hemolysis-in-gel (4,8,9,12); student's test was used to assess the significance of the differences observed.

Female BALB/cAnN mice (8-12 weeks of age) from NIH were used in all but one of the experiments to be described. Homozygous athymic nude (nu/nu) mice and phenotypically normal thymus-bearing littermate controls (nu/+ or +/+) were provided by Dr. Norman Reed, Department of Microbiology, Montana State University (13-16).

RESULTS

Prior treatment (priming) with a single injection of a marginally immunogenic (0.001-0.005 µg), or an optimally immunogenic (0.5 µg) dose of SSS-III, greatly reduced the capacity of mice to respond to an optimally immunogenic dose of antigen, given a few days or weeks later (Table I). In comparison to controls, priming with these doses of SSS-III resulted in a 65-98% reduction in the magnitude of the PFC response to subsequently administered antigen; similar reductions (39-96%) were also noted for mice primed with equivalent amounts of Pnc-III. Such unresponsiveness, which persists for several weeks or months after priming, was termed low-dose paralysis, in contrast to the longer-lasting high-dose paralysis regularly obtained with large doses (50-100 µg) of this antigen (4,5). Low-dose paralysis has been shown to be antigen-specific (6), not mediated by Ab produced as a consequence of priming (4,5), and is first demonstrable after an inductive or latent period of 2-3 days, regardless of the dose of antigen used for priming (4,5,6). The length of the inductive period closely approximates the time required for suppressor T cells to become activated and express their inhibitory effects following immunization with SSS-III (3).

An attempt was made to induce low-dose paralysis in both athymic nude and thymus-bearing littermate control mice (Table II). In the case of thymus-bearing mice primed with 0.005 µg of SSS-III produced a 70% decrease in the PFC response to 0.5 µg of antigen, given 3 days later; priming

TABLE I

PERCENT REDUCTION IN THE MAGNITUDE OF THE PFC RESPONSE TO 0.5 μg SSS-III IN
MICE PREVIOUSLY GIVEN A SINGLE INJECTION OF DIFFERENT AMOUNTS OF SSS-III OR
TYPE III PNEUMOCOCCI (Pnc-III)

Antigen Preparation	Priming Dose (μg/mouse)	Interval Between Priming and Immunization (days)				
		2	3	7	14	25
SSS-III	0.001	96.1±1.1[a]	-	-	95.7±0.8	98.1±0.1
	0.005	-	-	-	71.6±5.1	85.9±1.8
	0.5	65.1±3.3	-	-	88.7±1.0	97.3±0.4
Pnc-III	0.001[b]	-	39.0±16.8	79.6±9.7	-	-
	0.005	-	83.8±8.6	80.5±6.4	-	-
	0.01	-	95.1±1.5	89.5±3.9	-	-
	0.05	-	96.2±1.2	86.4±7.2	-	-

[a]Mean ± s- for 6-8 similarly treated mice; unprimed control mice produced 12,900 ±x1,300 PFC/spleen 5 days after immunization with 0.5 μg SSS-III.

[b]The doses of Pfc used are expressed in terms of their polysaccharide (SSS-III) content.

with the same low dose had no significant effect upon the capacity of nude mice to respond to subsequent immunization. Since nude mice do not differ greatly from thymus-bearing controls in their ability to respond to SSS-III (Table II: 2,14,17-19) and lack both types of regulatory T cells (2), these findings suggest that functionally active T cells are required in order to induce low-dose paralysis. If this is true, one would expect treatment with ALS or LDV, which results in the extensive depletion of T cells (2,11), to reduce significantly- if not abolish- the degree of low-dose paralysis obtained; this indeed occurs.

Mice make a weak PFC response to 0.005 μg of SSS-III (Table III, Group F) and priming with this dose reduces their capacity to respond to antigen given 3 days later (A vs. B, $p < 0.05$), but much less than that of unprimed mice given ALS at the time of subsequent immunization (C vs. D, $p < 0.001$).

Infection with LDV has been reported to result in the cytotoxic degeneration of lymphocytes in the thymus-dependent area of lymph node and spleen (11). Mice infected with LDV give a normal Ab response to SSS-III (Table IV A vs.C, $p > 0.001$), infection with LDV increases the capacity to respond to subsequently administered antigen (C vs.D, $p < 0.001$); the response obtained does not differ significantly from that of mice given only 0.5 μg of SSS-III (A vs.D, $p > 0.05$) (It should be noted that since commonly used adjuvants, e.g. bacterial lipopolysaccharide, pertussis vaccine, polynucleotides and Freund's complete adjuvant as well as X-ray treatment do not increase the Ab response to SSS-III (data not shown); it is unlikely that this effect can be attributed to an adjuvant effect on the part of ALS or LDV.) ALS-induced enhancement of the Ab response to SSS-III is also reduced in mice infected with LDV (data not shown). These findings suggest again that the abrogation of low-dose paralysis may be due to the depletion of T cells, and that priming with low-doses of SSS-III, besides decreasing the capacity of mice to respond to subsequent immunization, also reduces the degree of enhancement obtained upon treatment with ALS.

TABLE II

INABILITY TO INDUCE LOW-DOSE PARALYSIS TO SSS-III IN ATHYMIC NUDE MICE

| Mice | Treatment | | PFC/spleen | Probability Value[a] |
	Priming Dose (0.005µg)	Immunizing Dose[a] (0.5µg)		
Thymus-bearing littermates	-	+	3.534 ± 0.058[b] (3,400)	
	+	+	2.991 ± 0.124 (970)	<0.01
Athymic nude	-	+	3.354 ± 0.274 (2,260)	
	+	+	3.177 ± 0.177 (1,500)	>0.05

[a] Mice were immunized 3 days after priming. 5-6 mice 5 days after immunization; geometric

[b] Log_{10} PFC/spleen $\pm$ $s_{\bar{x}}$ for 5-6 mice 5 days after immunization; geometric means are in parentheses.

[c] Student's test.

497

TABLE III

ABROGATION OF LOW-DOSE PARALYSIS TO SSS-III IN MICE GIVEN ALS AT THE TIME OF IMMUNIZATION

Group	Treatment Priming Dose (0.005µg)	Immunizing Dose[a] (0.5µg)	ALS (0.5ml)	PFC/spleen[b]
A	-	+	-	4,107+0.067 (12,800)
B	+	+	-	3,337+0.065 (2,170)
C	+	+	+	4,349+0.126 (22,300)
D	-	+	+	5,554+0.029 (384,000)
E	+	-	+	2,891+0.152 (780)
F	+	-	-	<1.488+0.301[c] (<50)

[a]Mice were given 0.5µg SSS-III, with or without ALS, 3 days after priming with 0.005 µg SSS-III.

[b]$\log_{10}$ PFC/spleen $\pm$ s $_{\bar{x}}$ for 14-15 mice 5 days after immunization; geometric means are in parentheses.

[c]No PFC were detected in 7 of 15 mice examined; a value of 1 PFC/spleen was assigned to such mice.

TABLE IV

ABROGATION OF LOW-DOSE PARALYSIS TO SSS-III IN MICE GIVEN LACTIC DEHYDROGENASE VIRUS (LDV) AT THE TIME OF IMMUNIZATION

Group	Treatment		LDV^b (0.2ml)	PFC/spleen^c
	Priming Dose (0.005µg)	Immunizing Dose (0.5 µg)		
A	-	+	-	4.100 + 0.067 (12,600)
B	-	+	+	4.232 + 0.053 (17,000)
C	+	+	-	3.152 + 0.120 (1,400)
D	+	+	+	3,890 + 0.105 (7,800)

^{a}Mice were immunized with 0.5 µg SSS-III   3 days after priming with 0.005 µg SSS-III.

$^b10^8$ infectious units/ml given i.p.

^{c}Log$_{10}$ PFC/spleen $\pm$ s$_{\bar{x}}$ for 9-10 mice, 5 days after immunization with 0.5 µg SSS-III; geometric means are in parentheses.

499

DISCUSSION

Other studies have shown that suppressor T cells, activated during the course of an Ab response to SSS-III, first begin to express their inhibitory effects three days after immunization (3); such an interval closely approximates the time required for the induction of low-dose paralysis, a phenomenon which appears to be antigen-specific and T cell dependent (4-6). Furthermore, T cells seem to be much more efficient than B cells in their ability to respond to antigen (20, 21), and suppressor T cells act primarily by limiting the extent to which Ab-forming B cells proliferate following immunization (3). In view of these considerations one may conclude that suppressor T cells can be activated by low doses of antigen; the presence of such cells at the time of subsequent immunization imposes additional restraints upon the capacity of B cells to proliferate. Thus, fewer numbers of PFC are produced in response to an optimally immunogenic dose of antigen (low-dose paralysis). Aside from this effect, priming with low doses of antigen also impairs the ability of ALS to increase the magnitude of the Ab response to SSS-III. This could be the result of the inactivation of amplifier T cells, which are required in order to obtain such enhancement (1-3). In this context suppressor T cells have been shown to inhibit the activities of other types of T cells and consequently may contribute to the development of low-zone paralysis to "helper" T cell dependent protein antigens (6, 22-24). This implies that suppressor T cells may provide a homeostatic control mechanism for limiting the clone size of cell types of lymphoid cells; the relevance of such a control mechanism to the development of lymphoid cell malignancies and autoimmune disease has been discussed (3).

Although suppressor cells may be activated by low doses of antigen, there is no information to suggest that such cells cannot be activated by large doses of antigen as well. Indeed, the ability of all--including optimally immunogenic-- doses of SSS-III to induce paralysis implies that this is the case, and that the activation of suppressor T cells may be a natural consequence of immunization. However, the inability of ALS to abrogate high-dose paralysis (data not shown) indicates that other factors may contribute to the development of unresponsiveness following the administration of supra-optimal doses of this antigen. Besides the effects produced by activated suppressor T cells and the treadmill neutralization of Ab by excess circulating antigen (25, 26),

500

high dose paralysis appears to be largely the result of a central failure of the immune mechanism in which a decrease in the rate of Ab synthesis and release is an initial step in the development of unresponsiveness by B cells (5, 8). Thus, the development of an unresponsive state appears to be an extremely complex process in which, depending on the antigen dose and experimental procedure used, several-- rather than only one--mechanisms may be involved (6).

REFERENCES

1. Baker, P.J., Stashak, P.W., Amsbaugh, D.F., Prescott, B. and Barth, R.F., J. Immunol. 105:1581, 1970.

2. Baker, P.J., Reed, N.D., Stashak, P.W., Amsbaugh, D.F. and Prescott, B., J. Exp. Med. 137:1431, 1973.

3. Baker, P.J., Stashak, P.W., Amsbaugh, D.F. and Prescott, B., J. Immunol. 122:404, 1974.

4. Baker, P.J., Stashak, P.W., Amsbaugh, D.F. and Prescott, B., Immunol. 20:469, 1971.

5. Baker, P.J., Prescott, B., Barth, R.F., Stashak, P.W. and Amsbaugh, D.F., Ann. N.Y. Acad. Sci. 181:34, 1974.

6. Baker, P.J., Stashak, P.W., Amsbaugh, C.F. and Prescott, B., J. Immunol. In press.

7. Baker, P.J. and Stashak, P.W., J. Immunol. 103:1342, 1969.

8. Baker, P.J., Stashak, P.W., Amsbaugh, D.F. and Prescott, B., Immunol. 20:481, 1971.

9. Baker, P.J., Prescott, B., Stashak, P.W. and Amsbaugh, D.F., J. Immunol. 107:719, 1971.

10. Umbreit, W.W., Burris, R.H. and Stauffer, J.F., In Manometric Techniques, Burgess Publishing Co., Minneapolis, Minn., 1964.

11. Snodgrass, M.J., Lowrey, D.S. and Hanna, M.G., Jr., J. Immunol. 108:877, 1972.

12. Baker, P.J., Stashak, P.W. and Prescott, B., Appl. Microbiol. 17:422, 1969.

13. Aden, D.P., Reed, N.D. and Jutila, J.W. Proc. Soc.Exp. Biol. Med. 140:548, 1972.

14. Manning, J.K., Reed, N.D. and Jutila, J.W. Immunol. 108: 1470, 1972.

15. Reed, N.D. and Manning, D.D., Proc. Soc. Exp. Biol. Med. 143:350, 1973.

16. Manning, D.D., Reed, N.D. and Schaffer, C. F., J. Exp. Med. 138:488 , 1973.

17. Humphrey, J.H., Parrot, D.M.V. and East, J., Immunol. 7:419, 1964.

18. Davies, A.J.S., Carter, R.L., Leuchars, E., Wallis, V. and Detrick, F.M., Immunol. 19:945, 1970.

19. Howard, J.G., Christie, G.H., Courtenay, B.M., Leuchars, E. and Davies, A.J.S. Cell Immunol. 2:614, 1971.

20. Mitchison, N.A., In Cell Interactions and Receptor Antibodies in Immune Responses, edited by, O. Makela, A. Cross and T.V. Kosunen, Academic Press, New York, p. 249, 1971.

21. Mitchison, N.A., Rajewsky, K., and Taylor, R.B., In Developmental Aspects of Antibody Formation and Structure, edited by J. Sterzl and J. Riha, Academic Publ. House, Prague, Czechoslovakia, p. 547, 1970.

22. Gershon, R.K. and Kondo, K., Immunol. 18:723, 1970.

23. Gershon, R.K., Cohen, P., Hencin, R. and Liebhaber, S.A., J. Immunol. 108:586, 1972.

24. Zembala, M. and Asherson, G.L., Nature (Lond.). 244:227, 1973.

25. Howard, J.G., Ann. N.Y. Acad. Sci. 181:18, 1971.

26. Howard, J.G., Transplant. Rev. 8:50, 1972.

ARE SUPPRESSOR CELLS RESPONSIBLE FOR TOLERANCE
TO A SOLUBLE ANTIGEN?

David W. Scott
Department of Microbiology and Immunology
Duke University Medical Center
Durham, North Carolina   27710

It has become increasingly apparent to me at this
meeting that suppressor cells must be under genetic control,
at least at two levels: 1) the animals used in the experiments and 2) the animals doing the experiments. We have
investigated the possible role that suppressor cells may play
during the induction and/or maintenance of tolerance to
ultracentrifuged soluble sheep gamma globulin (ShIgSo) in
adult rats. In our early experiments we first wanted to determine whether any activation of lymphocytes, detectable by
stimulation of DNA, RNA or protein synthesis in vitro, occurred during tolerance induction. After a single 10 mg injection of ShIgSo, no detectable stimulation of lymphocytes by
these criteria and by the VSV assay for activation of T
lymphocytes occurred (1). Furthermore, we could never detect
any inhibitory (blocking?) activity of tolerant rat serum on
lymphocyte stimulation in vitro. The ability of cells from
tolerogen-treated rats to suppress the in vitro response of
sensitized lymphocytes to antigen was also determined in co-
cultivation experiments. In these experiments "tolerant"
cells in varying numbers are mixed with a constant number of
sensitized cells which are then cultured with antigen. No
suppression of the stimulation of DNA synthesis was detectable by this assay. It should be noted that larger numbers
of either tolerant or normal lymph node cells will cause a
marked non-specific suppression, which is probably analogous
to that described by Folch and Waksman (2).

We next examined an in vivo system to detect specific
suppressor cell activity in tolerance. In this system
tolerance is induced to a carrier protein (ShIgSo) and the
animals challenged with TNP-ShIg in adjuvant (Fig. 1). The
anti-TNP response measured in terms of PFC/10^6 lymph node
cells reflects ShIg carrier function. All our data so far
say that this correlates completely with T cell unresponsiveness. An example of this is shown in Fig. 2,
which shows the waning of carrier tolerance.   Animals
challenged at various intervals after the injection of

ShIgSo showed no waning of tolerance in terms of direct and indirect PFC for at least two months. By 4-6 months a gradual decline in the degree of unresponsiveness was seen. These data agree with the waning of tolerance in the thymus previously reported by Weigle and co-workers (3). We tested for suppression in an adoptive transfer system in 600 r irradiated rats, which received either no cells, tolerant cells or equal numbers of tolerant and normal cells. Table I shows that no suppressor cell activity was evident in these recipients when we measured tolerance in terms of carrier function.

TABLE I
ADOPTIVE TRANSFER OF CARRIER TOLERANCE

Spleen Cells Transferred (2x10^8)	TNP PFC[a]/Lymph Node	TNP PFC[a]/10^6 LNC
None	133 $\pm$ 19	83 $\pm$ 44
Tolerant[b]	12,300 $\pm$ 8,460	1,784 $\pm$ 394
Normal	212,000 $\pm$ 44,000	11,745 $\pm$ 1,543
Tolerant[b]+Normal	225,625 $\pm$ 46,561	7,475 $\pm$ 1,305

[a] All rats were exposed to 600r x-irradiation and challenged 5 days later with 200 μg TNP-ShIg/CFA i.d. Direct PFC determined 7 days after challenge.

[b] Two days after 10 mg ShIgSo i.v.

Furthermore, we could not demonstrate any effects of adult splenectomy or thymectomy or both on the induction or maintenance of tolerance, using this hapten-carrier model, with either ShIgSo as the carrier tolerogen or TNBS as a hapten-specific tolerogen. In these experiments the operations were performed either days or weeks before or after tolerogen injection.

Transfer of ShIgSo or TNBS tolerant spleen or thymus cells to normal adult rats did not produce a specific suppressor effect (4). In contrast, a nonspecific inhibition of responsiveness to TNP-ShIg challenge was repeatedly observed in rats receiving <u>normal</u> lymphocytes a few days before challenge.

Finally, we have been unable to break tolerance (to ShIgSo) by transferring normal lymphoid cells to rats rendered tolerant 2 weeks to 2 months previously. This effect could be due to suppressor cells or to remaining super-tolerogen. Attempts to remove remaining tolerogen with passive antibody one week prior to cell transfer did not result in reversal of tolerance, nor did it allow normal cells to break tolerance. The failure to break tolerance with normal syngeneic cells could be due to the non-specific suppression I described above (in which normal lymphoid cells inhibit the response of normal rats). Therefore, we are presently testing the specificity of this system.

We would conclude at present time that "tolerodominant" pathway to tolerance in our system is either not through specific suppressor cells or, if caused by suppressors, they do not act at the level of hapten-carrier cell co-operation. The possibility that there are quantitative strain differences in the levels of suppressors is presently being investigated as reason for these results.

REFERENCES

1. Scott, D.W., <u>J. Immunol.</u> <u>111</u>:789, 1973.

2. Folch, H. and Waksman, B.H., <u>Cell.Immunol.</u> <u>9</u>:12, 1973.

3. Weigle, W.O., Chiller, J.M. and Habicht, G.S., <u>Transplant. Rev.</u> <u>8</u>:3, 1972.

4. Ha, T-Y., Waksman, B.H. and Treffers, H.P., <u>J. Exp. Med.</u> <u>139</u>:13, 1974.

Figure 1.

INDUCE TOLERANCE TO:	CHALLENGE	ASSAY	MEASURE FUNCTIONAL TOLERANCE IN: *
Ultracentrifuged Carrier (X)	Hapten-Carrier (H-X)	Hapten-Specific PFC	Carrier (X) Specific Helper Cells (T Cells)
Hapten-Isologous Carrier (H-Self)	Hapten-Carrier (H-X)	Hapten-Specific PFC	Hapten-Specific PFC Precursors (B Cells)

Examples:

1) Sheep gamma globulin (ShIgSo)	TNP-ShIg in CFA	TNP PFC	ShIg-Specific T Cells
2) TNP-rat gamma globulin	TNP-ShIg in CFA	TNP PFC	TNP-Specific B Cells

*Tolerance in other populations may exist but is not measured.

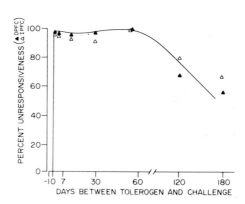

Fig. 2. Waning of carrier tolerance. Rats were injected with 10 mg ShIgSo and challenged at various times thereafter with TNP-ShIg in adjuvant. PFC (to TNP) were performed six days after challenge. The solid line is redrawn from the data of Chiller and Weigle.

STIMULATION OF SPECIFIC SUPPRESSOR T CELLS BY THE TERPOLYMER L-GLUTAMIC ACID[60]-L-ALANINE[30]-L-TYROSINE[10] IN GENETIC NONRESPONDER MICE

Baruj Benacerraf, Judith A. Kapp and Carl W. Pierce

Department of Pathology
Harvard Medical School
Boston, Massachusetts 02115

It has become increasingly apparent in the last few years that T cells play a crucial role in the regulation of immune responses (1). Thus, antigen may activate not only carrier-specific T cells capable of providing helper function for development of antibody responses of various Ig classes by B cells, but also, under the appropriate conditions, may activate T cells capable of suppressing specific immune responses (2-5). In some documented cases of specific immunological tolerance, these "suppressor T cells" appear to function by suppressing the activities of helper T cells (4), or T cells which mediate cellular immunity (5).

Studies of immune responses which are controlled by histocompatibility-linked Ir genes have demonstrated an absence of antigen specific helper T cell function and T cells concerned with cellular immunity in genetic non-responder animals (6). Although the failure of nonresponder animals to develop immune responses to an antigen, the response to which is under Ir gene control, can be attributed to this lack of specific helper T cells or T cells which mediate cellular immunity, it appeared relevant to explore whether such an an antigen could nevertheless stimulate specific suppressor T cells as originally proposed by Gershon et al (7).

In earlier studies of the immune response of inbred mice to the terpolymer L-glutamic acid[60]-L-alanine[30]-L-tyrosine[10] (GAT), we have demonstrated that antibody responses to this antigen are controlled by an Ir gene(s) which maps in the I region of the H-2 complex (8). Mice bearing $H-2^{a,b,d,f,j,k,r,u,v}$ haplotypes behaved as responders and synthesized specific antibody to GAT, whereas mice bearing $H-2^{n,p,q,s}$ haplotypes were nonresponders and developed no antibody response to GAT (9,10). Both responder and nonresponder mice, however, produced anti-GAT antibodies when immunized with GAT complexed to the immunogenic carrier methylated bovine serum albumin (MBSA), indicating the functional capacity of GAT-specific B cells in nonresponder animals.

In previous reports we have described a technique for the detection of primary GAT-specific IgG plaque-forming cell (PFC) responses in mouse spleen cell cultures (11). Analogous to the data from <u>in vivo</u> studies, spleen cells from both responder (H-2a,b,d,k) and nonresponder (H-2p,q,s) mice developed IgG PFC responses specific for GAT after incubation with GAT-MBSA, but only spleen cells from responder mice develop GAT-specific IgG PFC responses to GAT.

The antibody responses to both GAT and GAT-MBSA are T cell-dependent (12). Furthermore, spleen cells from GAT-primed, irradiated responder mice are able to provide GAT-specific helper T cell function for B cell responses to GAT, while no GAT-specific helper T cell function could be demonstrated in spleen cells from GAT-primed, nonresponder mice (12). These data suggested that the defect in genetic nonresponder mice is indeed the failure of their T cells, after interaction with GAT, to provide appropriate helper T cell function for the initiation of the B cell response to GAT. The antibody response to GAT <u>in vitro</u> provides therefore a suitable system to explore the possibility that GAT-specific suppressor T cells are present and function in nonresponder animals. Accordingly, we have investigated whether GAT could induce specific tolerance in nonresponder mice. We have observed that injection of GAT not only fails to elicit a GAT-specific PFC response in nonresponder mice, but also specifically decreases the ability of these mice to develop a GAT-specific PFC response to a subsequent challenge with GAT-MBSA (13) to which control mice respond with an excellent anti-GAT antibody response. This suppressive effect may be obtained with very small doses of GAT (0.1 µg in Maalox), is observed as early as 3 days after GAT injection and is still detectable 5 weeks after GAT administration. Injection of nonresponder DBA/1 or SJL mice with GAT also renders their spleen cells unable to develop a GAT-specific response when incubated with GAT-MBSA <u>in vitro</u>, although their response to sheep red blood cells (SRBC) is equivalent to that of spleen cells from normal DBA/1 or SJL mice (13).

A summary of some of these experiments is presented in Figure 1. On day 0, nonresponder C57Bl/6 (H-2b) and nonresponder DBA/1 (H-2q) mice were injected i.p. with 10 µg GAT in Maalox-pertussis or with Maalox-pertussis alone. On day 3, both normal control mice and the GAT-primed mice were injected i.p. with GAT-MBSA, containing 10 µg GAT, in Maalox-pertussis. All mice were sacrificed 7 days later and their spleens examined for GAT-specific IgG PFC. Pre-injection of responder C57Bl/6 mice with GAT caused no decrease in their immune responses to GAT-MBSA. However, 10 µg GAT caused a decrease in the GAT-specific immune response of nonresponder DBA/1 mice from a geometric mean of 7,800 PFC/spleen to a geometric mean of 620 PFC/spleen. (Two hundred PFC/spleen is the lowest number of PFC/spleen detectable by this assay). Although not shown, injection of Maalox-pertussis alone on day 1 caused no decrease in GAT-specific PFC responses to GAT-MBSA in either the responder or nonresponder strains of mice. Furthermore, injection of 10 µg GAT in Maalox-pertussis on day 0 did not decrease the primary immune re-sponse to SRBC injected i.p. on day 3 in either of the strains of mice (not shown). We concluded that the failure of nonresponders to develop a GAT-specific PFC response to GAT is not merely a failure to recognize GAT determinants. Quite the contrary, nonresponder mice do react to these determinants and after an encounter with GAT, nonresponder mice are less able to produce GAT-specific antibody upon immunization with GAT-MBSA.

To analyze the mechanism involved in the unresponsive-ness induced by GAT in nonresponder mice, we then investi-gated: 1) the immunocompetence of separated T and B cells from spleens of nonresponder mice previously rendered un-responsive by injection of GAT; and 2) the effects of T and B cells from unresponsive mice on the development of GAT-specific PFC responses by normal nonresponder spleen cells stimulated with GAT-MBSA (14). We have shown that B cells from nonresponder DBA/1 mice rendered unresponsive by GAT in vivo can respond in vitro to GAT-MBSA if exogenous, carrier-primed T cells are added to the cultures as shown in Figure 2. A comparison of PFC responses in spleen cell cultures from normal and GAT-primed DBA/1 mice demonstrates that just simply removing the spleen cells from the GAT tolerant mouse does not restore the ability of these cells to respond to GAT-MBSA.

Normal B cells or spleen cells from GAT-MBSA-primed, irradiated DBA/1 mice (T cells) were added to cultures of spleen cells from GAT-primed DBA/1 mice to determine the immunocompetence of B and T cells from tolerant mice. GAT-MBSA-primed irradiated T and B cells prepared by treatment of normal spleen cells with anti-Θ serum and complement, did not develop GAT-specific PFC responses when cultured separately with GAT-MBSA, but developed a GAT-specific response when cultured together with antigen showing that both populations were functional. Addition of normal B cells to the GAT-primed spleen cells failed to restore responsiveness to GAT-MBSA. Thus, the specific unresponsiveness of these spleen cells is not due merely to an inactivation or elimination of GAT-specific B cells by in vivo exposure to GAT. If that were the case, normal B cells should cooperate with carrier (MBSA)-specific T cells present in the spleen cells of GAT-primed mice and such cultures would be expected to develop a PFC response to GAT-MBSA.

Addition of 10^7 irradiated GAT-MBSA-primed helper T cells to cultures of otherwise unresponsive spleen cells from GAT-primed mice did restore the GAT-specific immune response to GAT-MBSA. Thus, B cells from unresponsive mice are not themselves unresponsive, but can be induced to develop a GAT response to GAT-MBSA provided additional MBSA helper T cells are used. We can conclude from these experiments that priming with GAT renders T cells of the nonresponder mice unable to provide adequate helper cell function for the B cell response.

We then examined spleen cells from GAT-primed nonresponder mice for the presence of active suppressor cells. Spleen cells from GAT-primed mice specifically suppressed the GAT-specific PFC response of spleen cells from normal DBA/1 mice incubated with GAT-MBSA. This suppression disappeared after pretreatment of GAT-primed spleen cells with anti-theta serum plus complement or x-irradiation, suggesting that the suppressor cell was a radiosensitive T cell. The results of these experiments are presented in Figures 3 and 4. Identification of the suppressor cells as T cells was confirmed by the demonstration (Figure 5) that the suppressor cells were confined to the fraction of lymphocytes recovered from anti-mouse immunoglobulin columns which contained most if not all of the theta-positive cells, a few contaminating B cells and a few nonimmunoglobulin-bearing cells or null cells.

Data presented in the experiments thus far have shown that the generation of suppressor T cells in nonresponder mice depends upon previous exposure to GAT. The findings that mice injected with GAT fail to respond to a subsequent challenge with GAT-MBSA, but respond normally to a subsequent injection of SRBC and that cultures containing GAT-induced suppressor cells are nevertheless able to respond to SRBC suggests, but does not prove, that the suppression is antigen-specific. Since the demonstration of suppression involves exposure to GAT-MBSA, it is possible that GAT-MBSA may be required to induce active suppressors in cultured spleen cells from mice previously primed with GAT. Therefore, the specificity of the suppressive activity must be examined by the addition of both GAT-MBSA and SRBC to cultures containing normal and GAT-primed spleen cells. Such an experiment is presented in Figure 6. All spleen cell cultures responded to SRBC and GAT-primed spleen cells did not inhibit the normal spleen cell response to SRBC. Addition of GAT-MBSA to cultures of normal spleen cells stimulated by SRBC did not inhibit the development of anti-SRBC PFC responses nor was the response inhibited if GAT-primed spleen cells were present. Therefore, the suppressor cells elicited by GAT inhibit only GAT-specific B cell responses.

The demonstration that nonresponder mice injected with GAT, the response to which is under Ir gene control, do not develop an antibody response to GAT and become specifically unresponsive to a subsequent challenge with GAT-MBSA and that this unresponsiveness is the result of an active suppressive process mediated by T cells, raises important questions concerning the mechanism of Ir gene regulation of the immune response. The first question is whether the generation of suppressor T cells in nonresponder mice is unique to this system or may be generalized to other systems and species where the response to the antigen is under the control of histocompatibility-linked Ir genes. Experiments are in progress to resolve this important issue.

What are the implications of the demonstration of GAT-specific suppressor T cells in nonresponder animals for the function of Ir genes and their products? We can offer these alternatives:

1) One could postulate that nonresponder animals develop both GAT-specific suppressor and helper T cells, but that the suppressor T cells predominate. However, we feel that this is an unlikely possibility since we have so far been unable to demonstrate GAT-specific T cell helper activity for nonresponder B cells in nonresponder animals even when we took advantage of the considerably greater sensitivity to x-irradiation of suppressor T cells compared to helper T cells. Thus, GAT-primed, irradiated nonresponder DBA/1 cells have never been able to function as GAT-specific helper T cells for nonresponder B cells in anti-GAT responses in vitro.

2) The second hypothesis is that suppressor T cells are a normal component of all immune responses, in responder and nonresponder animals, but that Ir genes determine the presence or absence of helper T cells specific ·for the antigen and are not involved in the regulation of suppressor cells. However, since GAT specifically induces suppressor T cells in nonresponders it would be necessary to postulate two separate, antigen-specific recognition systems for helper and suppressor T cells, respectively, with only the former under Ir gene control.

3) The last hypothesis and the one which we feel is the most attractive postulates that T cells have the potential of developing into helper or suppressor cells. The manner of interaction of antigen with GAT-specific T cell receptor would determine whether the cell develops as a helper or suppressor cell. In a nonresponder animal the absence of the critical Ir gene would limit the differentiation of the T cells after interaction with antigen to suppressor cells and not to helper cells or cells mediating cellular immunity.

Since suppressor T cells have been shown to be responsible for many states of specific tolerance at the T cell level (2-5), H-linked Ir genes could thus be intimately concerned with the development of tolerance or immunity. The manner in which a gene product with antigen recognition capacity in T cells could perform this function in responder and nonresponder mice is a matter for speculation. Several possible mechanisms may be involved. If the Ir gene product functions as an antigen receptor on T cells, the strength of the binding and the amount of antigen bound by different Ir gene products could account for the differences between responder and nonresponder T cells which would then result in the generation of helper versus suppressor T cells according to this interpretation. Alternatively, the Ir gene products in responders could affect the interaction of a spatially related receptor molecule on the T cell membrane with antigen. This interaction would be critical for the stimulation of helper, but not of suppressor T cells. The observations that equal numbers of thymocytes from responder and nonresponder mice bind antigens such as (T,G)-A--L (15) or GAT (16), but that only T cells from primed responder animals are able to be stimulated by (T,G)-A--L to incorporate ^{3}H-thymidine (17) is in agreement with this last hypothesis.

ACKNOWLEDGMENTS

We thank Ms. Fern DeLaCroix for excellent technical assistance and Ms. Candace Maher for secretarial help in preparation of the manuscript. This work was supported by Grant AI-09920 from the National Institutes of Health. Dr. Pierce is a recipient of a U. S. Public Health Service Research Career Development Award from the National Institute of Allergy and Infectious Diseases.

REFERENCES

1. Katz, D.H. and Benacerraf, B. Adv. Immunol. 15:1, 1972.

2. Gershon, R.K. Contemp. Topics in Immunobiol. 3:1, 1974.

3. Tada, T. and Takemori, T. J. Exp. Med. In press, 1974.

4. Basten, A. This volume.

5. Phanuphak, P., Moorehead, J.W. and Claman, H.N. J. Immunol. 112:849, 1974.

6. Benacerraf, B. and McDevitt, H.O. Science 175:273, 1972.

7. Gershon, R.K., Maurer, P.H. and Merryman, C.F. Proc. Nat. Acad. Sci. USA. 70:250, 1973.

8. Dunham, E.K., Dorf, M.E., Shreffler, D.C. and Benacerraf, B. J. Immunol. 111:1621, 1973.

9. Martin, J.W., Maurer, P.H. and Benacerraf, B. J. Immunol. 107:715, 1971.

10. Merryman, C.F. and Maurer, P.H. J. Immunol. 108:135, 1972.

11. Kapp, J.A., Pierce, C.W. and Benacerraf, B. J. Exp. Med. 138:1107, 1973.

12. Kapp, J.A., Pierce, C.W. and Benacerraf, B. J. Exp. Med. 138:1121, 1973.

13. Kapp, J.A., Pierce, C.W. and Benacerraf, B. J. Exp. Med. In press, 1974.

14. Kapp, J.A., Pierce, C.W., Schlossman, S.F. and Benacerraf, B. J. Exp. Med. In press, 1974.

15. Hämmerling, G. and McDevitt, H.O. J. Immunol. 112:1734, 1974.

16. Kennedy, J., Unanue, E.R. and Benacerraf, B. Manuscript in preparation.

17. Lonai, P. Fed. Proc. 32:993, 1973. (Abstract).

18. Schlossman, S. F. and Hudson, L. J. Immunol. 110:313, 1973.

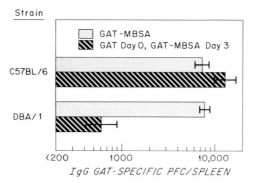

Fig. 1. Effect of GAT on responses to GAT-MBSA by responder and nonresponder mouse strains. 10 µg of GAT in Maalox and pertussis was administered i.p. on day 0 to C57Bl/6 (responder) and DBA/1 (nonresponder) mice. On day 3 GAT-MBSA containing 10 µg GAT in Maalox and pertussis was injected i.p. to these and control mice. Mice were sacrificed 7 days later and the IgG GAT-specific PFC/spleen determined. Values are geometric means of the responses of 8 to 12 mice. Brackets indicate standard error of the mean.

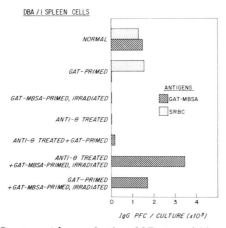

Fig. 2. Restoration of the GAT-specific response in cultures of GAT tolerant spleen cells by syngeneic, irradiated, GAT-MBSA-primed spleen cells. DBA/1 mice were immunized with 10 µg GAT in Maalox and pertussis i.p. 15 days prior to culture initiation. Mice primed with GAT-MBSA received 10 µg GAT as GAT-MBSA in Maalox and pertussis 32 days prior to x-irradiation with 800 R and culture initiation. 10^7 normal cells or cells treated with anti-Θ serum and C, 10^7 GAT-primed cells, and 10^7 GAT-MBSA-primed cells from irradiated donors were cultured separately or together as indicated. Cultures were harvested after 5 days incubation with 10^7 SRBC or 5 µg GAT as GAT-MBSA and the GAT-specific IgG PFC response/culture determined.

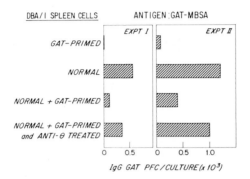

Fig. 3. Effect of spleen cells from GAT-primed animals on the PFC response of normal DBA/1 spleen cells to GAT-MBSA in vitro. GAT-primed mice received 10 µg of GAT in Maalox 3 days (experiment I) or 4 days (experiment II) prior to culture initiation. Cell numbers used, antigen dose and culture conditions are the same as those in Fig. 2.

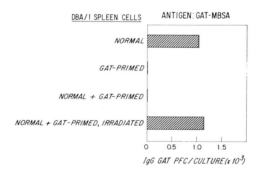

Fig. 4. Radiation sensitivity of suppressor T cells. GAT-primed mice were immunized with 10 µg GAT in Maalox 11 days before culture initiation. Cell numbers used, antigen dose and culture conditions are the same as those in Fig. 2.

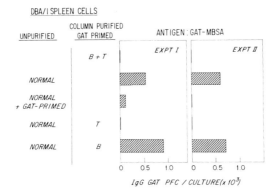

Fig. 5. Suppressive activity of column purified T cells from GAT-primed nonresponder mice. Mice were primed with 10 μg GAT in Maalox 3 days before culture initiation. Sephadex G-200 columns to which rabbit anti-mouse Fab had been conjugated were used to fractionate T and B spleen cells (as described in References 14 and 18). The cell populations were examined by immunofluorescence for Ig bearing cells with the following results: Exp. I, 85% of B cells and 0% of T cells stained for mouse Ig; Exp. II, 96% of B cells and 7% of T cells stained for mouse Ig. Cell numbers used, antigen dose and culture conditions are the same as those in Fig. 2 with the exception that 5×10^6 T and/or B cells were added to cultures as indicated.

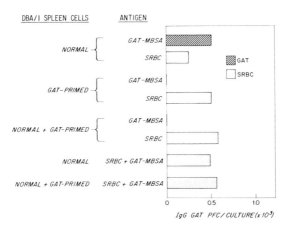

Fig. 6. Antigenic specificity of suppressor T cells stimulated by GAT in nonresponder mice. Mice were primed with 10 μg GAT in Maalox 11 days before culture initiation. Cell numbers, antigen dose and culture conditions are the same as those in Fig. 2.

MECHANISM OF ALLOTYPE SUPPRESSION IN MICE

Leonore A. Herzenberg, Charles M. Metzler

Leonard A. Herzenberg

Department of Genetics
Stanford University School of Medicine
Stanford, California 94305

Within the last year or two immunologists have begun to focus on the role of thymus-derived (T) cells as regu-lators of antibody production and the immune response in general. Previously, the few studies which demonstrated suppressive effects of T cells on antibody responses were considered either suspect or irrelevant (sometimes even by the investigators doing the studies). Now, however, the number of well-documented instances of T cell suppression has increased to the point where it is becoming necessary to determine not whether, but how, suppressor T cells interact with B cells and cooperator T cells in response to antigen. (See articles in this volume.)

We have been working with a system in which we can generate a T cell population in a hybrid mouse which suppresses production of γG_{2a} immunoglobulins carrying one of the two parental allotypes (reviewed in 1). This system is rather special in that we have thus far been able to demonstrate the suppressor cells in only one hybrid, SJL x BALB/c. Nonetheless, the information on the characteristics of suppressor cells and the methodology for working with them which we have gained with these studies have made this system a useful model for suppression studies in addition to its intrinsic value.

Generally, we use progeny from the cross of SJL male x BALB/c female mice and study suppression of the paternal (Ig-1b) allotype which is carried on γG_{2a} globulins. Sup-pressed mice are obtained either by exposing very young hybrids (0-3 weeks) to anti-Ig-1b allotype anti-serum (primary suppression) or by transfer of lymphoid tissue from primary suppressed mice to two-week old normal F_1's (secondary suppression).

The suppression is an active (or dominant) phenomenon, i.e. lymphocytes from suppressed animals suppress Ig-1b production by normal spleen cells. It may be measured in mixture-transfer experiments where lymphocytes from suppressed donors are mixed with spleen cells from normal syngeneic donors and transferred to irradiated recipients. Decrease of either Ig-1b antibody-forming cells (Ig-1b anti-DNP-PFC) or serum Ig-1b level have been used as indices for suppression.

The age of onset and extent of suppression is variable in primary suppressed mice (i.e., those exposed to maternal antibody). Basically, there are three categories into which these mice fall. A few percent never initiate production of Ig-1b. Most do produce some allotype between three and five months of age but cease production before six months. The allotype levels in these mice generally remain below detectability after six months, although a small proportion of mice "break" suppression and produce Ig-1b, usually at a low level and for a short period of time. The remainder of exposed mice show allotype levels similar to the second group as young adults, but the allotype production does not become completely suppressed at six months of age. Many of these latter mice are partially suppressed in that their allotype production maintains at a low level throughout life.

(Donor mice for transfer experiments are taken from either of the first two categories and tested for serum Ig-1b levels just before transfer to be certain of complete suppression.)

The mechanism for partial suppression has not been studied directly as yet, although it may represent a good vehicle for determining whether the allotype suppressor T cell functions as a regulator of immunoglobulin synthesis. Data presented below from titration studies with suppressor cells taken from fully suppressed donors suggest this may be the case. However, the picture is more complicated in that the intensity of the suppression appears to be related not only to suppressor dose but to the balance of activities between suppressor and cooperator populations.

The data in Figs. 1 and 2 show that the intensity of suppression is correlated with the dose of suppressor lymphoid tissue. In Fig. 1 the serum Ig-1b levels of normal F1's given varying numbers of suppressor spleen cells at two weeks is presented as a function of age of animals. Those mice receiving the largest cell dose (1.5×10^7) are completely suppressed. More than 90% never produce any detectable Ig-1b. Those receiving an intermediate dose (5×10^6) produce Ig-1b but remain partially suppressed throughout life. While they never cease allotype production entirely, their serum levels always stay below normal. Those mice receiving the lowest cell dose (10^6) show serum levels which are roughly within normal range. (A non-injected control group was not included with this particular experiment.)

In Fig. 2 Ig-1b levels are given as a function of time after transfer of mixtures of a constant number of normal F_1 cells with varying numbers of cells from spleens of suppressed F_1's. With no suppressor cells added, the normal cells establish Ig-1b production and serum levels remain high throughout the life of the recipient. When the mice receive suppressor cells in addition to normal cells, there is an initial burst of allotype synthesis followed by a fall in serum allotype level. The final level obtained is progressively lower as the suppressor dose increases. Thus, in both cases, the intensity of suppression depends on the size of the suppressor population in a given animal.

Indications that "cooperating" T cells also play a role in determining the intensity of suppression come from studies with suppression of production of antibody marked with Ig-1b allotype (Ig-1b anti-DNP) in a hapten-carrier system. These show that there is a marked antagonism between suppressors and cooperators such that either increasing the number of cooperators or decreasing the number of suppressors will result in a greater Ig-1b anti-DNP-PFC response. (2)

The data in Table I show that the Ig-1b adoptive secondary response to the DNP-KLH is completely suppressed by 10^7 cells from suppressed spleen. In this experiment 1.2×10^7 DNP-KLH-primed normal spleen cells were mixed with varying doses of unprimed suppressor cells and transferred to irradiated (600 R) BALB/c animals. Recipients were challenged with DNP-KLH on day 1 after transfer and sacrificed for estimation of PFC on day 7. As the data in the table show, the lowest dose of suppressed spleen had no affect on the Ig-1b Pfc response, intermediate doses partially suppressed, and the highest dose suppressed completely.

TABLE I

SUPPRESSION OF Ig-1b ANTI-DNP RESPONSE

DNP-KLH 1° Normal Spleen x 10⁶	Unprimed Spleen		PFC/10⁶		
	Normal x 10⁶	Suppressed x 10⁶	Direct	Ig-1a +Ig-4a	Ig-1b
12	10	–	34	3800	400
12		1.1	29	4300	410
12		3.3	40	3300	170
12		6.7	40	2300	120
12		10	42	3300	17

100 μg alum-pptd DNP-KLH + 2×10^9 B. pertussis injected i.p. 1-3 months prior to transfer.

10 μg DNP-KLH boost i.v. 1 day after transfer.

Donors: (SJL x BALB/c)F₁; recipients BALB/c irradiated (600R) ~18 hours prior to transfer.

To examine the interaction between suppressors and cooperators, we moved to a heterologous hapten-carrier system so that cooperator dose could be varied. DNP-KLH-primed normal F_1 spleen was used as the source of DNP-primed B cells. Ovalbumin-primed normal F_1 spleen was used as the source of cooperators. Spleens from suppressed F1 mice (as above) provided the source of suppressor cells. Irradiated (600 R) BALB/c recipients were challenged one day after transfer with DNP-ovalbumin. PFC were measured on day 7 as before.

Two separate experiments with the heterologous hapten-carrier system are presented in Table II (in each case three doses of carrier-primed spleen was used). As the data shows, when no suppressor cells were added, the number of Ig-1b PFC increases with increasing numbers of cooperators. Formation of these PFC is completely suppressed, regardless of cooperator dose, when transferred recipients also received a large number of suppressor cells. Suppression is partially reversed, however, in recipients of smaller numbers of suppressor cells and larger numbers of cooperators.

Thus, the extent of suppression of Ig-1b PFC anti-DNP appears to depend on the balance between the activity of carrier-primed T-cooperator population and the activity of the suppressor population. In the presence of suppressors, more cooperators are needed to achieve a PFC response of a given level. Similarly, in the presence of larger numbers of cooperators, more suppressors are needed to achieve a given level of suppression.

The mechanism of the suppressor-cooperator antagonism is difficult to infer from these types of experiments. These data could equally well be interpreted as fitting either a model which postulates a competition between suppressor and cooperator for a site on a DNP antibody-forming cell precursor or a model which sees the suppressor as acting on the B cell after or before the cooperator has started it on the road to antibody production. In the latter case, the antagonism would depend on increasing numbers of cooperators "turning on" increasing numbers of B cells, therefore, requiring more suppressors for equivalent suppression. Another model which fits the data would postulate a direct T-T interaction prior to B cell stimulation. Whatever the case, it is clear that any mechanism for suppression must take into account the cooperator-suppressor antagonism.

TABLE II

ANTAGONISM BETWEEN SUPPRESSOR

AND COOPERATOR T CELLS

	Unprimed Suppressed Spleen (x 10^6)	Ovalbumin (Carrier) 1^0 Normal Spleen * (x 10^6)		
		1	3	10
Expt. 1	0 **	23	72	246
	1	0	0	64
	3	0	0	0
		2.7	8	24
Expt. 2	0	80	290	330
	1.6	0	45	50
	4	0	0	0

* All animals received 12 x 10^6 hapten-primed (DNP-KLH) spleen cells together with carrier-primed spleen and unprimed suppressed spleen as indicated. Carrier-primed animals received 100 μg alum precipitated ovalbumin i.p. 4 to 8 weeks before transfer. Hapten primed animals: See legend for Table I. Recipients (600 R) irradiated BALB/c were boosted with 10 μg DNP-ovalbumin 1 day after transfer.

** 0 means <5 ppm.

There is another aspect of suppression, not necessarily directly related to the suppressor cooperator antagonism, which I would like to bring up at this point. Suppressor T cells are found in all lymphoid tissues of the mouse, even thymus and bone marrow. Localization of suppressors in these latter tissues raise interesting questions with respect to what is known about the overall distribution of T cells in the tissues.

With respect to thymus it is not unreasonable to ask how the suppressor cells get there. As data in Table III shows, 10^7 thymocytes suppress about as well as 10^7 spleen cells. (Parathymic nodes were removed.) Since the thymus is thought of as primarily an exporter of T cells and since cells with immunologic memory are seldom found in the thymus, the existence of specific suppressor activity is unexpected.

The finding of suppressor activity in the bone marrow is even more surprising considering the notoriously low T cell content of bone marrow. It has been shown to be sensitive to anti-Thy-1 treatment (1) and therefore, meets the standard criterion for a T cell. Quantitatively, the activity of bone marrow is about equal to suppressor activity of spleen suggesting that the few T cells in bone marrow are highly enriched for suppressors.

To test for this enrichment directly, we isolated T cells from bone marrow and spleen by nylon wool passage and compared their activity. As the data in Table IV show, the suppressor activity per T cell is roughly the same (or slightly greater) in the original tissue and the isolated T population. However, the bone marrow T cell population has considerably more suppressive activity per T cell than the splenic T cell population (e.g. compare 4×10^3 T cells isolated from bone marrow with 6.4×10^5 T cells isolated from spleen).

It is not clear why bone marrow T should be enriched for suppressor activity. It may be that suppressor cells home to the bone marrow because of the presence of large numbers of Ig-1b precursors. It may also be that the high suppressor activity in bone marrow represents not so much a homing phenomenon as the absence of other T cell types (e.g. GVH precursors) which may be selectively excluded from bone marrow. Neither of these explanations is particularly satisfactory, and I raise the question here in the hope of stimulating discussion which could lead to some experiments which might help to explain this finding.

TABLE III

SUPPRESSOR CELLS IN LYMPHOID TISSUES

Normal Donor		Suppressed Donor	No. of	Ig-1b levels (mg/ml) weeks after transfer					
Spleen	Tissue	No. of Cells Transferred	Recip.	1	2	3	4	6	8
10^7	-	-	3	.24	>.38	>.5	>.5	>.5	>.5
"	Spleen	10^7	4	<.04	.01	<.01	<.01	<.01	<.01
"	=	10^6	4	.4	.13	<.03	<.01	.02	.04
"	Thymus	10^7	4	.02	<.01	<.01	<.01	<.01	<.01
"	=	10^6	4	>.3	>.3	>.32	.12	.15	.08

See legend for Figure 2 for details of transfer.

TABLE IV

SUPPRESSOR T CELLS IN SPLEEN AND BONE MARROW

Normal (SJL x BALB/c) Spleen	Suppressed[1] (SJL x BALB/c) Tissue	Treatment[2]	# of cells transferred Total (x 10⁶)	T-cell content[3] (x 10⁶)	No. of Recip.	Mean Serum Ig-1b (mg/ml)[5] weeks after transfer						
						1	2	3	4	6	8	10
1.2×10^7	—	—	—	—	4	>.5	>.5	>.5	>.5	>.5	>.5	>.5
"	spleen	—	10	2.3	4	>.2	.1	—	—	—	—	—
"	"	nylon	4	3.2	3	.1	.05	—	—	—	—	—
"	"	—	3	0.7	4	.1	.1	.09	<.05	—	—	—
"	"	nylon	0.8	0.64	4	>.4	>.5	>.5	>.4	.06	<.07	<.04
"	bone marrow	—	9	0.05	4	.2	.1	.08	<.05	—	—	—
"	"	nylon	1	0.05	4	>.2	>.3	.1	—	—	—	—
"	"	—	1.3	0.006	4	>.4	>.4	>.5	.1	<.08	<.04	—
"	"	nylon	0.1	0.004	4	>.2	>.3	>.2	.1	—	<.05	—

1 Donors were SJL x BALB/c hybrids over 6 months of age exposed perinatally to maternal anti-Ig-1b.
2 Treated cell suspension passed through nylon wool to remove B cells.
3 T cell content determined by fluorescent staining.
4 Recipients were 600 R irradiated BALB/c mice.
5 Ig-1b levels determined by immunodiffusion. (-) = <0.01 mg/ml serum.

ACKNOWLEDGMENTS

This work was supported by N.I.H. grants HD-02187-12 and CA-04681-15.

The present address of Dr. Charles M. Metzler is at the Department of Pathology, Yale University School of Medicine, New Haven, Connecticut, 06150.

REFERENCES

1. Herzenberg, L.A. and Herzenberg, L.A, In <u>Contemporary Topics in Immunobiology</u>, Volume 3, edited by M.D. Cooper and N.L. Warner, Plenum Press, New York, p. 41, 1974.

2. Metzler, C.M. and Herzenberg, L.A., in preparation.

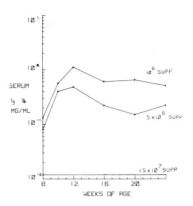

Fig. 1. Transfer of suppressor cells to young syngeneic F_1 mice. Donors of spleen cells were completely suppressed SJL x BALB/c F_1 mice over 6 months of age exposed perinatally to maternal anti-Ig-1b. Recipients were 2 week old normal SJL x BALB/c F_1 mice. Cells were injected i.p. Recipients were not irradiated. Ig-1b levels in serum were determined by radioimmune assay.

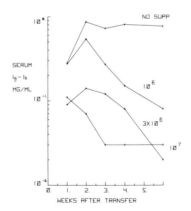

Fig. 2. Dose dependence of suppression in mixture-transfer assay. Recipients are 600 R irradiated BALB/c mice. All recipients receive 1.2×10^7 normal F_1 cells in addition to graded numbers of spleen cells from suppressed donors, i.e. SJL x BALB/c F_1 mice over 6 months of age exposed peri-natally to maternal anti-Ig-1b. Cell suspensions were mixed immediately prior to transfer. Serum Ig-1b level determined by radioimmune assay.

REMARKS ON ALLOTYPE SUPPRESSION IN RABBITS

Rose G. Mage

Laboratory of Immunology
National Institute of Allergy and Infectious Diseases
National Institutes of Health
Bethesda, Maryland 20014

INTRODUCTION

Since a recent review of allotype suppression is available (1), I shall try to concentrate in this discussion on what we know about the induction and maintenance of the suppressed state in rabbits and to compare and contrast the rabbit and mouse models. The work of Herzenberg and co-workers (2 and this volume) clearly indicates that in SJL x BALB/c F1 mice, active suppression of the paternal Ig-1b allotype occurs via specific suppressor T cells. I know of no direct evidence that this is the mechanism for the maintenance of the chronic suppressed state in rabbits.

COMPARISONS OF THE SUPPRESSION PHENOMENON IN MICE AND RABBITS

Compensation.

The allotype which is suppressed in the SJL x BALB/c mice, (Ig-1b in Herzenberg's nomenclature (2); MuA2 in Cinader's nomenclature (3); "unassigned 2" in the Lieberman and Potter nomenclature (4)) is believed to reflect antigenic determinants present on the Fc portion of one sub-class of IgG. Lieberman and Potter have not assigned the "2" marker to a heavy chain sub-class since myeloma proteins carrying this specificity are not yet available. Thus, it is not firmly established that the Ig-1b or "2" is the true allelic form of Ig-1a or $G^{1,6,7,8}$ (4). In Ig-1b suppressed mice compensatory increases in the amounts of the BALB/c Ig-1a allotype are not observed, but it is conceivable that it is not the alternative allelic form. In rabbits the allotypic markers which have classically been studied (5) are on kappa-type light chains or on the variable portion of heavy chains (6). Heterozygous rabbits at the a and b loci compensate by production of the alternative "allelic" form so that IgG levels in the suppressed rabbits are indistinguishable from normal. It should be noted that the alternative forms of a and b allotypic markers in rabbits may not be simple alleles either. If total suppression of kappa-type light chain is achieved in homozygotes at the b locus,

there is compensatory production of lambda-type light chains.
The lambda and kappa-type light chains are controlled by the
c and b loci which are not closely linked. In contrast to
this compensation by the product of an unlinked locus, total
suppression of a allotype expression results in increased
expression of V_H regions with distinct allotypic markers
such as x32 and y33 controlled by genes closely linked to
the a locus (4). The increased production of these V_H
forms, which are normally expressed in low concentrations,
leads to total IgG concentrations which are essentially
normal (1).

$C\gamma$ markers.

A chronic form of suppression has not yet been observed
for markers on the Fc (A14 and A15) (7, 8) or hinge region
(A11) (9) of rabbit IgG. Some delay in attainment of adult
levels of paternal Fc allotype may occur similar to that
observed when allotype suppression is attempted with mouse
strains other than the SJL x BALB/c (10). It is probable
that an initial step in the establishment of chronic allotype suppression in rabbits is the interaction of anti-allotype antibody with the allotype as it exists on membrane-
bound immunoglobulin of B cell precursors. Such potential
target cells are present in the peripheral blood, spleens
and appendixes of newborn rabbits (11). If the virgin B
cells in neonatal rabbits do not express γ chains on their
surface, appropriate targets for suppressing antibody may
not be present. The allotypic markers which have been successfully suppressed in rabbits would be present on membrane-
associated as well as circulating IgM.

Transient expression.

In SJL x BALB/c mice suppressed for expression of the
Ig-1b allotype, there are occasional bursts of re-expression
followed by apparent complete suppression again (3, 12).
The only similar observation in rabbits is illustrated in
Fig. 1. If we examine total IgG and allotype concentrations,
we observe that once some suppressed allotype is being produced, fluctuations in total IgG levels are mirrored by
fluctuations in total levels of the suppressed allotype.
The proportion of suppressed allotype expressed as a percentage of the IgG concentration always rises with time and
never decreases significantly. We have never observed re-
version to total nonexpression of the suppressed allotype
in the very large numbers of suppressed rabbits we have
examined during the last 10 years.

Cell surface Ig with suppressed allotype.

In the rabbit we have correlated the escape from total suppression with the appearance of lymphocytes bearing membrane-associated immunoglobulin with the suppressed allotype (11, 13). After a period of total absence of lymphoid cells with detectable membrane Ig of the suppressed allotype (11, 13), there is a period during which increasing proportions of Ig-bearing cells with suppressed type are observed. Although these cells may be the potential precursors of Ig-producing cells, the percentage of serum IgG with suppressed allotype remains disproportionately depressed. It is during this period when potential precursors may be present that it is particularly tempting to invoke a suppressor cell with an active regulatory role. However, as mentioned earlier, we have no direct evidence for the existence of such a cell. The fact that these cells do not appear to lead to productive B cells in proportion to their frequency suggests that they may be functionally different from the normal Ig-bearing B cell of adult rabbits. Indeed, their proliferative responses to anti-b5 antiserum are markedly subnormal both as judged by blast transformation and by DNA synthesis (14). Similar observations were reported by Sell in 1968 for cells of suppressed heterozygotes (15). There may be some intrinsic block in their capacity to differentiate, or they may simply represent virgin B cells which do not compete effectively with the large numbers of lambda-bearing memory cells which have undoubtedly been established in these animals.

Release from allotype suppression.

In the mouse model it has recently been reported that allogeneic thymus cells abrogate the suppression (3). It will be of considerable interest to learn if elicitation of a graft versus host reaction can produce such a striking result in rabbits. Release from allotype suppression in vitro has recently been reported by Louise Adler (16). In her system spleen cells from b4-suppressed heterozygous rabbits gave primary in vitro responses to T2 phage which were of the maternal allotype, indicating that the mechanism for allotype suppression and compensatory production of the alternate allotype in vivo continued to operate in culture. Release from suppression was observed when a concentration of antibody to the maternal type which partially suppressed the maternal response was added to cultures. We will need more complete information about the system before this important new observation of release can be interpreted in terms of mechanisms. Introduction of the suppressed antigen alone, either in vitro (16) or in vivo (17), does not abrogate suppression. It is only during the early initiation stages of allotype suppression in rabbits that introduction of sufficient quantities of antigen of the suppressed type can halt the establishment of the chronic suppressed state (9, 18). We have interpreted the neutralization of suppression during neonatal development to simply indicate that the continued presence of suppressing antibody in the milieu of differentiating target cells is required. The mechanism by which immunoglobulin precursors are prevented from re-emerging during chronic allotype suppression appears to clearly differ from that operating during the initiation stages in both the mouse and rabbit models. The levels of expression during "escape" and in partially neutralized rabbits (9, 18) indicate to me that the final level of expression of a suppressed allotype in rabbits may well represent the net result of a variety of antagonistic suppressive and stimulatory cells and/or mediators which are those that normally govern the differentiation and clonal expansion of B cells.

REFERENCES

1. Mage, R.G., In Current Topics in Microbiology and Immunology, edited by N. Jerne, Springer-Verlag, Heidelberg, 63:131, 1974.

2. Herzenberg, L.A., Chan, E.L., Ravitch, M.M., Riblet, R.J. and Herzenberg, L.A., J. Exp. Med. 137:1311, 1973.

3. Cinader, B., Koh, S.W. and Kuksin, P., Cell. Immunol. 11:170, 1974.

4. Mage, R., Lieberman, R., Potter, M. and Terry, W.D., In The Antigens, edited by M. Seal, Academic Press, N.Y., p. 299-376, 1973.

5. Dray, S., Nature. 195:677, 1962.

6. Mage, R.G., Young, G.O. and Dray, S., J. Immunol. 98: 502, 1967.

7. Mage, R.G., Annals N.Y. Acad. Sci. 190:203, 1971.

8. Mage, R.G., Federation Proceedings. In press.

9. Lowe, J.A., Cross, L.M. and Catty, D., Immunol. 25:367, 1973.

10. Herzenberg, L.A., Herzenberg, L.A., Goodlin, R.C. and Rivera, E.C., J. Exp. Med. 126:701, 1967.

11. Harrison, M.R. and Mage, R.G., J. Exp. Med. 138:764, 1973.

12. Jacobson, E.B. and Herzenberg, L.A., J. Exp. Med. 135:1151, 1972.

13. Harrison, M.A., Mage, R.G. and Davie, J.M., J. Exp. Med. 137:254, 1973.

14. Harrison, M.R., Elfenbein, G.J. and Mage, R.G., Cell. Immunol. 11:231, 1974.

15. Sell, S., J. Exp. Med. 128:341, 1968.

16. Adler, L.T., Fed. Proc. 33:808, 1974 (abstr. 3398).

17. Dubiski, S. and Fradette, K., Proc. Soc. Exp. Biol. Med. 122:126, 1966.

18. Young-Cooper, G.O. and Mage, R.G., Immunol. In press, 1974.

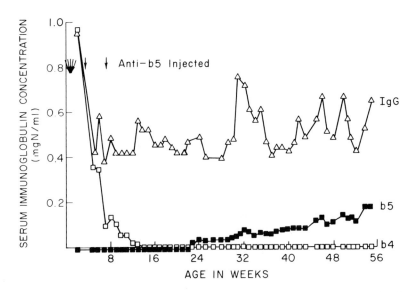

Fig. 1. The serum immunoglobulin concentrations during the first year of life of a homozygous b5 rabbit. The animal received approximately 16 mg of anti-b5 antibody protein in five injections during the first week, 8.5 mg on day 24 and 4.2 mg on day 52. During the escape period fluctuations in the concentrations of the suppressed allotype mirror fluctuations in total IgG levels.

GENERAL DISCUSSION - SESSION V

ACTIVITY OF SUPPRESSOR CELLS AS A MECHANISM OF TOLERANCE

Byron Waksman, Chairman

MITCHELL: Mage and Herzenberg both mentioned Cinader's evidence that a GVH reaction breaks allotype suppression. Can we hear Cinader's data to enable us to assess whether this is simply an increase of Ig-1b above a certain level of detectability which is mirrowed by a comparable increase in the amount of Ig-4b for example?

CINADER: The GVH reaction increases the IgM levels and IgG levels of normal hybrid mice. In suppressed animals it results in a more dramatic increase and, finally in normal values of circulating allotype concentrations. The now suppressed allotype is increased as in a normal animal. The GVH effect is thus not allotype specific--unlike the suppressor effect. There is a cyclic (diphasic) variation with time of allotype concentration in suppressed GVH animals which might be interpreted as a consequence of the persistence of suppressor cells (Cell Immunology. 11: 170, 1974)

BRITTON: Is it conceivable to summarize this morning's session on suppressor T-cells that their action is either specific or non-specific, that their activity is either directed against themselves, against other T-cells or against B-cells and that their activity can be overcome by the mere injection of an immunizing dose of a different antigen, making them completely unimportant for the important issue; namely, maintenance of self-tolerance?

GERSHON: Sven's question can be answered quite succinctly-- No! Because something is hard to demonstrate experimentally, does not mean that under physiological conditions it is not playing an important role.

WAKSMAN: Rather than leave the discussion at this point, let me take a moment to illustrate the fact, established by Folch in several recent papers, that splenic suppressor cells in several systems are adherent to glass wool. I showed earlier a slide demonstrating that when spleen cells are stimulated with increasing doses of conanavalin A, there is marked suppression of DNA synthesis without any visible reduction of early RNA or protein synthesis.

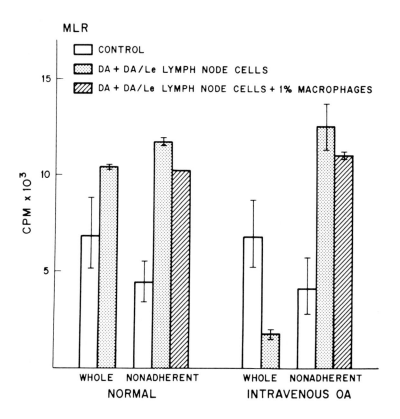

Figure 3: Five day MLR obtained with mixtures of DA and DA/Le lymph node cells. The reaction is suppressed with cells from an animal given 100 mg. ovalbumin 24 hours earlier, but this suppressor effect is removed by passing the test cells through glass wool. From Bash, J. and Waksman, B.H. In preparation.

In this slide (Fig. 3), you see the suppression of mixed lymphocyte reactivity in spleen cells from a rat given a massive dose of i.v. ovalbumin 24 hours earlier. Removal of glass wool-adherent cells restores

the remaining cells (about 50% of the total) to a normal level of responsiveness (Bash and Waksman, unpublished). The significant cell in this system is not
the macrophage, since readdition of normal or activated
macrophages does not restore the suppressor effect.

The demonstration that our "weakly adherent" cell
is a T-cell is shown in Fig. 4. Mitomycin-C-treated
whole spleen cells suppress the PHA response of non-
adherent cells, but fail to do so if obtained from a
doubly thymus-deprived donor (Folch and Waksman, J. Immunology, in press). Please remember that the use of
anti-Θ and similar markers is validated by tests in
similarly deprived mice. We feel therefore, that this
is an acceptable preliminary demonstration of the point.

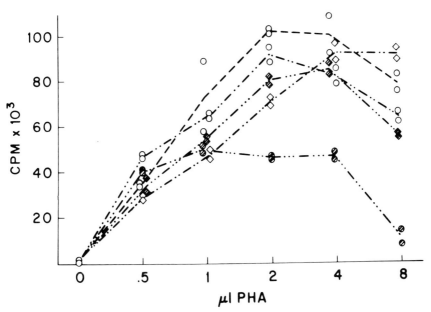

Figure 4. Dose-response curve with PHA and cell mixtures
containing 2x10⁶ nonadherent (glass wool-passed) DA
rat spleen cells plus 2x10⁶ mitomycin C-treated additional cells as follows: O---, none; O-..-.., non-
adherent normal spleen; ⊘-...-..., whole normal spleen;
◇-..-.., nonadherent spleen from thymus-deprived donor;
◆-...-..., whole spleen from same donor. From Folch,
H. and Waksman, B.H. J. Immunology. In press.

SUPPRESSIVE ACTIVITY OF ANTIBODY AND ANTIGEN-ANTIBODY COMPLEXES

BERNHARD CINADER, CHAIRMAN

IS THERE A UNIFYING CONCEPT FOR DIVERSE MODELS OF TOLERANCE INDUCTION?

Erwin Diener

The MRC Transplantation Group and
the Department of Immunology
The University of Alberta, Edmonton, Alberta, Canada

INTRODUCTION

Reviewing the contents of various symposia held over the past years on immunological tolerance reveals the fact that most of what we know about the subject is still phenomenological in nature. Attempts to extrapolate from a multitude of parameters drawn from in vivo experiments has led to a number of theories on cellular mechanisms of tolerance induction which have many important aspects in common but which also often contradict each other. We must agree that the enigma of the mechanisms underlying tolerance can only become unraveled by studies carried out at the level of the immunocompetent cell. Fortunately, tissue culture techniques have provided us with a very powerful tool to take the single lymphocyte to task about its means of communicating with an environment that can be maintained within a high degree of uniformity in terms of antigen concentration. Unfortunately, an in vitro milieu is not necessarily analogous to in vivo conditions, a possibility which demands careful interpretation of data. We, nevertheless, can assume that any reaction an immunocompetent cell is induced to display in vitro may potentially also occur in vivo; it is up to the experimentor to verify the presence or absence in the animal of environmental conditions to which he exposes the cells in the test tube.

I shall attempt in this presentation to compile some of the key findings from in vitro studies on tolerance induction and to discuss them in the light of what we know about tolerance in vivo. It is hoped that we will be able to delineate two major aspects of the tolerance phenomenon: First, the environmental aspects in the animal's lymphoid system that mediate tolerance, and second, the tolerance induction mechanisms at the level of immunocompetent cell. The mediating mechanisms may be many fold and quite different depending on the type of tolerance we look at (i.e. high-zone tolerance, low-zone tolerance, tolerance mediated by suppressor cells and by antigen-antibody complexes). The question is: Do the various mechanisms merge into a common path of action? Perhaps I may convince you that they do, provided the following assumption is made: Both immunity and tolerance induction have qualitatively the same triggering signal in common which is mediated by each individual antigen specific receptor. It is the sum total of such signals per immunocompetent cell that decides whether tolerance or immunity is induced.

IN VIVO MECHANISMS THAT MEDIATE TOLERANCE

Structural components.

It is uniformly accepted that the reticuloendothelial system (RES) plays a regulatory role in the immune performance of an animal. Its function of antagonizing tolerance induction is well known and has been the subject of extensive discussion in a previous Brook Lodge meeting (1). An antigen which is presented in such a form that it readily and rapidly stimulates the RES is less likely to be tolerogenic, hence, the ease with which tolerance may be induced in newborn animals where phagocytosis is minimal and antigen may freely diffuse through the tissue (2). An interesting genetic aspect of the phenomenon has recently been reported by Das and Leskowitz (3) who showed that the degree of susceptibility to tolerance induction correlates with a mouse strain's capacity for phagocytosis. But are there aspects of the RES apparatus which provoke tolerance--rather than immune induction? Some time ago Ada and Parish (4) suggested such a role may be played by the lymphoid follicles of lymph node cortex and the splenic white pulp. Here, antigen is retained by adhering to cell surface membranes rather than be being phagocytosed. Antigen in such follicles, if present in a high enough local concentration, could initiate tolerance as lymphocytes pass by. According to this interpretation, the immunological state of an animal at a given point in time after administration of antigen is a reflection of antigen distribution between two anatomical sites; within macrophages on one hand and in lymphoid follicles on the other. Since lymphoid follicles are the sites of the B cell rather than the T cell compartment, this mechanism would primarily account for B cell tolerance. The attractiveness of the hypothesis lies in the fact that it has introduced the possibility that a surface-bound matrix of antigenic epitopes when interacting with an immunocompetent cell may render it tolerant. As I shall discuss in more detail later on, such a matrix depends on the presence of antibody as a link between the cell surface and the antigen.

Humoral mediators.

The possible significance of humoral mediators in some forms of in vivo tolerance has been suggested by the in vitro work of Diener and Feldmann (5). They provided an experimental model whereby antigen-antibody complexes act as specific immunosuppressants at the level of the immunocompetent cell. This form of tolerance required the presence of a critical ratio of antigen to antibody concentration (excess of antigen over antibody) (6, 7) and could be achieved with immunogenic as well as subimmunogenic amounts of antigen complexed with antibody (8). Although the tolerance obtained in these experiments was interpreted as an effect on B cells, further evidence has established that antigen-antibody (AG-AB) complexes may also induce T cell tolerance (9). The phenomenon of AG-AB-induced tolerance is quite in agreement with the previously discussed aspects of structural mediators of tolerance. It is, thus, conceivable that optimally tolerogenic AG-AB complexes may readily exert their tolerogenic effect when bound to cell surfaces such as those of dendritic cells in lymphoid follicles. Indeed, in conditions of tumor or allograft enhancement and in tetraparental chimaeras, the target cells themselves may carry a tolerance-inducing matrix on their surface consisting of soluble target cell antigen complexed with antibody. Fig. 1 shows different possibilities by which a matrix may be formed at these sites. The fact that blocking factors have been suggested to consist of antigen-antibody complexes (10, 11, 12) supports this notion. A unique concept which implies antibody as a mediator of tolerance to histocompatibility antigens has been introduced by Ramseier and Lindenmann (13). They have demonstrated that antibodies can be raised against lymphocyte receptors specific for a histocompatibility antigen which they called anti-recognition structure (RS) antibody. The therapeutic potential of such antibodies has been demonstrated by the fact that it effectively inhibited graft versus host reaction in experimental situations (14). Anti-RS antibodies are expected to play a significant role in tolerance control of lymphoid chimaerism.

Cells as the mediators of tolerance induction.

Evidence is now abundant which implies some forms of tolerance to be mediated and maintained by specific suppressor cells (15, 16). I shall now briefly describe some experiments by my colleagues, Drs. Jirsch and Kraft and myself (17) which demonstrate the existence of suppressor cells in allograft enhancement. The experimental model makes

545

use of a heterotopic cardiac allograft whereby a fetal heart
from 18 day old BALB/c mice is transplanted into the subcutaneous ear tissue of adult CBA recipients (18). Graft
function is monitored by specialized electrocardiography
which differentiates the electrical activity generated by
the adult host heart from that of the graft (Fig. 2). Graft
rejection is judged by cessation of the graft-induced pattern. In order to obtain permanently-established allografts
across the major histocompatibility barrier, lethally
irradiated mice bearing a cardiac allograft were given purified populations of syngeneic stem cells so that differentiation toward immunocompetence would occur in the presence of
alloantigens. It turned out that best success in obtaining
allografts surviving permanently was when bone marrow cells
were mixed with large spleen cells at a ratio of $10^5:2 \times 10^6$
cells per mouse, whereas repopulation with fractionated or
unfractionated bone marrow without the presence of spleen
cells always caused rejection of 100% of allografts by 10
weeks (Fig. 3). The 25% of animals that maintained their
allografts permanently were examined for the presence of
cell-mediated immunity to the allograft antigen, the presence of serum-blocking factors and the ability of their
lymph node cells to transfer tolerance. In the first of
these tests, spleen cells from normal and tolerant mice were
compared for their ability to become sensitized in vitro to
BALB/c mastocytoma cells and to subsequently effect ^{51}Cr
release from these target cells. Table I shows that CBA
mice considered tolerant to BALB/c heart grafts demonstrated
full reactivity to BALB/c alloantigens in vitro and were
thus immunocompetent. However, our search for blocking factors in the serum of such mice has altogether failed. Even
though blocking of effector cells was not detected in sera
from tolerant mice, it appeared evident that some mechanism
was preventing in vivo expression of allograft immunity. We,
therefore, attempted to inhibit in vivo allograft immunity
by transferring small numbers of lymph node cells from tolerant mice along with the reconstituting inoculum of bone
marrow cells which on its own would cause allograft rejection. The data in Fig. 3 show a dramatic difference between
the two treatments (p<0.01); transfer of lymph node cells
from tolerant donors led to adoptive tolerance, whereas
rejection of the allograft occurred upon transfer of either
bone marrow alone or bone marrow plus normal lymph node cells.

TABLE I

COMPARISON OF SPLEEN CELL ACTIVITY FROM
TOLERANT AND NORMAL MICE IN VITRO

Treatment	% ^{51}Cr Release
Normal CBA spleen + mastocytoma cells in vitro	31.9 ± 6.9
Normal CBA spleen tissue culture	3.7 ± 2.4
Normal BALB/c spleen tissue culture	2.2 ± 1.9
CBA spleen (fresh)	5.7 ± 1.9
BALB/c spleen (fresh)	4.5 ± 2.1
Tolerant CBA spleen + mastocytoma cells in vitro	31.7 ± 6.1

Figures listed represent the release of ^{51}Cr from labelled BALB/c mastocytoma cells effected by spleen cells from normal and tolerant CBA mice.

Students' paired T test-

1) Normal CBA + in vitro mast versus tolerant CBA + in vitro mast; p>0.5.

2) Normal CBA + in vitro mast versus normal CBA tissue culture; p<0.005.

3) Normal CBA + in vitro mast versus fresh CBA; p<0.01.

The experiments described demonstrate that transplantation tolerance established across a strong histocompatibility barrier in the absence of lymphoid chimerism may be transferred with lymphocytes. In agreement with similar findings regarding tolerance of humoral immunity (16), these data suggest the existence of an active state of cell repression. Although we have as yet failed to demonstrate the presence of serum-blocking factors in tolerant mice, it is postulated that such factors are operative, possibly at quite low concentrations and are in fact, produced by the very cells that could transfer the state of allograft tolerance in vivo. Since in our experiments allograft enhancement was strain-specific (a CBA mouse tolerant to BALB/c allograft would reject a graft from a C57 mouse), it is tempting to furthermore postulate that the enhancing factor is an antigen-antibody complex. The antibody in such a complex could conceivably derive from B cells (5) or T cells (IgX, specific helper function) (9).

THE IMMUNOCOMPETENT CELL
THE TARGET OF TOLERANCE-MEDIATING MECHANISMS

Whatever the mediating mechanisms of tolerance induction, their target is the immunocompetent cell. Thus, any common mechanism which invokes the various phenomena of in vivo tolerance should be detectable on the surface membrane of this cell. To be more specific, the channel through which tolerance is brought about is represented by a set of antigen receptors; the manner in which these receptors interact with a ligand determines whether tolerance or immune induction will occur. I shall restrict myself in this paragraph to the discussion of tolerance-inducing at the B cell level since it is this cell we are most familiar with from in vitro experimentation. There are two main schools of thought regarding the role of antigen receptors in tolerance and immunity: One opinion holds that one and the same receptor may convey discriminatory signals to the cell, depending on whether or not the interacting ligand carries tolerogenic or immunogenic properties. Some have suggested a subdivision of tolerance-inducing signals, one for high-zone and one for low-zone tolerance (38). A second, more recent opinion, holds that the receptor acts merely as an antigen-focussing device and that cell triggering takes place via parts of the membrane other than the antigen receptor (19).

Since the evidence for or against the two theories is about equally circumstantial, I shall allow myself a biased

opinion in favor of the hypothesis that triggering or immunity or tolerance is at least in part conveyed by immunoglobulin receptors for antigen. Indeed, Dr. Pernis and I
have provided some evidence that interaction of surface immunoglobulin receptors with a ligand has to involve certain
distinct portions of the receptor molecule (20). Thus,
triggering of receptor re-synthesis within a period of 3 to
6 hours following receptor capping by anti-rabbit anti-allotype immunoglobulin was only observed when the anti-allotype
antibody was directed against parts of the $F(ab')_2$ portion
of the IgM receptor molecule (anti-a1; anti-b4); no such
stimulation occurred, however, when receptor binding involved
the constant region of the μ chain and an allotypic marker
associated with the hinge region of the receptor (anti-Ms3;
anti-Ms4) (Table II). In support of some of these data is
work by Frensdorff et al (21) who showed that in vitro exposure of rabbit lymphocytes heterozygous for allotype markers
b^5/b^9 to anti-b^9 antibody would stimulate these cells to
secrete increased amounts of b^9-antibody upon subsequent
transfer to irradiated recipients of allotype b^4/b^4. These
findings are, furthermore, in agreement with autoradiographic
studies on antigen-binding cells of the mouse which showed
that tritium-labelled polymerized flagellin (^3H POL) would
readily induce receptor reformation at increased density
following capping (22, 23). In contrast, anti-mouse immunoglobulin antibodies (which are mainly directed against antigens of the Fc portion) have been reported to lack the stimulatory capacity for such receptor re-synthesis (24). The
above findings thus favor those molecular theories which
postulate that antigen receptors mediate triggering signals
independently from each other, perhaps by antigen-induced
allosteric changes (25).

CONDITIONS AT THE SINGLE CELL LEVEL
WHICH BRING ABOUT TOLERANCE INDUCTION

Much evidence from in vivo and in vitro studies empha-
sizes the importance of both the dose and/or the quality of
the antigen as the parameters influencing the conditions
for the induction of tolerance. In the following part of
this communication, I shall concentrate on in vitro evidence
for this statement.

TABLE II

STIMULATORY EFFECT OF ANTI-ALLOTYPE ANTIBODIES ON THE FORMATION OF SURFACE IMMUNOGLOBULINS BY RABBIT LYMPHOCYTES*

Time of Incubation (Hours)	Temperature (C°)	Antibody	Cells Labelled /10³ Cells Screened	Antibody	Cells Labelled /10³ Cells Screened	Antibody	Cells Labelled /10³ Cells Screened
0.5	4	anti-al†	74	anti-b4†	44	anti-Ms3†	71
2.0	37		100		179	Ms4	33
3.0	37		129		200		72
4.5	37		290		276		41
10.5	37		132		196		18

*A representative experiment out of 4 with similar data but somewhat different timing of incubation at 37°C. Considering all 4 experiments, the differences between groups (anti-al; anti-b4) and group (anti-Ms3; anti-Ms4) are statistically significant ($p<0.01$).

†Cells incubated with Rhodamine-conjugated antibody after capping had been induced with unlabelled antibody. The percentage of caps in all groups was between 80 and 95%.

The antigen dose.

Certain antigens such as polymerized flagellin (POL)
(26) or DNP conjugated to POL (27) exert immunogenic as well
as tolerogenic properties in vitro. Which of these two
properties is to be expressed depends entirely on the dose
of the antigen to which immunocompetent cells are exposed.
As for POL, dose response curves have shown that an only
ten-fold increase in the antigen concentration over the
immunogenic dose results in tolerance induction within about
3 hours of exposure of mouse lymphocytes to the antigen (26).
Furthermore, tolerance could not only be induced upon incubation of cells with this antigen at a temperature of 37°C
but also at 4°C. It was concluded that tolerance depended
on the binding of critical amounts of antigen to the surface
of relevant immunocompetent cells. This was further substantiated at the functional level in experiments in which
the cell-bound antigen was removed by treatment with proteolytic enzymes (28). Trypsinization of lymphocytes, if carried out within the first 2 days of the tolerant state,
resulted in immunity. Beyond the 2 to 3 day mark, tolerance
was irreversible. More recently, we have obtained further
direct evidence in support of the above interpretation. The
use of bio-synthetic tritium-labelled POL (^{3}H POL) has made
it possible to directly follow the early events that take
place on the surface of antigen-binding cells (22). Autoradiography of such cells in combination with functional
assays has shown that the population of between 20 to 50
antigen-binding cells per 10^6 lymphocytes not only reforms
surface receptors after they have been stripped by capping,
but also undergo transformation into blast cells within 12
to 24 hours (23). To prevent removal of antigen by capping,
the antigen-binding experiments were carried out at 4°C.
After washing the cells were processed for autoradiography.
Figure 5 shows the correlation of the grain count distribution profile within populations of antigen-binding cells
after incubation for 1 hour in the presence of 200 ng/ml,
1 μg/ml, 5 μg/ml, 10 μg/ml and 20 μg/ml of ^{3}H POL, doses
from 5 to 20 μg being tolerogenic in vitro. The number of
antigen-binding cells reached a definite plateau with increasing antigen concentration. This suggests that POL-
binding cells comprise a distinct population of a limited
size. There also occurred a shift in the grain count distribution profile from low grain counts at immunogenic, to
high grain counts at tolerogenic antigen concentrations. As
has been demonstrated with anti-gamma globulin antibody,
^{3}H POL also causes cap formation in the majority of antigen-
binding cells. Unlike anti-immunoglobulin caps, however,

^{3}H POL caps are shed from the cell rather than pinocytosed (23). Although we have conclusively shown that antigen capping per se plays no part in the immune triggering process (29), it may, nevertheless, act as a safe-guard against cell paralysis. This notion derives from the fact that under conditions of tolerance induction, antigen capping fails to take place. Since the amount of antigen bound to a lymphocyte is also a function of time, one may argue from a teleological point of view that capping ought to remove antigen from the cell surface before it had accumulated tolerance-inducing amounts.

The quality of the antigen.
It is well known from in vivo work that, apart from the antigen concentration, a further parameter which affects the induction of tolerance resides in the quality of the antigen. In vitro experiments have demonstrated a direct relationship between the tolerance-inducing capacity of an antigen and its immunogenicity (5). This is in direct contrast to observations made from in vivo experiments where the capacity of an antigen to induce tolerance is inversely related to its immunogenic potency. Thus, polymerized flagellin was found to express both high immunogenicity as well as tolerogenicity in vitro, whereas the same antigen was immunogenic in vitro but failed to induce in vivo tolerance. Monomeric flagellin (Mol. wt. 40,000) and "fragment A", a cyanogen-bromide digest of flagellin (Mol. wt. 18,000) (30) which share the same major antigenic determinants with POL, have been found to act as relatively weak immunogens both in vivo and in vitro but acted as tolerogens in vivo only (4). These facts have led to the conclusion that the induction of tolerance in vivo to a weak immunogen such as fragment A requires a mediating mechanism which is absent under in vitro conditions of the experiments described above. In our attempts to reconcile the two opposing sets of data, it is useful to remember that POL has a higher binding energy to an immunocompetent cell than have monomeric flagellin or fragment A due to a large number of antigenically identical determinants along a linear backbone. We reasoned that similar conditions might be achieved if say fragment A was presented to the immunocompetent cell in the form of an antigen-antibody complex. This hypothesis has, indeed, been realized experimentally when it was shown that such complexes when formed at a particular concentration ratio between antigen and antibody were capable of rendering mouse spleen cells tolerant in vitro to a subsequent challenge with POL (6, 7). The fact that such antigen-antibody-mediated tolerance could

only be achieved with bivalent F(ab¹)2 but not with monovalent Fab¹ is in support of the proposed mechanism whereby
antigen and antibody become focussed on the surface receptors of immunocompetent cells (31). Since the antigen-
antibody ratio proved critical in the formation of tolerogenic complexes, it was possible to render cell populations
tolerant in vitro in the presence of antigen concentrations
which, in the absence of antibody, were immunogenic or subimmunogenic. Recently, the above theoretical concept referring to the increased binding energy of appropriately-shaped
antigen-antibody complexes over that of antigen alone has
been further documented by Niederer (32).

A UNIFYING CONCEPT

In the preceding chapter I have attempted to provide
evidence in support of the hypothesis that the conditions at
the level of the immunocompetent cell's surface which bring
about tolerance may be reduced to a single parameter, namely,
the number of interactions between antigen recognition sites
and their corresponding determinants on the antigen molecule.
The more antigen attaches to the cell, the more likely it is
to induce tolerance, provided it causes antigen receptors to
become cross linked. This necessity for receptor cross
linking, at least when dealing with B cells, is also emphasized in studies by Feldmann who showed that B cell tolerance
in vitro to DNP only occurred if there were a large number
of DNP groups conjugated per unit of polymeric flagellin
(27). Clearly, there must exist a threshold level of antigen receptor interactions which marks the transition of an
immunogenic stimulus to a tolerogenic one. This then rein-
troduces the problem mentioned earlier; that of signal discrimination by the immunocompetent cell. Basically, there
are two possibilities: The simplest one calls for the
existence of one type of signal for both immunity and tolerance to be transmitted to the cell. It is irrelevant
whether such a signal reaches the cell's interior directly
via the receptor molecule or via intermediary steps involving membrane components. The observed antigen dose dependence of immunity and tolerance induction thus refers to the
sum total of individual interactions that are necessary for
either event to take place. Another theory proposes a two-
signal hypothesis to account for discrimination between a
tolerogenic and an immunogenic stimulus (25). According to
this theory, induction of immunity in a B cell requires the
recognition of at least two antigenic determinants. One
determinant binds to the antigen receptor on the immuno-

competent cell. As in the above hypothesis, the binding energy released in this interaction is thought to cause an allosteric change in the antigen receptor. However, this signal is tolerogenic unless counteracted by a second signal that results from interaction of the second antigenic determinant with so-called associative antibody. Associative antibody is regarded as a specific helper factor produced by thymus-derived (T) cells. For thermodynamic reasons it is argued that an immunocompetent cell will receive a mixture of tolerogenic and immunogenic signals and that the decision for the cell to undergo either paralysis or immune induction depends on the ratio between the sum total of individual paralytic signals and that of inductive signals. This hypothesis does not readily agree with the fact that the small fragment A of flagellin or DNP when conjugated to POL below a certain density fail to induce tolerance, while they would be expected to deliver the initial signal in the same manner as POL. Attempts to explain the tolerogenic potency of POL on grounds of its apparent independence of T cells are complicated by the finding that such independence applies to some strains of mice but not to others (33). Furthermore, tolerance to the same POL could be induced with equal ease in mouse strains that do or do not express thymus dependence of their immune response to this antigen.

In my interpretation of the different models of tolerance induction, I have attempted to focus on a common mechanism at the cellular level which intimately concerns both the triggering of immunity and of paralysis. This, I have proposed, is the case by assuming that both phenomena depend on the sum total of individual triggering signals. The important point here is that the sum total of such signals must meet certain threshold requirements: the threshold for paralysis of the cell would always be higher than that for immune triggering. As I have discussed earlier in this meeting, these thresholds for the two immune phenomena must reflect the metabolic state of the immunocompetent cell and may be subject to fluctuations under physiological conditions. One such condition may be controlled by glucosteroid hormones (34) as I have outlined in my contribution as a discussant. Once agreed upon a common pathway of immunity and tolerance induction, one is faced with the difficult task of fitting the various tolerance-mediating mechanisms into the scheme. I have attempted to do this by showing that the conditions of tolerance induction at the level of the immunocompetent cell in terms of antigen receptor cross linking may be met by either polymeric antigens carrying repeating determinants of a given specificity or by antigen-antibody complexes of defined three dimensional configuration. These complexes may be active either in free solution or by being bound to the surface of specialized cells of the RES or, in the case of tumor or allograft enhancement, to the target cells. In such complexes the ligand for the antigen may comprise B cell-derived conventional antibody or T cell-derived specific helper factor. As has been suggested by Feldmann and Nossal (9), complexes containing T cell-derived helper factor may well account for those tolerance models which depend on suppressor T cells. Although most of the more direct experimental data I have referred to concern B cell tolerance, there is no a priori reason to assume that T cells follow different mechanisms of tolerance induction. There is, nevertheless, evidence from in vivo (35, 36) and in vitro work (9) which suggests that T cells become tolerized under conditions at which B cells remain responsive. This may be interpreted as a reflection of differences between B and T cells in their triggering threshold for immunity and paralysis. Considering then the possibility that mechanisms for B cell and T cell tolerance are basically similar, one might conclude that B cell-derived antibody, when complexed with antigen under appropriate conditions, could equally well become tolerogenic for T cells as for B cells. Indeed, this possibility argues for the existence of suppressor B cells as regulators of cell-mediated immunity.

SUMMARY

It has been attempted to center the various means by which tolerance is brought about around a common requirement for its induction at the level of the immunocompetent cell. It is suggested that tolerance results from antigen-receptor interactions in excess of what is regarded as optimal for immune induction. These requirements are ideally met by polymeric antigens. Non-polymeric antigens may require humoral mediators such as antibody to assume tolerance inducing properties in the form of antigen-antibody complexes. Such complexes derive their antigen-ligand from either B suppressor cells (classical antibody) or from T suppressor cells (antigen-specific T cell factor) and may be effective in free solution or when bound to cell surfaces of the RES, to tumor cells or to cells of an allograft.

ACKNOWLEDGMENTS

Part of this work was supported by the Canadian Medical Research Council and by the National Institute of Health, U.S.A., # 1 RO1 AI11595-01.

REFERENCES

1. Immunological Tolerance, Proceedings of an International Conference, Brook Lodge, edited by M. Landy and W. Braun, Academic Press, N. Y., London, 1969.

2. Nossal, G.J.V. and Mitchell, J., In Thymus, Experimental and Clinical Studies; CIBA Foundation Symposia, edited by G.E.W. Wolstenholme and R. Porter, London, Churchill, 1966.

3. Das, S. and Leskowitz, S., J. Immunol. 112:107, 1974.

4. Ada, G.L. and Parish, C.R., Proc. Nat. Acad. Sci. U.S.A. 61:556, 1968.

5. Diener, E. and Feldmann, M., Transplant. Rev. 8:76, 1972.

6. Feldmann, M. and Diener, E., J. Exp. Med. 131:247, 1970.

7. Diener, E. and Feldmann, M., J. Exp. Med. 132:31, 1970.

8. Feldmann, M. and Diener, E., Immunol. 21:387, 1971.

9. Feldmann, M. and Nossal, G.J.V., Transplant. Rev. 13:3, 1972.

10. Sjögren, H.O., Hellström, I., Barsal, S.C., Hellström, K.E., Proc. Nat. Acad. Sci. 68:1372, 1971.

11. Wright, P.W., Hargreaves, R.E., Barsal, S.C., Bernstein, I.D. and Hellström, K.E., Proc. Nat. Acad. Sci. 70:2539, 1973.

12. Baldwin, R.W., Price, M.R. and Robius, R.A., Int. J. Cancer. 11:527, 1973.

13. Ramseier, H. and Lindenmann, J., Transplant. Rev. 10: 57, 1972.

14. Joller, P.W., Nature. New Biol. 240:214, 1972.

15. Gershon, R.K., Cohen, P., Hencin, R. and Liebhaber, S., J. Immunol. 108:586, 1972.

16. McCullagh, P., J. Exp. Med. 132:916, 1970.

17. Jirsch, D.W., Kraft, M. and Diener, E., Transplant. In press.

18. Jirsch, D.W., Kraft, N. and Diener, E., Cardiovasc. Res. In press.

19. Continho, A. and Möller, G., Nature. New Biol. 245:12, 1973.

20. Diener, E., Pernis, B., Lee, K-C, Langman, R.E., Kraft, N. and Paetkau, V.H., In Control of Proliferation in Animal Cells, Cold Spring Harbor Symposium, 1972. In press.

21. Frensdorff, A., Jones, P.P., Berwald-Netter, Y. and Cebra, J.J., Science. 171:391, 1971.

22. Diener, E. and Paetkau, V.H., Proc. Nat. Acad. Sci. U.S.A. 69:2364, 1972.

23. Kraft, N., Diener, E., Lee, K-C and Shiozawa, C. In preparation.

24. Taylor, R.B., Philip, W., Duffus, H., Raff, M.C. and de Petris, S., Nature. New Biol. 233:225, 1971.

25. Bretscher, P.A. and Cohn, M., Nature. 220:444, 1968.

26. Diener, E. and Armstrong, W.D., J. Exp. Med. 129:591, 1969.

27. Feldmann, M., J. Exp. Med. 135:735, 1972.

28. Diener, E. and Feldmann, M., Cell. Immunol. 5:130, 1972.

29. Lee, K-C, Langman, R.E., Paetkau, V.H. and Diener, E., Europ. J. Immunol. 3:306, 1973.

30. Parish, C.R., Wistar, R. and Ada, G.L., Biochem. J. 113:501, 1969.

31. Feldmann, M. and Diener, E., J. Immunol. 108:93, 1972.

32. Niederer, W., Immunol. 26:137, 1974.

33. Langman, R.E. In preparation.

34. Diener, E. and Lee, K-C. In preparation.

35. Chiller, J.M., Habicht, G.S. and Weigle, W.O., Proc. Nat. Acad. Sci. 65:551, 1970.

36. Chiller, J.M., Habicht, G.S. and Weigle, W.O., Science. 171:813, 1971.

37. Wegmann, T.G., Hellström, I. and Hellström, K.E., Proc. Nat. Acad. Sci. 68:1644, 1971.

38. Nossal, G.J.V., In Immunological Tolerance, Proceedings of an International Conference held at Brook Lodge, edited by M. Landy and W. Braun, p. 53-70, 1968.

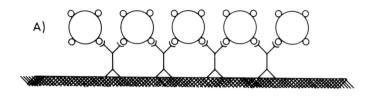

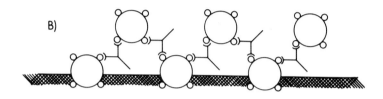

Fig. 1. Mediator mechanisms of tolerance:
Antigen-antibody complexes form a matrix of antigenic determinants on cell surfaces.

a) on dendritic cells of lymphoid follicles. The complex binds to cell surface receptors for the Fc-portion of Ig molecules.

b) on cells of an allograft or on tumor cells. The complex binds to alloantigens or tumor-specific antigens on the cell surface. The same antigen is released by the cell as a product of membrane turnover and thus, participates in the formation of antigen-antibody complexes.

Note: Depending on the density and distribution of antigenic determinants in the matrix, immunocompetent cells may become stimulated, paralyzed or temporarily blocked.

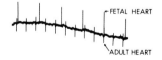

Fig. 2. Electrocardiogram obtained from a mouse bearing a fetal heartgraft in one ear:
Note the distinct pattern due to the function of the graft.

559

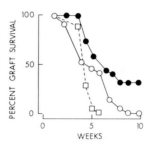

Fig. 3. Graft survival as a percentage of mice bearing detectable allografts two weeks after transplantation:

Recipient Mouse:	CBA/Hi (H-2k)
Heart Graft:	BALB/c (H-2d)
Reconstituting cells:	CBA/Hi

-o- 0.1 x 10^6 normal bone marrow cells (32 mice)

-•- 0.1 x 10^6 normal bone marrow cells plus 2 x 10^6 large spleen cells (10 mice)

-□- 0.1 x 10^6 normal bone marrow cells plus 2 x 10^6 small spleen cells (17 mice)

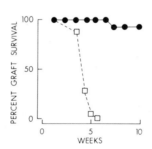

Fig. 4. Transfer of tolerance with lymph node cells from tolerant donors:

Irradiated CBA/Hi mice were given 0.1 x 10^6 syngeneic bone marrow cells and 1 to 10 x 10^6 tolerant lymph node cells.

-•- with tolerant lymph node cells

-□- with normal lymph node cells or spleen cells

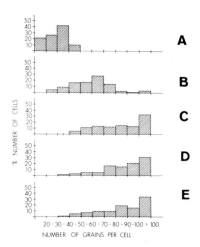

<u>Fig. 5.</u> <u>Grain count distribution profiles of normal</u>
<u>mouse spleen cells binding tritiated polymerized flagellin</u>:

Cells were incubated <u>in vitro</u> at 4°C for 1
hour in the presence of different concentrations of antigen:

a)   200 ng/ml

b)   1 µg/ml

c)   5 µg/ml

d)   10 µg/ml

e)   20 µg/ml

The number of antigen-binding cells in each
group per 10^6 nucleated cells was: 5, 53, 37, 50 and 37.
Significant difference between group a) and all the other
groups. At least 3 x 10^6 cells were screened for each group.

DISCUSSION FOLLOWING ERWIN DIENER

PAUL: In the capping experiments in which different resynthesis results were obtained depending on the precise
specificity of the antibodies which were used, can you
give us more details on the anti-immunoglobulin
reagents which you utilized?

DIENER: First, I would be careful to use the term "resynthesis"; we have no evidence that receptor re-appearance
has to do with re-synthesis. The reagents were anti-
allotype antibodies prepared according to standard techniques by Drs. Kelus and Pernis.

FELDMANN: Erwin, you mentioned that in tolerance to POL at
at 20 µg/ml there was no cap information. With DNP-POL
at 10 µg we have found capping. Do you know the threshold for inhibition of cap formation in tolerance induction?

DIENER: There are two important points in answer to your
question: (1) To observe inhibition of capping with
a dose of 10 µg, the incubation time of cells with antigen has to be long enough to allow equilibration of
binding. In our hands this is 2 hours. (2) Inhibition of capping in virgin cells is less effective
than in cells which have passed through the first capping cycle and have expressed new receptors.

MITCHELL: Erwin Diener indicated that tolerogenic (large)
quantities of antigen would freeze the receptors on
POL-reactive B cells and yet in the experiments with
Pernis, large amounts of anti-Fab allotype sera in the
rabbit induced a cleansing and resynthesis of surface
Ig. Can these two observations be brought together?

DIENER: I don't think they can be brought together since we
don't know the comparable concentrations for the two
ligands in question, which might inhibit capping. It
has however been shown by others (Raff, Taylor) that
capping of receptors can be inhibited by high concentrations of anti-receptor antibody.

G. MÖLLER: Did you induce Ig synthesis when you reacted
lymphocytes with anti-Fab?

DIENER: No.

G. MÖLLER: I want to emphasize that no one has been able to induce Ig synthesis by reacting lymphocytes with anti-Ig of a variety of specificities and a variety of concentrations. Thus, there is no evidence that Ig cross-linking induces a signal for Ig synthesis.

DIENER: Receptor re-appearance as I have described it can of course not be equated with re-synthesis.

E. MÖLLER: But you have not shown that any signal for activation has been delivered through the Ig receptor.

DIENER: In the sense of mitogenic activation not. However, as far as receptor re-formation after capping is concerned, we have shown that anti-allotype against the V-region of the μ chain or the constant region of the L-chain activates these processes.

LESKOWITZ: Erwin, your failure to see capping with high to tolerogenic doses may be due to a failure to get cross-linking much as in antigen excess complexes--that is, each receptor would have its own antigen molecule with no cross-linking possible. In that case, you might see capping if antibody was added.

DIENER: As far as polymer is concerned, I don't think your comment is valid. Here the cross-linking is mediated by the polymer "backbone", not by antibody.

BENACERRAF: Does your data on grain counts with POL refer to low dose or high dose tolerance?

DIENER: These data refer to the difference in cell-bound antigen between immunogenic and high-zone tolerogenic conditions.

HELLSTRÖM: Do you have any evidence that the suppressor cells you are transferring in your heart allograft tolerance model produce "blocking factors", in vivo or in vitro?

DIENER: Although we have so far not been able to demonstrate "blocking factor", we assume they exist. We think it is for technical reasons that we have so far not been able to demonstrate their presence.

HUMPHREY: Can you show that very low levels of POL with low levels of antibody result in binding of amounts of POL comparable to those bound in tolerogenic conditions? And were the numbers of binding cells similar?

DIENER: We have started to do these experiments but have no results available yet.

BLOCKING FACTORS IN TUMOR IMMUNITY
AND ALLOGRAFT TOLERANCE

K.E. Hellstrőm, I. Hellstrőm, P.W. Wright and I.D. Bernstein

Departments of Pathology and Microbiology
University of Washington Medical School
and Division of Immunology,
Fred Hutchinson Cancer Research Center
Seattle, Washington 98195

We will summarize some evidence that "blocking factors"
are present in the serum of animals and human patients with
growing tumors as well as in the serum of rats which are
operationally tolerant to skin allografts; the blocking
factors being detected by their ability to specifically
inhibit ("block") lymphocyte mediated cytoxic reactions in
vitro. The molecular nature of the blocking factors will
be discussed, and their role in vivo will be commented on.
Since an extensive review in this area has been recently
published (1), we will make this paper short and will delete
most references covered by the review.

Blocking factors in tumor immunity.
In most systems studied -- although not in all of them-
lymphocytes from animals and human patients with growing
tumor have been found to be capable of killing cultivated
cells from the respective neoplasms, as assayed by the
microcytoxicity test (1). This test involves the seeding
of tumor cells in plastic plates, exposing them to experimental group (or control) lymphocytes during 30-40 hours and
counting the number of tumor cells remaining attached to
the plate. Lymphocyte reactivity measured in this way and
expressed as the minimum ratio between lymphocytes and target cells producing significant killing can be as high in
tumor-bearers as in individuals whose tumors have been removed. It is commonly lower in the tumor-bearers, however
(1).

The finding that lymphocyte reactivity can be detected
also in many individuals with growing tumor led us to study
whether tumor-bearer serum can abrogate lymphocyte-mediated
cytotoxic reactions to tumor antigens. The results from
such studies were published in 1969 (2) and have since been
confirmed and extended (see e.g. 1, 3-9), and it is now clear
that serum from animals and human patients with growing

tumors can, indeed, inhibit the cytotoxic effect of lymphocytes reactive to the respective neoplasms. The blocking
effect is specific; control sera of various kinds, including
sera from individuals with tumors of "other" antigenicity,
do not block.

The blocking activity can be detected by pre-incubating
either the target cells or the lymphocytes with serum followed by washing before they are mixed with each other (1).
Most of the early work was performed by pre-incubating the
target cells, while we now (since 1972) routinely add the
serum to the mixture of lymphocytes and target cells (except
when the effect on either cell type is studied).

Blocking activity is generally not seen when sera are
tested from individuals free of tumor (1). There have,
however, been a few exceptions when sera from animals whose
tumors had spontaneously regressed were found to block
lymphocyte-mediated reactivity (9-11). Hayami et al found,
for example, that sera from Japanese quails, whose Schmidt-
Ruppin Rous virus-induced sarcomas had spontaneously regressed, could sometimes block lymphocyte-mediated cytotoxicity to Rous sarcoma cells when tested at certain dilutions
(10,11). Since Amos et al (12) and Klein (13) have reported
that sera enhancing tumor allografts in mice can interact
with the tumor cells and release an "immunosuppressive substance", Hayami et al studied whether regressor sera blocking cytotoxicity to Rous sarcoma cells at the target cell
level might do so by interacting with the tumor cells and
releasing some factor, e.g. an antigen-antibody complex preventing the cytotoxicity of the effector cells (11). Fig. 1
illustrates an experiment on this. It shows that blocking
factors capable of acting on the effector cells can, indeed,
be detected after incubation of the tumor cells with the
immune serum.

Most sera from animals and human patients, whose tumors
have been removed or which have spontaneously regressed,
lack blocking activity. Many of these sera are, instead,
"unblocking", i.e. they are capable of cancelling the
blocking effect of tumor-bearer serum (1). The unblocking
effect is specific. It is mediated by an antibody to tumor
cell antigens and can be selectively removed by absorption
with the respective neoplastic cells.

Figure 2 summarizes the rather scarce information available about the nature of the blocking factors. As shown

in the figure, the blocking factors appear to be of two kinds: antigen-antibody complexes and free antigens. Under the conditions most tests have been performed, there is rather little evidence for blocking by free antibody. The experiment shown in Fig. 1 indicates, however, that antibodies can, at some dilutions, interact with tumor cells so that blocking factors inhibiting effector cell reactivity are formed. Furthermore, hyperimmune sera often prevent target cell killing (14); this is perhaps by covering their foreign antigens.

More knowledge about the nature of the blocking factors is obviously needed. Are these factors, indeed, antigen-antibody complexes and not just mixtures, and, if so, what kind of complexes are they and what is the nature of the antigens which block? Information on this could, in addition to being a prerequisite for understanding the mechanisms of the blocking effect, lead to the establishment of radioimmunoassays. Such assays would be useful for the simple quantitation of the blocking factors (e.g. in human patients).

As emphasized already, the major point of attack of the blocking factors appears to be the effector cell, and there is evidence that both T and B cell reactivity can be blocked. This is illustrated in Fig. 3. As also shown in the figure, the concentration of blocking factors is higher in the local microenvironment of a growing tumor than elsewhere in the organism (1). This may, at least partially, explain "concomitant tumor immunity", i.e. the commonly observed finding that a tumor can grow at its primary site while the tumor-bearing individual rejects a challenge dose of cells from the same tumor given elsewhere (15,16). At the site of the challenge, the neoplastic cells may be destroyed by circulating from blockade by antigen (or complexes) and/or from deletion of reactive cells, could further contribute to the local growth of the tumor.

Most work on blocking serum factors has been performed with the 30-40 hrs. microcytotoxicity assay, and studies involving short term assays (e.g. the 3-8 hrs Cr^{51} test) are needed to further dissect their action. There is evidence that the immune response to tumor antigens detectable with the macrophage migration inhibition test (17), and the mixed leukocyte culture (MLC) assay (18) can be also blocked by tumor-bearer serum. Using the former technique, Halliday found that peritoneal cells from tumor-bearing mice are commonly non-reactive by themselves and can specifically prevent peritoneal cell populations from tumor-free, immune mice to react (17). This is reminiscent of the suppressor cell activity, discussed much at this conference, but the similarity may, of course, just be coincidental.

It is interesting that Halliday found that supernatants from peritoneal cells derived from tumor-bearing animals had blocking activity, and that serum from immune animals, un-blocking in microcytotoxicity experiments, could specifically restore reactivity to cell populations derived from tumor-bearing mice (17). Although the molecular nature of Halliday's blocking factor is unknown, his findings are compatible with the notion that complexes (or free antigens) are involved.

Somewhat similar findings have been made on Rous sarcomas in Japanese quails using the microcytotoxicity assay (10). In this system where tumor-bearer lymphocytes have not been detectably cytotoxic, these were found to suppress the cyto-toxic effect of reactive lymphocytes (from quails whose tumor had spontaneously regressed), except when the regressor quails had been bursectomized and so made unable to form antibodies. Lymphocytes from tumor-bearing quails were not tested for their ability to release blocking factors in cul-ture. Nelson and Pollack have found, however (19), that spleen cells from tumor-bearing mice can often release block-ing factors when cultivated in vitro. Analysis of this re-lease of blocking factors (following upon production?), e.g. with respect to the nature of the cells involved, is of potential interest.

The correlation between blocking serum activity in vitro and tumor growth in vivo has been repeatedly stressed (see e.g., 1 and 20). It has thus been pointed out that serum which blocks lymphocyte-mediated cytotoxicity to tumor cells in vitro can enhance tumor growth in vivo, that animals with blocking serum are more susceptible to small tumor trans-plants than are animals whose sera do not block, and that tumor-bearing animals, whose sera were originally blocking, if given unblocking antibodies, often demonstrate a delayed tumor growth and sometimes even tumor regression.

Likewise, studies on human patients have established a correlation between a blocking serum activity in vitro and the presence of tumor growth in vivo (1). Patients who are clinically free of tumor following surgery, but whose sera are blocking, have been shown to have a higher risk for recurrency than similar patients whose sera do not block (21). Since the blocking factors contain tumor antigens as one part, these data are simplest explained by concluding that patients whose post-surgery sera blocked had (more) tumor on board (1). The data can thus not be taken as proof that blocking factor facititate human tumor growth in vivo. They are, nevertheless, important because of the potential they have for the monitoring of human patients. The prospect for a practically feasible manner in which to perform such monitoring will increase when simpler assays for blocking factors become available.

The ability of tumor cells to release antigens which block lymphocyte-mediated cytotoxicity and/or form complexes which do so may provide an important escape mechanism for neoplastic cells from immunological control (1); whether it is the most important one in unknown. The possibility should be considered that some tumor antigens detected in vitro may appear to be weak (or nonexistent) in vivo just because they are particularly good blockers (alone or as part of complexes). We would now like to discuss some preliminary data of I. and K.E. Hellström (22) leading us to suspect that this may, indeed, be the case with respect to some, probably embryonic, antigens which are shared by many tumors.

Lymphocytes from multiparous mice are commonly cytotoxic to syngeneic tumor cells, but not to normal syngeneic fibroblasts, as tested for the microcytotxicity assay (23-25). It is believed that this is because the pregnant animals are sensitized to embryonic antigens present in the tumors; one cannot exclude, however, that the common antigens are associated with some virus (oncogenic or non-oncogenic). We have been able to confirm the observation of a tumoricidal effect of lymphocytes from multiparous mice, using as targets both methylcholanthrene-induced sarcomas of recent origin and cells transformed to neoplasia in vitro from (non-neoplastic) 3T3 fibroblasts of BALB/c origin; the in vitro transformed cells were all derived from the same clone 3T3 cells, which was then used as a control (22). Table I summarizes an experiment of this kind.

The demonstration of Baldwin et al (25) that serum from multiparous mice can block the cytotoxic lymphocyte effect could be confirmed, and a blocking effect at both the effector and the target cell level was seen. Absorption of serum with transformed cells, but not with normal BALB/c fibroblasts or non-transformed 3T3 cells removed the blocking activity (Table II), indicating that the blocking factors were specific and were at least partially antibodies (22).

TABLE I

ONE EXPERIMENT SHOWING THE CYTOTOXIC EFFECT OF 150,000 LYMPH NODE CELLS/WELL FROM MULTIPAROUS BALB/c MICE ON BALB/c CELLS. LYMPH NODE CELLS FROM AGE MATCHED VIRGIN BALB/c FEMALES USED AS CONTROL.

Target Cells	Percent Cytoxicity
MCA sarcoma #1315	47.4
MCA sarcoma #1321	38.7
3T3 Mol. sarc. virus transformed	54.5
3T3 spont. transformed	30.6
3T3 SV40 transformed	42.4
3T3 control	-1.4
Adult BALB/c fibroblasts	-8.0

Mice immunized in the classical way against the unique antigens of individual methylcholanthrene-induced sarcomas (by transplanting tumor cells, letting them grow out into a nodule and then removing that) were found to have blocking serum factors which could abrogate the cytotoxic effect of lymphocytes from multiparous mice (22). The same mice did not have any blocking serum activity against the unique antigens of the tumor used for immunization, and they have transplantation resistance to that tumor but not to different methylcholanthrene-induced sarcomas. The findings are thus compatible with the notion that the common embryonic antigens are better inducers of blocking serum activity than are the unique ones; this may, or may not, explain why they are not good transplantation antigens <u>in vivo</u>. A few data on this are presented in Table III.

TABLE II

BLOCKING ACTIVITY OF SERUM FROM MULTIPAROUS BALB/c MICE
AFTER ABSORPTION WITH SYNGENEIC TUMOR (OR CONTROL) CELLS.
THE BLOCKING ACTIVITY WAS CALCULATED AS THE ABILITY OF
SERUM TO ABROGATE THE CYTOTOXIC EFFECT OF LYMPHOCYTES
FROM MULTIPAROUS BALB/c MICE.

Target Cells	Serum absorbed with	%Blocking activity
MCA sarcoma #1315	MCA sarcoma #1315	-16.8
	MCA sarcoma #1321	33.1
	Adult BALB/c fibroblasts	92.1
MCA sarcoma #1321	MCA sarcoma #1315	40.3
	MCA sarcoma #1321	20.8
	Adult BALB/c fibroblasts	115.8
MCA sarcoma #1315	3T3 Mol. sarc. virus transformed	14.7
	3T3 control	64.7
3T3 Mol. sarc. virus transformed	3T3 Mol. sarc. virus transformed	-3.0
	3T3 control	73.0

TABLE III

BLOCKING ACTIVITY OF SERUM FROM MICE WITH MCA SARCOMA #1315
(OR FROM WHICH THIS TUMOR HAD BEEN REMOVED). SERA WERE
TESTED IN COMBINATION WITH LYMPH NODE CELLS FROM MULTIPAROUS
SYNGENEIC MICE AND FROM MICE SENSITIZED TO THE TUMOR SPECIFIC
ANTIGENS OF SARCOMA #1315.

	% blocking serum activity in combination with lymph node cells from	
Serum Donor	Multiparous BALB/c	BALB/c immunized to #1315
BALB/c carrying growing #1315	41;65 (2 tests)	106
BALB/c whose #1315 tumor was removed and which were 10 days later challenged with #1315. The serum was harvested 8 days after this challenge. These mice were resistant to #1315.	91	5
BALB/c whose #1315 tumor was removed and which were 10 days later challenged with #1321; the serum was harvested 8 days after this challenge. These mice accepted the grafted #1321 cells.	40;34 (2 tests)	NT

Blocking factors in allograft tolerance.

We will now discuss some work showing that cytotoxic
lymphocytes and blocking serum factors can be seen in operationally defined allograft tolerance; with operational
tolerance we mean the ability of neonatally inoculated animals to specifically and permanently (i.e. for more than 100
days) accept skin allografts from the tolerated strain. We
are not going to take up early work demonstrating blocking
serum effects in mice, dogs and human patients since this
work has been reviewed (1). Rather we will discuss recent
findings which were made by studying W/Fu rats, neonatally
inoculated with BN or (BN x W/Fu) F_1 cells and so rendered

capable of accepting BN skin grafts for more than 100 days.

Rats rendered tolerant to skin allografts were found, almost without exception, to have circulating blood lymphocytes capable of reacting in microcytotoxicity tests against cells carrying the "tolerated" antigens, and they also have blocking serum factors abrogating that effect (26-28). These findings are different from those of Beverly et al in mice according to which cellular reactivity and blocking activity were seen only in partially tolerant animals where tolerance was induced by inoculation of too few cells to establish permanent chimerism (29).

Most, although not all, of the rats studied in our earlier work had lymphocytes with a weak but consistent reactivity against the tolerated antigens in MLC assays and in assays for graft versus host reactivity in vivo (28); this was seen in spite of the fact that tolerance had been induced by inoculating the W/Fu rats with 40×10^6 BN bone marrow cells, a cell dose derived from the studies of Billingham and Silvers (30). For this reason we decided to study rats in which tolerance had been induced with even higher doses, and we have lately followed a protocol used by Elkine (31) involving the neonatal inoculation of W/Fu rats with 80×10^6 (W/Fu x BN)F$_1$ bone marrow and spleen cells. In difference to the rats previously tested, these animals have only occasionally shown any reactivity in MLC assays (32). Nevertheless, both a specific lymphocyte-mediated cytotoxicity against BN cells and a specific blocking serum activity could be detected, and there was no evidence that the reactivity was lower than that seen in rats with positive MLC (32). The cytotoxic lymphocyte effect appeared to be dependent upon a T cell function, since it could be removed by incubation with anti-T sera (33). All these rats continue to maintain skin grafts (now for more than 150 days) and they do, like the rats previously studied by us, accept second and third skin grafts; thus, they seem to fulfill stringent criteria for tolerance.

Experiments have been performed similarily to those done in tumor systems to approach the molecular nature of the blocking factors. They indicate that the blocking factors demonstrated in tolerant sera are antigen-antibody complexes (34) with the antibody part of the complexes being IgG immunoglobulin (35). The complexes have been shown to act at both the effector and the target cell level, while a smaller fraction split off from them by ultrafiltration at ph 3.1 believed to antigen, was found to act only at the effector cell level (34).

The most crucial question at this time is what role in vivo the blocking factors seen in allograft tolerance may play. Are they preventing graft rejection by those lymphocytes which have been shown to be cytotoxic in vitro or do both the cytotoxic lymphocytes and the blocking factors seen in tolerant rats lack relevance in vivo? We do not know the answer to these questions, and must, therefore, keep a careful attitude vis-à-vis the meaning of the in vitro observations. It is interesting, however, that animals spontaneously losing tolerance, which happened in some of the rats in our early work (when tolerance was induced with 4×10^7 BN cells), regularly lost detectable serum activity before the grafts were rejected (26). Furthermore, breakage of tolerance induced by inoculation of large doses of syngeneic lymphocytes, immune or nonimmune, was found to be preceded by disappearance of the blocking serum factors (27). These findings are compatible with the notion that blocking serum factors play an important role in maintaining the tolerant state, but they do not prove it.

We sould finally like to mention some recent experiments of Wright and Bernstein on in vitro sensitization of lymphocytes (36). They show that lymphocytes from normal and from skin graft immunized W/Fu rats can be specifically immunized in vitro to BN antigens and so rendered cytotoxic to BN cells (additional cytotoxic cells are generated from the immune populations) following a MLC response to these antigens. This was not seen with lymphocytes from W/Fu rats tolerant to BN. They neither reacted in the MLC assays nor formed any additional cytotoxic cells in spite of the fact that the "tolerant" lymphocytes were specifically cytotoxic to BN cells when harvested directly from the rats. A simple conclusion may be that different lymphocyte populations vary with respect to the tolerance mechanisms involved, and that the cell populations involved in the generation of new cytotoxic cells (subsequent to proliferation) are either deleted in the tolerant rats or suppressed in a stable manner. It becomes important, then, to consider the mechanisms of tolerance induction and maintenance with respect to individual antigens to the cell populations involved and to various lymphocyte functions rather than with respect to the whole animal. Such considerations may help to avoid controversies as to the role of clonal deletion and suppression mechanisms for the maintenance of allograft tolerance (see 37 for discussion).

SUMMARY

Sera from tumor-bearing animals and human patients and rats operationally tolerant to skin allografts, contain factors which can prevent lymphocytes from specifically destroying cultivated cells carrying the relevant antigens and which appear most often to be antigen-antibody complexes. The blocking factors seem to play an important role in facilitating tumor growth in vivo, and the ability of tumors to induce the formation of such factors may be of fundamental importance for their escape from immunological control. The role of blocking factors in maintaining allograft tolerance is less clear.

ACKNOWLEDGMENTS

The authors' work was supported by grants CA 10188 and CA 10189 from the National Institutes of Health, by grants IC-56D from the American Cancer Society and by contract NIG NCI E 71-2171 from the Solid Virus Tumor Program of the National Cancer Institute.

REFERENCES

1. Hellström, K.E. and Hellström, I., Adv. Immunol. 18:209, 1974.

2. Hellström, I., Hellström, K.E., Evans, C.A., Heppner, G.H., Pierce, G.E. and Yang, J.P.S., Proc. Nat. Acad. Sci. 68:1345, 1971.

3. Sjögren, H.O. and Borum, K., Cancer Res. 31:890, 1971.

4. Jagarlamoody, J.M., Aust, J.C., Tew, R.H. and McKhann, C.F., Proc, Nat. Acad. Sci. 68:1346, 1971.

5. Baldwin, R.W., Glaves, D. and Pimm, M.V., In Progress in Immunology, edited by B. Amos, Academic Press, New York, p. 907, 1971.

6. Currie, B.A. and Basham, D., Brit. J. Cancer. 26:427, 1972.

7. Youn, J.K., LeFrancois, D. and Barski, G., J. Nat. Cancer Inst. 50:921, 1973.

8. Jose, D.G. and Skvaril, F., Int. J. Cancer. 13:173, 1974.

9. Skurzak, H.M., Klein, E., Yoshida, T.O. and Lamon, E.W. J. Exp. Med. 135:997, 1972.

10. Hayami, M., Hellström, I., Hellström K.E. Int. J. Cancer. 12:667, 1973.

11. Hayami, M., Hellström, I., Hellström, K.E. and Lannin, D., Int. J. Cancer. 13:43, 1974.

12. Amos, D.B., Cohen, T. and Klein, W.J. Jr., Transplant. Proc. 2:68, 1970.

13. Klein, W.J. Jr., J. Exp. Med. 124:1238, 1971.

14. Feldman, J., Adv. Immunol. 15:167, 1972.

15. Southam, C.M., Progr. Exp. Tumor Res. 9:1, 1967.

16. Gershon, R.K., Carter, R.L. and Kondo, K., Nature. 213:674, 1967.

17. Halliday, W.J., Cell. Immunol. 3:113, 1972.

18. Vanky, F., Stjernswärd, J., Klein, G. and Nilsonne, V., J. Nat. Cancer Inst. 47:95, 1971.

19. Nelson, K. and Pollack, S. Submitted for publication.

20. Sjögren, H.O. and Bansal, S.C., In Progress in Immunology, edited by B. Amos, Academic Press, New York, p. 921, 1971.

21. Hellström, I. and Hellström, K.E., Cancer. In press.

22. Hellström, I. and Hellström, K.E. To be submitted for publication.

23. Brawn,R.R., Int. J. Cancer. 6:245, 1970.

24. Dierlam, P., Anderson, N.G. and Coggin, J.H., In Pro-
    ceedings of the First Conference and Workshop on Embry-
    onic and Fetal Antigens in Cancer, edited by
    N.G. Anderson and J.H. Coggin, Oak Ridge, Tenn., p.203, 1971.

25. Baldwin, R.W. and Embleton, M.J., Int. J. Cancer. 13:43,
    1974.

26. Bansal. S.C., Hellström, I., Hellström, K.E. and
    Sjögren, H.O., J. Exp. Med. 137:590, 1973.

27. Bansal, S.C., Hellström, I., Hellström, K.E. and
    Wright, P.W., Transplant. 16:610, 1973.

28. Wright, P.W., Bernstein, I.D., Hamilton, B., Gluckman,
    J.C. and Hellström, K.E., Transplant. In press.

29. Beverley, P.C.L., Brent, L., Brooks, C., Medawar, P.B.
    and Simpson, E., Transplant. Proc. 5:679, 1973.

30. Billingham, R.E. and Silvers, W.K., In Foundations of
    Immunobiology Series. Prentice-Hall, Inc., Englewood
    Cliffs, N.J., 1971.

31. Elkins, W.L., J.Exp. Med. 137:1097, 1973.

32. Wright, P.W., Bernstein, I.D., Hamilton, B.L. and Hell-
    ström, K.E. Manuscript in preparation.

33. Wright, P.W., Djeu, J., Mattison, R.A., Bernstein, I.D.
    and Hellström, K.E. Manuscript in preparation.

34. Wright, P.W., Hargreaves, R.E., Bansal, S.C., Bernstein,
    I.D. and K.E., Proc. Nat. Acad. Sci. 70:2539, 1973.

35. Wright, P.W., Hargreaves, R.E., Bernstein, I.D. and
    Hellström, I., J. Immunol. 112:1267, 1974.

36. Wright, P.W. and Bernstein, I.D. Manuscript in prepara-
    tion.

37. Elkins, W.L., Hellström, I. and Hellström, K.E., Trans-
    plant. In press.

38. Hellström, I. and Hellström, K.E., Int. J. Cancer. 4:
    587, 1969.

39. Sjögren, H.O., Hellström, I., Bansal, S.C. and Hellström, K.E., Proc. Nat. Acad. Sci. 68:1372, 1971.

40. Baldwin, R.W., Price, M.R. and Robins, R.A., Int. J. Cancer. 11:527, 1973.

REGRESSOR SERUM BLOCKING AT TARGET CELL LEVEL, NOT AT LYMPHOCYTE
LEVEL, INTERACTS WITH TARGET CELLS TO PRODUCE BLOCKING FACTOR:

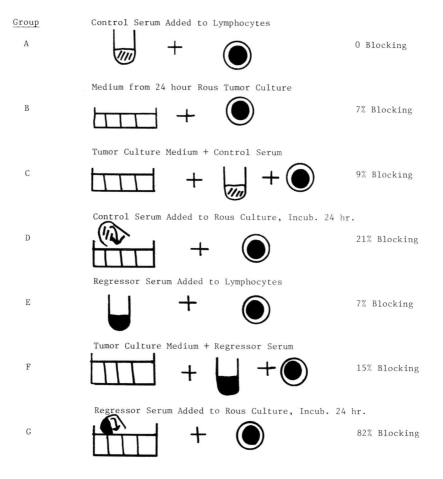

Group

A   Control Serum Added to Lymphocytes   0 Blocking

B   Medium from 24 hour Rous Tumor Culture   7% Blocking

C   Tumor Culture Medium + Control Serum   9% Blocking

D   Control Serum Added to Rous Culture, Incub. 24 hr.   21% Blocking

E   Regressor Serum Added to Lymphocytes   7% Blocking

F   Tumor Culture Medium + Regressor Serum   15% Blocking

G   Regressor Serum Added to Rous Culture, Incub. 24 hr.   82% Blocking

ON THE NATURE OF BLOCKING FACTORS

A.   Blocking activity of serum from mice with Moloney sarcomas specifically
     removed by <u>absorption</u> with Moloney sarcoma cells (Hellström + Hellström,
     1969).

B.   Blocking activity of serum from mice with Moloney sarcomas undetectable
     after adding Goat <u>anti</u> mouse <u>IgG</u> to the blocking serum (Hellström +
     Hellström, 1969).

C.   Blocking activity of serum from mice with Moloney sarcomas detected in
     <u>7s</u> fraction (Hellström + Hellström, 1969).

D.   Amicon filtration at pH 3.1 of blocking serum (Sjögren, Hellström,
     Bansal, Hellström, 1971).

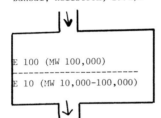

<u>E10-E100 mixture = AG-AB complex (?)</u>
<u>E10 = Antigen (?); E100 = Antibody (?)</u>

E10 + Lymphocytes: <u>Blocks</u>
E10 + Target Cells: No Blocking
E100 + Lymphocytes: No Blocking
E100 + Target Cells: No Blocking
<u>E10-E100 mixture</u> + Lymphocytes: <u>Blocks</u>
<u>E10-E100 mixture</u> + Target Cells: <u>Blocks</u>

E 100 (MW 100,000)

E 10 (MW 10,000-100,000)

E.   Prepared tumor <u>antigens</u> from rat hepatomas can specifically block
     lymphocyte mediated cytotoxicity <u>(at the lymphocyte level)</u>. <u>Mixtures</u>
     of such antigen and specific antibodies can block at both the <u>lymphocyte</u>
     <u>and the target cell level</u> (Baldwin, Price, Robins, 1973).

Tentative Conclusion:

     Antigen can block, antigen-antibody complexes can block; blocking
by complexes appear to be more "important" than blocking by free
antigen, but it is quite possible that blocking by free antigen plays
a very large role at the site of a growing tumor. The point of attack
of the blocking factors appears to be the <u>effector cell</u>, although they
can <u>bind to the tumor</u> and are present at the site of a growing tumor
in a higher concentration than in the bloodstream.

References:

Hellström, I. and Hellström, K.E., <u>Int. J. Cancer.</u> <u>4</u>:587, 1969.

Sjögren, H.O., Hellström, I., Bansal, S.C. and Hellström, K.E.,
     <u>Proc. Nat. Acad. Sci.</u> <u>68</u>:1372, 1971.

Baldwin, R.W., Price, M.R. and Robins, R.A., Int. J. Cancer. <u>11</u>:527, 1973.

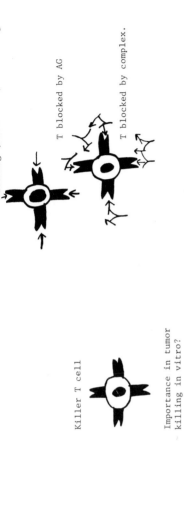
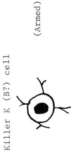

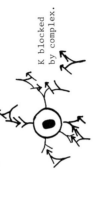
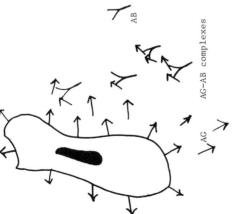

Blocking (inhibition) of killing.

T blocked by AG

T blocked by complex.

K blocked by AG

K blocked by complex.

Killer T cell

Importance in tumor killing in vitro?

Killer K (B?) cell

(Armed)

Unblocking antibodies tie up free antigen as well as antigen forming AG-AB complexes, so it cannot block lymphocyte mediated killing.

AB

AG-AB complexes

AG

Tumor cell. Releases antigen. More antigen apparently released after contact with antibodies. High local concentration of AG and AG-AB complexes.

581

DISCUSSION FOLLOWING KARL-ERIK HELLSTRÖM

BENACERRAF: Do you interpret your observation that you can cause skin rejection in tolerant animals by transferring competent lymphocytes and that this phenomenon is associated with the loss of blocking factors that the animals were indeed tolerant. The transferred cells can be interpreted to have formed antibody to eliminate the immune complexes as well as having generated cytotoxic T cells. The animals were therefore at least partially tolerant.

HELLSTRÖM: I think these results are simplest interpreted that the animals in which tolerance was broken had some cell populations which were reactive (the cytotoxic cells we observed in vitro, cells producing the antibody part of the blocking factors) and some cell populations which were either not reactive at all or whose reactivity was decreased quantitatively (due to a deletion or very effective suppressor type mechanism). The cells breaking tolerance may have either generated new cytotoxic cells and/or cells having an amplifying effect in vivo or they may have acted primarily by forming more antibodies, changing the nature of circulating antigen-antibody complex from those which could block to complexes which could not (the serum of these rats might even have become unblocking). We have not yet done experiments trying to distinguish between these alternatives. Our original data gives no support for the notion that more cytotoxic cells were generated from the cells inoculated to break tolerance, but before one has also used a short term assay (like the Cr^{51} Test) to study that, we cannot exclude that this had happened.

GERSHON: Sjögren originally used splenectomized animals for in vivo deblocking studies. Do you have any further information on what role the spleen may be playing in either the production or mode of action of blocking or deblocking factors?

HELLSTRÖM: Splenectomy depresses blocking serum activity, and this was the reason for Sjögren to splenectomize the animals which he then further treated by giving unblocking antibodies. The effect of splenectomy is, however, most clearly seen when performed before inoculation of animals with tumor cells. When it is done on tumor-bearing animals, the effects are marginal.

GERSHON: You say prior splenectomy diminished the production of blocking factors while post-splenectomy does not diminish the production once it has started. This is similar to the data I presented yesterday with the mode of action of suppressor spleen-seeking T cells in the absence of antibody production.

HELLSTRÖM: Of course, one interesting possibility is that the molecules released by your suppressor spleen cells and "our" blocking factors are essentially the same. I found Marc Feldmann's provocative observation that supernatants of suppressor cells contained IgT-antigen complexes most interesting in this respect. Some old observations of Hapmer comes to my mind in this context. He found, in agreement with Martinez, that neonatal thymectomy of mammary tumor virus containing mice decreased the frequency of spontaneous mammary carcinomas. A few mice got such tumors, however, even when thymectomized. The serum from such mice had a lesser blocking activity than that from controls with tumors; the controls had been sham-thymectomized neonatally.

BRITTON: The ease by which you abrogate transplantation tolerance in your rats (i.e., by injection of 20 x 10^6 normal syngeneic lymph-node cells) does not that argue against suppressor cells being responsible for your type of transplantation tolerance?

HELLSTRÖM: Maybe it does, but I do not at all think that it excludes a suppressor mechanism. Such a mechanism may provide a delicate balance which is fairly easily disturbed. The doses we used for tolerance abrogation in rats were the same as employed by Billingham and others in the past (20 x 10^6 immune cells, 40 x 10^6 non-immune cells) and these doses regularly broke tolerance. On the other hand, it is the experience of at least some that allograft tolerance in mice is not always that easily broken by inoculation of lymphoid cells.

G. MÖLLER: The correlation between blocking factors and tumor recurrence after surgery is a necessary consequence of the system and does not in any way indicate that blocking factors contribute to tumor development. Since the patients get tumors because all tumors were not removed, there will be synthesis of antigens and of

specific antibodies which you detect as blocking factors. The correlation is intrinsic in the system.

HELLSTRÖM: I certainly agree with you on that. This does
not, of course, diminish the potential importance of
these findings since the demonstration of evidence of
a growing tumor, before it is clinically apparent, by
using an immunological technique can be practically
very important. Why I say that blocking factors to
tumor antigens play a role in facilitating tumor growth
in vivo is primarily because of the demonstration that
inoculation of rats with serum blocking (polyoma)
tumor-cell destruction in vitro could enhance tumor
growth in vivo, and the finding that unblocking antibodies, reversing the blocking effect in vitro and in
vivo could inhibit tumor growth when given in vivo. The
correlative data obtained on human patients are in
agreement with the notion that the blocking factors
facilitate tumor growth in vivo, but do not at all prove
it for the reasons you mentioned.

LESKOWITZ: Following up on Göran Möller's question, could
you say whether the blocking factor found in patients
with no detectable tumor is physicochemically the
same or different from that isolated from patients with
tumors.

HELLSTRÖM: So far, there is no evidence they are any different, but one needs to know more about the physicochemical nature of the blocking factors before this question
can be conclusively answered.

SMITH: The question of whether tumor antigen acts directly
upon effector T lymphocytes is perhaps more complex
than we have realized. In our assay using carefully
washed peripheral lymphocytes, lymph node cells, or
spleen cells taken from MCA tumor-bearing animals, are
treated with varying concentrations of KCL-solubilized
tumor membranes. Proliferation is assessed over a 13
day period as in an MLC. We found stimulation occurs
when a 40-50000 MW material is used whereas equally
specific inhibition of ongoing DNA synthesis in such
cell subpopulations occurs when fractions having average MW below 30,000 and above 10,000 are used. This
system involves no added antitumor antibody.

Addition of tumor-bearing serum does however give

inhibition (=blocking). While it would appear that we are dealing with a purely antigen-mediated effect, as Hellstrom has described in his inhibition or blocking studies, we cannot exclude the possibility that B-cells present in the cell mixtures secrete small amounts of high affinity antibody thus the effects do indeed require that antigen be in form of a complex. The fact that higher MW material actually overcomes inhibition and stimulates may then be due to stimulation of a separate subset of tumor responsive cells.

ANTIBODY-MEDIATED TOLERANCE

Gregory W. Siskind, Marc E. Weksler and Gary Birnbaum

Division of Allergy and Immunology
Department of Medicine
Cornell University Medical College
New York, N.Y. 10021

Immunological tolerance, if defined in operational terms, refers to a specific depression of antibody synthesis as a result of previous exposure to antigen. So defined, a variety of different states of specific tolerance can be envisioned. It has been clearly demonstrated that a tolerant state can exist as a result of specific inhibition of either or both T lymphocyte or B lymphocyte function (1). Other types of tolerant states must also be considered. It is well known that passively administered antibody will specifically depress the immune response to concomitantly injected antigen (2). Antibody-mediated suppression has furthermore been shown by Bystryn, Graff and Uhr (3) to operate in vivo as a control mechanism in the normal immune response. Most studies dealing with antibody-mediated suppression support the concept that antibody acts by binding antigen, and thus blocking its interaction with potential antibody-forming cells and/or causing its rapid elimination from the host. Consistent with this interpretation is our data indicating that high affinity passive antibody is far more effective in causing suppression than is low affinity passive antibody (4). Our further observation (5, 6) that suppression preferentially affects low affinity antibody formation is also consistent with this hypothesis.

In view of these observations it may be predicted that if an animal were immunized in such a manner as to elicit the synthesis of relatively small amounts of high affinity antibody, then the animal would exhibit a depressed response to a subsequent attempt at immunization. That is, the presence of small amounts of circulating antibody would be expected to suppress the animal's immune response upon subsequent challenge. Such an animal would be called "tolerant" by the classical definition, although the mechanism of the tolerant state is the synthesis of high affinity antibody. Several previous workers have described states of immune depression which appeared to be directly mediated by circulating antibody (7, 8).

We have been studying a state of specific immunological tolerance which appears to be mediated by the production of small amounts of moderately high affinity antibody as a result of the "tolerizing" injection of antigen. In this system tolerance to 2,4-dinitrophenylated-bovine gamma globulin (DNP-BGG) is induced in inbred mice (LAF$_1$; Jackson Laboratories, Bar Harbor, Maine) by a single intravenous injection of 0.5 mg DNP-BGG. Such animals show an 80% reduction in their indirect plaque-forming cell PFC response to 0.5 mg DNP-BGG in complete Freund's adjuvant (CFA) five days later. It should be noted that the tolerance-inducing antigen preparation is a highly substituted protein (57 DNP groups per molecule) with a tendency to aggregate and partially precipitate from solution in normal saline at neutral pH. The antigen was not ultracentrifuged or in any way treated so as to render it free of aggregates. Such an antigen preparation would generally be regarded as highly immunogenic.

Based upon inhibition of PFC by DNP-ε-amino-n-caproic acid (DNP-EACA), a high avidity subpopulation of anti-DNP antibody-forming cells can be detected at one and at two weeks after immunization with antigen in CFA in the tolerant but not in the normal animals. Mice injected only with 0.5 mg DNP-BGG intravenously show a small but definite direct (2,200) and indirect (8,300 PFC/spleen) anti-DNP PFC response five days after antigen injection. The response was of moderate affinity.

Lethally irradiated syngeneic mice reconstituted with spleen cells from tolerant animals were not tolerant when immunized with DNP-BGG in CFA. In fact, recipients of cells from tolerant animals showed a greater PFC response of higher avidity than was observed in recipients of cells from untreated controls. Moderate numbers of normal spleen cells injected into tolerant animals failed to alter the tolerant state. The above data are all consistent with the hypothesis that tolerance in this experimental model is the result of the synthesis of small amounts of relatively high affinity antibody in response to the tolerance-inducing injection of antigen.

It may be predicted that antibody-mediated tolerance, such as described above, would be hapten-specific. To test this prediction, mice tolerized with DNP-BGG were immunized with either DNP-BGG or DNP-rabbit serum albumin (DNP-RSA). There was an 89% depression of the direct and an 83% depression of the indirect anti-DNP PFC response to DNP-BGG. In contrast, there was only a 17% depression of the direct and a 33% depression of the indirect anti-DNP PFC response to DNP-RSA. Thus, the tolerant state was found to have a significant degree of carrier specificity. Carrier specificity is usually associated with T cell functions. However, it should be borne in mind that serum antibody also has considerable carrier specificity in the sense that anti-hapten antibody binds the hapten-immunizing carrier complex with greater affinity than it binds either the free hapten or the hapten on a different carrier (9). Thus, circulating antibody might well show carrier specificity in antibody-mediated suppression. Mice injected with mouse anti-DNP-BGG antibody showed a 98% suppression of direct and a 99% suppression of indirect PFC response to DNP-RSA. Thus, the carrier specificity observed in the tolerant animals is consistent with the hypothesis that the tolerance is mediated by serum antibody.

In conclusion, we have characterized a state of specific immunological tolerance which was induced in adult mice by a single intravenous injection of a soluble, although presumably somewhat aggregated antigen. The data suggest that this tolerance state is mediated by the production of relatively high affinity serum antibody as a result of the tolerance-inducing injection of antigen. Tolerance in this experimental model appears to be the consequence of a normal immune response to an immunogenic antigen.

ACKNOWLEDGMENTS

This work was supported in part by research grants from the U.S.P.H.S., N.I.H. numbers AM-13701 and CA-13339. Dr. Gregory W. Siskind is a Career Scientist of the Health Research Council of the City of New York under Investigatorship I-593.

REFERENCES

1. Chiller, J.M., Habicht, G.S. and Weigle, W.O., Science. 171:813, 1971.

2. Uhr, J.W. and Möller, G., Advanc. Immunol. 8:81, 1968.

3. Bystryn, J.C., Graff, M.W. and Uhr, J.W., J. Exp. Med. 132:1279, 1970.

4. Walker, J.G. and Siskind, G.W., Immunology. 14:21, 1968.

5. Siskind, G.W., Dunn, P. and Walker, J.G., J. Exp. Med. 127:55, 1968.

6. Heller, K.S. and Siskind, G.W., Cell. Immunol. 6:59, 1973.

7. Crowle, A.J. and Hu, C.C., J. Immunol. 103:1242, 1969.

8. Asherson, G.L., Zembala, M. and Barnes, R.M.R., Clin. Med. 123:689, 1966.

9. Paul, W.E., Siskind, G.W. and Benacerraf, B., J. Exp. Med. 123:689, 1966.

IgE ANTIBODY-SPECIFIC ABROGATION OF AN ESTABLISHED IMMUNE RESPONSE IN MICE BY MODIFIED ANTIGENS

Michael K. Bach and John R. Brashler

Department of Hypersensitivity Diseases Research
The Upjohn Co.
Kalamazoo, Michigan 49001

We have employed the model described by Levine and Vaz (1) for the elicitation of a boostable IgE response in mice to seek methods for the specific abrogation of an establish- ed IgE immune response. Our approach was based on the ob- servations by Parish (2, 3) that acetoacetylated antigens are tolerogenic with respect to humoral antibody production while at the same time inducing a cell-mediated immune res- ponse. This may point to a change in the way T cells res- pond to the antigen. In addition, Okumura and Tada (4, 5) have presented evidence that T cells control and regulate the IgE response in rats. Our hope, therefore, was that acetoacetylated antigens, by affecting the T cell response to the antigen, might be useful in abrogating the reagin response. We would like to present results which demonstrate that it is possible to specifically block IgE production in DBA/1 mice in response to booster, low dose immunizations with ovalbumin (OA) by treating the OA-primed animals with acetoacetylated ovalbumin (AcAc-AO).

Acetoacetylated-OA was prepared by the slow addition of the calculated volume of an acetone solution of diketene to a solution of OA in 0.05 M borate buffer pH 8.2 with stir- ring (2). The pH was maintained by addition of alkali. After standing at room temperature overnight and exhaustive dialysis, the degree of acetoacetylation was estimated by determining the absorption at 540 nm of the $FeCl_3$ complex (6), using a molar extinction coefficient of 371 for the acetoacetyl-ferric chloride complex.

Production of IgE was initiated by the injection of 1 μg OA complexed to 1 mg aluminum hydroxide gel, i.p. Subse- quent booster injections were given at 4 week intervals by the same route, using the same doses of antigen and adjuvant. Bleedings by the orbital sinus were collected serially 8-10 days after each booster injection. Two tenths of a ml of blood were obtained from each of 5 animals and the sera from these were pooled and stored at $-85^{\circ}C$ until use. Treatment with AcAc-OA was, in general, by the intravenous route and was given as three 1 mg doses of the antigen on alternate days beginning 4 weeks after the initial immunization. The titers of IgE antibody to OA were estimated by the PCA titration in Sprague Dawley rats (7). The total antibody content of the sera was estimated by Osler's modification of the Farr technique (8) using ^{125}I-labelled OA.

A series of acetoacetylated OA preparations were evaluated for their effect on the capacity of primed mice to produce IgE on subsequent challenge with unsubstituted or dinitrophenyl-substituted OA complexed to aluminum hydroxide gel (Table I).

There was no IgE produced which cross-reacted with acetoacetylated BSA. Although not shown in the table, the same was also true when hemagglutinating antibodies were estimated with sheep erythrocytes passively sensitized with AcAc-OA, OA or AcAc-BSA.

Since tolerance induction usually requires the i.v. administration of antigen in soluble form, the effect of the intravenous administration of the various AcAc-OA preparations was examined (Table II). Two effects were noted: 1) When unsubstituted OA or OA with a low level of acetoacetylation were used, a large number of mice died in anaphylaxis and 2) With the more highly substituted AcAc-OA, there was a rapid increase in titer about a week after the treatments; this was followed by an apparent paralysis or tolerance when subsequent i.p. challenges of antigen bound to aluminum hydroxide were given. In all subsequent experiments AcAc-OA having an average substitution of 11-13 acetoacetyl groups per mole (73 - 87% of the free amino groups) was used. For convenience the effect will be referred to as "tolerance" although it is recognized that the mechanism of unreactivity has not been defined.

Even a single 1 mg dose of AcAc-OA caused a 70% reduction in IgE titer when the response of the animals during a subsequent challenge with OA was compared to that of untreated, challenged controls. Two 1 mg doses caused essentially a 100% inhibition and further doses up to a total of 5 given over intervals of 1 to 4 days between treatments had the same effect. Maximum inhibition was achieved when a cumulative dose of 0.4 mg AcAc-OA or greater was given in 3 or 4 doses spaced one to two days apart. A single 0.1 mg dose or five 0.01 mg doses resulted in a 50% inhibition. Administration of AcAc-OA by the i.v. route resulted in the greatest inhibition of IgE production upon challenge with OA while the subcutaneous route was somewhat less effective. Treatment by the intramuscular or intraperitoneal routes was considerably less effective. On the other hand three 1 mg doses of unsubstituted OA given without aluminum hydroxide i.p. consistently caused more tolerance than the same dose of AcAc-OA given by any route. It will be recalled that when unsubstituted OA was given to these sensitized animals by the i.v. route, it caused anaphylaxis and the death of the animals.

One of the features of the mouse model for IgE production is that it is possible to maintain the mice with boostable and high IgE titers for many months and many cycles of booster immunization. We were interested to know if the suppression of IgE production would persist over the useful period of IgE production in this model system. As seen in Fig. 1, the "tolerogenic" effect of AcAc-OA persisted through at least three booster immunizations over a total period of 180 days when the treated groups were subjected to a second round of i.v. treatments with AcAc-OA after the first booster immunization with OA. Without this second round of treatments with AcAc-OA (Fig. 2), "tolerance" lasted through two rounds of booster immunizations, but by the time of the third round (day 126), the titer of the "tolerant" group was nearly the same as the titer of the control group even though no antigen had been injected into either group since day 88. There was no inhibition of IgE production during booster immunization in "tolerant" mice at the third round of immunization. This "escape from tolerance" is somewhat related to the dose of antigen or modified antigen which was used during the original treatments. Animals which received five treatments with 0.01 mg AcAc-OA per treatment "escaped" by the time of the fourth treatment with antigen, i.e. the second treatment after the "tolerizing" treatments. Animals receiving five treatments with 0.1 or 1 mg of AcAc-OA per treatment, on the other hand, were protected through an additional booster immunization before their IgE titers rose to the level of the controls.

TABLE I

IMMUNOGENICITY OF AcAc-OA

Groups of mice were immunized with 1 μg AcAc-OA in 1 mg Al (OH)$_3$, challenged 28 days later with the same preparation and finally, challenged a third time with 1 μg DNP-OA + 1 mg Al (OH)$_3$ on day 56.

Immunogen / PCA Challenging Antigen	DAY 28 DNP OA	28 OA	28 AcAc⊕ BSA	38 DNP OA	38 OA	38 DNP BSA	38 AcAc⊕ BSA	56 DNP OA	66 DNP OA	66 DNP BSA	66 AcAc⊕ BSA
DNP OA	65	<10		560	970	232		378	1800	2930	
AcAc 2.1 OA	116			1120				325	930		
AcAc 6.7 OA	91			540				162	930		
AcAc$_{10.9}$ OA	18	<10	<25	530	460	<10	<10	232	1820	23	<10
AcAc$_{12.7}$ OA	25			540				135	800		
OA*	40							40	650		

*This group was not reimmunized until day 56.

⊕AcAc 12.5 BSA was used for challenge.

594

TABLE II

EFFECT OF DEGREE OF ACETOACETYLATION ON THE INHIBITION OF SUBSEQUENT IgE ANTI-OA PRODUCTION IN OA-PRIMED MICE TREATED WITH AcAc-OA.

Treatment (Day 28-32)	DAY 38	56	66[+]
None	---	40	650
OA*	217	100	340
AcAc $_{2.1}$ OA*	58	24	41
AcAc $_{6.7}$ OA**			
AcAc$_{10.9}$ OA	1040	75	122
AcAc$_{12.7}$ OA	420	100	240

+10 days after challenge with 1 μg OA and 1 mg Al $(OH)_3$ i.p.

*Only one mouse survived; the rest died in anaphylaxis.

**All the mice in this group died from anaphylaxis.

Since maintenance of tolerance usually requires the persistence of antigen at low doses, we examined the duration of the "tolerant" state in the AcAc-OA-treated mice in the absence of intervening exposure to booster immunizations with antigen. The results of one such experiment are summarized in Table III. In this experiment the animals were primed with OA and then treated with a "tolerizing" regimen of AcAc-OA after various intervals. At least 2 months could elapse between the first exposure to antigen and the treatment to induce "tolerance". However, when three months were allowed to elapse, most of the "tolerizing" effect of the treatment seemed to have been lost.

TABLE III

PERSISTENCE OF THE PROTECTIVE EFFECT OF A SINGLE COURSE OF OA-
PRIMED MICE WITH AcAc-OA IN THE ABSENCE OF FURTHER EXPOSURE TO OA

All treated mice received three, one mg doses of AcAc-OA on alternate days beginning
as shown. Controls for each treatment group received their first booster immunization
on the day treatments were begun, and pre- and post-boost bleeds on the controls were,
therefore, approximately 1 month earlier than those from the treated groups.

Day of Treatment	Day of Challenge		PCA Units		% of Control Increase*
			Pre-Boost	Post-Boost	
49	77	Control	475	830	
		Treated	210	322	31
63	105	Control	526	1520	
		Treated	250	450	20
91	133	Control	294; 800**	2500; 1590**	
		Treated	330; 500**	1190; 1000**	39; 63**

* % of control increase = $\dfrac{\text{(PCA post-boost - PCA pre-boost) treated}}{\text{(PCP post-boost - PCA pre-boost) control}} \times 100$

** Data from a separate experiment which differed in that controls were first challenged
on the actual day on which treated groups were challenged.

Attempts were made to find correlations between the antibody content of the sera of animals at the time of booster immunization and the response of the animals to the immunization. Despite technical difficulties with the passive hemagglutination reaction using OA as the antigen, sera of animals which had been treated with AcAc-OA had hemagglutinating antibody titers 5 to 10 times those of the boosted controls in several experiments. The persistence of these high titers did not generally coincide with the persistence of "tolerance" in the same animals even though the high hemagglutinating antibody titers seemed to persist for long periods of time. Using the Osler modification of the Farr technique to measure total OA-specific antibody, both these values were uniformly highest early following treatment with AcAc-OA or following the first booster immunization in the boosted controls. The antibody content then declined to a relatively stable lower level. Figure 3 is a representative example of these relationships using the results from only one "tolerizing" treatment in three different experiments.

There was, thus, no correlation between the hemagglutinating antibody titer, the total or high affinity antibody content or the IgE response of the respective animals to booster immunization. The well known (9) difficulty in radioiodination of OA to high specific activity prevented us from carrying out any more detailed analyses of the composition of the OA-specific antibodies in these sera.

We tested the possibility that "tolerance" induction after treatment of mice with AcAc-OA was due to suppression of the IgE response by other circulating immunoglobulins further (10, 11). Mice were primed with OA and 2 days before the first booster immunization they were injected i.v. with up to 100 μl of a mouse serum pool containing 0.6 mg/ml of OA-specific antibody. The serum pool had been obtained from mice three months after treatment with AcAc-OA and after repeated booster immunizations to which the mice had not responded. Not only did these treatments fail to prevent IgE production upon booster immunization, the titers of the sera from the treated mice resembled the titers of the late bleeds of the immunized control animals in that the characteristic drop in IgE titer 4 weeks after booster immunization was abolished.

The "tolerogenic" effect of treatment of the mice with AcAc-OA was antigen-specific. Simultaneous or subsequent induction of an IgE antibody response to dissociated keyhole limpet hemocyanin (KLH) was unaffected by the treatments. On the other hand and contrary to our predictions, the effect was not at all unique to acetoacetylated antigen. Of a series of some 13 chemically-modified OA derivatives, all were more or less tolerogenic provided the native structure of OA was sufficiently modified to reduce its antigenicity. Thus, a number of preparations in which the available amino groups of lysine were substituted by relatively large groups were tolerogenic regardless of the charge or hydrophobicity of these groups; if the degree of substitution was small or if the substituting groups were small (e.g. acetyl groups), the treated animals died in anaphylaxis. Modification of the arginyl or tryptophanyl residues of OA also resulted in "tolerogenic" preparations even when the lysine residues were left intact. Death by anaphylaxis during "tolerizing" treatment correlated with the presence in the animals of high circulating titers of a heat-sensitive 2-mercaptoethanol-sensitive antibody which, from all indications, represents mouse IgE. It did not correlate with the presence of even very high titers of circulating precipitating or total antibodies. For this reason we have not been able to induce "tolerance" in mice which had already received a booster immunization of OA by treating them subsequently with AcAc-OA.

The mechanism of the "tolerogenic" effect of the AcAc-OA treatments remains unclear. Operationally, high doses of modified antigen were required to produce the effect. Levine and Vaz (1) reported that primary immunization of mice with high doses of antigen complexed to aluminum hydroxide tends to result in lower titers of IgE and in loss of the ability to evoke a boostable response. We have confirmed these observations. It is, therefore, possible that the induction of tolerance by high doses of modified OA is analogous to the non-boostable response which is seen when the primary immunization is with a similarly high dose of antigen. In practice, the difference between "high" dose and "low" dose immunization is actually quite small. It should be recalled that 3 to 5 treatments with 10 μg given i.v. can constitute the "high" dose while 1 μg complexed to aluminum hydroxide which presumably remains around much longer is a "low" dose.

Recent observations on the life expectancy of different functional subgroups of T cells (12) may afford an explanation for our observed effects: We postulate that one way to achieve "tolerance" is by the net induction of "suppressor" T cells while induction of IgE synthesis depends on stimula-

tion of the IgE-specific helper T cells. Immunization with
low doses of antigen activates the helper cells without
activating the suppressor cells, thus, resulting in a net
increase in the level of circulating IgE. Feedback effects
of the circulating immunoglobulins cause the induction of
suppressor cells or the inhibition of the IgE-producing cells
directly, resulting in a gradual decrease in the level of
circulating IgE. The IgE-specific "memory" cells remain
intact; however, a repeated induction of the suppressor cells
by this route causes the gradual elimination of the suppressor cells precursor pool so that after several cycles of low
dose booster immunization, IgE production becomes chronic
and no longer displays the decreased titers between booster
immunizations. When immunization is with high doses of antigen, the suppressor cells are directly activated along with
all the available helper cells. The interactions which follow result in the relative elimination of the helper cells
and retention of the suppressor cell function, thus, producing a transient, non-boostable IgE response which was
equated with "tolerance" in the model system we have been
describing. Finally, the passive administration of late
serum from "tolerant" mice bypasses the need to generate the
immunoglobulins which inhibit the suppressor cells and thus,
effects a suppressor cell depletion early in the course of
these chronic immunizations. Obviously, there is no evidence
in the work we have presented to support this theory, and a
number of alternatives can be envisioned. The theory is
being presented as a point for discussion in the hope that
it will lead to the formulation of further experiments.

It is too early to speculate on the practical applicability of the "tolerogenic" phenomenon we have described.
In the clinical situation patients are generally seen after
the equivalent of more than one booster exposure to the
allergen to which they are responding. Before application
can be considered, therefore, it will be necessary to devise
means of abrogating the IgE response not only after a priming immunization but after booster immunizations as well.
As already mentioned, attempts to achieve this have not been
successful up to now. Thus, until less antigenic preparations and/or better protective maneuvers can be devised,
this study will have to remain in the realm of mouse medicine.

REFERENCES

1. Levine, B.B. and Vaz, N.M., Int. Arch. Allergy. 39:156, 1970.

2. Parish, C.R., J. Exp. Med. 134:1, 1971.

3. Parish, C.R., J. Exp. Med. 134:21, 1971.

4. Okumura, K. and Tada, T., J. Immunol. 106:1019, 1971.

5. Okumura, K. and Tada, T., J. Immunol. 107:1682, 1971.

6. Marzotto, A., Pajetta, P., Galzinga, L. and Scoffone, E., Biochem. Biophys. Acta. 154:450, 1968.

7. Bach, M.K. and Brashler, J.R., Immunol. Communic. 2: 85, 1973.

8. Osler, A.G., In Methods in Immunology and in Immuno-chemistry, edited by C.A. Williams and M.W. Chase, Academic Press, N.Y., Vol. 3, p. 73, 1971.

9. McConahey, P.J. and Dixon, F.J., Int. Arch. Allergy. 29:185, 1966.

10. Tada, T. and Okumura, K., J. Immunol. 106:1002, 1971.

11. Strannegard, O. and Belin, L., Immunology. 18:775, 1970.

12. Feldbush, T.L., Cell. Immunol. 8:435, 1973.

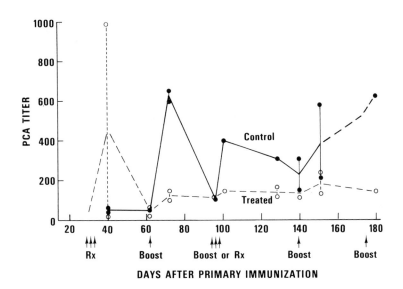

Fig. 1. Persistence of the protective effect of repeated i.v. administration of AcAc-OA to DNP-OA-primed mice during subsequent booster immunizations with DNP-OA. Results are combined from two separate experiments.

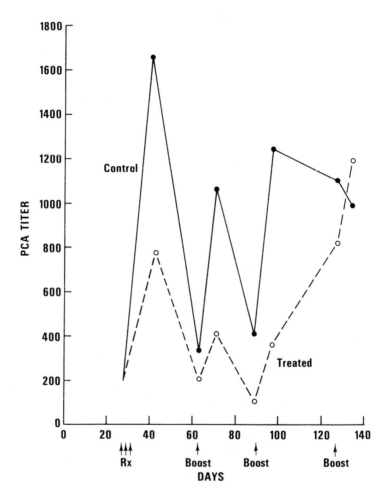

Fig. 2. Persistence of the protective effect of treatment with AcAc-OA in OA-primed mice during subsequent challenges with OA. Results are combined from three experiments.

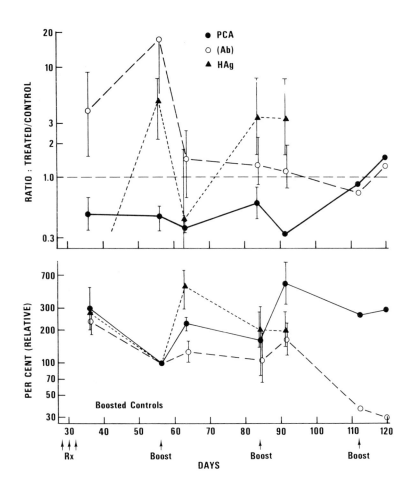

Fig. 3. Effect of treatment of OA-primed mice with AcAc-OA on the IgE, hemagglutinating and total antibody titers during subsequent challenges with OA. Results from three separate experiments are combined using the data from the boosted controls on day 56 as 100% (relative) in each case. HAg is hemagglutinating antibody; (Ab) is total antibody concentration.

GENERAL DISCUSSION - SESSION VI

SUPPRESSIVE ACTIVITY OF ANTIBODY
and ANTIGEN-ANTIBODY COMPLEXES

Bernhard Cinader, Chairman

WAKSMAN: We should remember the observations of Voisin who, in a series of papers extending from 1958 to the present, incriminated certain specific immunoglobulin classes as responsible for tolerance to tumor or transplantation antigens and for enhancement. These proved to be either IgG1 or IgA in a variety of systems. One wonders whether the fact that these are non-complement-fixing is in some way significant.

HELLSTRÖM: It was good you brought attention the fact that Voisin was the one who said, before most of the rest of us, that blocking type mechanisms can exist in operationally-defined allograft tolerance. As to Voisin's report, however, that antibodies with enhancing or blocking properties are of the IgA class, unable to bind complement, I think it is important to point out that others like Tokuda, Fahey and Hildemann, also studying the nature of enhancing antibodies in mice did not come to that conclusion: their evidence was that the molecules were IgGγ2, which can bind complement. In the tumor systems studies by ourselves, Baldwin and others there is evidence that sera with cytotoxic antibodies active in the presence of complement become blocking in vitro following addition of antigen suggesting (but not proving) that the blockers are antigen-antibody complexes and that antibodies of a class normally binding complement can form a part of such complexes.

WAKSMAN: Voisin employed several types of column separation and compared antibody activities in each fraction, measured by several serological techniques, with ability to enhance tumor growth. It seems clear from this work that there are several types of antibody, e.g. IgM, which do not act in this manner.

E. MÖLLER: You must distinguish between the antibody Voisin found in skin graft tolerant mice, and the enhancing antibody. As a matter of fact, the antibody present in tolerant mice was only revealed by an indirect

605

technique, which could be explained by its being an antigen-antibody complex.

G.MÖLLER: It is important to distinguish between enhancement and complex-induced tolerance of the type Diener and Feldmann try to convince us is an important mechanism. In animals receiving passive antibody (enhanced animals), tumors grew because the lymphocytes were not turned off and it could easily be demonstrated in a variety of systems that the cells in antibody-treated animals be-haved as normal lymphocytes. In the hypothesis of Diener-Feldmann it is claimed that the cells are turned off.

WAKSMAN: I well remember Göran's elegant study on this ques-tion. At the time they were done, it seemed vital to distinquish afferent, central, and efferent forms of enhancement. The Möller data bear only on the question of afferent blocking, whereas the Voisin and Hellstrom work has to do mainly with central and efferent effects.

DIENER: We should keep in mind that enhancement in its original sense means no more than enhanced growth of a tumor or prolonged acceptance of an allograft under conditions in which immune rejection is expected.

BRITTON: Spleen cells from mice carrying an allogeneic transplant (embryonic heart) do reveal cytotoxic cells after 4 days in vitro culture but not if tested directly after in vivo harvest. I would like to ask Erwin Diener what is the organ nature (T or B?) of this re-vealed cytotoxic cell and is it identical in nature with the cytotoxic cell found in the immune animal? I sug-gest that this is not the case but that in vitro in-cubation may allow for alloantibody formation which causes antibody induced cell-mediated cytotoxicity. Such a mechanism would not be operative in vivo in graft rejection as the effector cell is a non-circulating one.

DIENER: I have said that our heart-allograft tolerant mice have immunocompetent spleen cells which, as in normal mice, can be induced in vitro to become effector cells. These effector cells have shown to be active in the in vitro killing of mastocytoma target cells.

PAUL: I wish to address a question to both Marc Feldmann and Erwin Diener. Can you tell us 1) what concentrations of

a characterized complex of antigen and purified antibody are required to achieve T lymphocyte and B lymphocyte tolerance, 2) for how long these complexes must
be present, and 3) whether these conditions are apt
to be achieved in the milieu of lymphocytes in vivo?

FELDMANN: That is a difficult question to answer. Our old
work on tolerance to POL could be made to work with 20
ng/ml of antigen and appropriate, approximately equivalent concentration of antibody. But what we really
need to know is the amount at the cell surface, and that
has not yet been quantitated.

DIENER: We have to stress that in our model, a blocking
complex behaves optimally when the ratio of antigen
to antibody is about 1:3. Such a complex is an open
system which keeps increasing its size as long as
appropriate amounts of antigen and antibody are available. We understand that if such a complex starts to
build up on the surface of an immunocompetent cell, it
will in time cover up as many receptors as must occur
under conditions of high-zone tolerance.

DRESSER: Does Professor Benacerraf think the phenomenon of
immune-deviation (Borek, Asherson) is an example of a
blocking factor acting within the B-system?

BENACERRAF: The phenomenon you are referring to is that
originally described by Dvorak and Asherson and termed
immune deviation. That phenomenon was interpreted then
as selective tolerance in a class of immunoglobulins.
We feel today that a more appropriate interpretation
would be that different classes of immunoglobulins are
differently susceptible to the regulatory activities
of helper and suppressor T cells which are induced by
different modes of immunization.

LESKOWITZ: I've always had a fond spot for the Diener-Feldmann antigen-antibody aggregate model since it is the
only molecular model we have. But I have a conceptual
difficulty in understanding it in relation to antigens
such as serum proteins. Since a particular T cell has
only one kind of receptor on its surface, the protein
antigen having no repeating units will be effectively
monovalent in respect to this T cell. Therefore in
order to build up a complex, the antigen would have to
react with one T cell then another and another in order

to build a complex such as you get with a polyvalent serum. This seems like a very inefficient process <u>in vivo</u>.

FELDMANN: I agree that complexes of antigen and antibody formed with antibody released by B cells or IgT released by T cells would probably be small with monomeric antigens, unless multiple lines of cells are present. At the moment we do not know the size of complexes needed to suppress T cells compared with B cells. The fact that T cells are suppressed by monomeric antigens alone, and are more sensitive to complex-induced suppression would suggest that small complexes may be sufficient to tolerize T cells.

DIENER: In answer to your question I refer to our review in <u>Transplant. Rev.</u> 8:76, 1972 where we try to explain the problem you mentioned. According to our model it is possible to build an antigen-antibody complex on an immuno-competent cell by antibody of different specificity than that of the receptor on the cell. This would work, provided both antigenic specificities are on the same carrier.

TAYLOR: Further to Dr. Leskowitz's remark on tolerance to monomeric proteins; if it is true that one can get tolerance with the hapten ABA-tyrosine, then it would not be necessary to have any kind of complex at all.

LESKOWITZ: Tolerance by monovalent ABA conjugates since they are transient in nature may involve a different mechanism of some sort such as receptor blockade by the monovalent antigen alone.

SUMMARY AND POTENTIAL THERAPEUTIC APPLICATIONS

BARUJ BENACERRAF, CHAIRMAN

GENERAL DISCUSSION - SESSION VII

Baruj Benacerraf, Chairman

BENACERRAF: The final General Discussion should attempt to
identify what has been established concerning the phenomenology and mechanisms of specific immunological tolerance, what are the major unresolved issues and what
approaches appear most promising to answer these questions.

We must also ascertain realistically whether our
understanding of tolerance phenomena and of their
mechanisms can begin to be successfully applied to the
treatment of clinical problems, and whether the systems
or tools have been developed in the laboratory which
can be used to suppress undesirable and harmful specific immune responses. In this respect, it is already
apparent that as far as B cell tolerance is concerned,
a type of molecule of which the random linear copolymer
of D-glutamic acid and D-lysine (D-GL) is a typical
example, can be used successfully in an appropriate
dose range to tolerize primary and memory B cells specific for determinants covalently bound to it. These
molecules are characterized by: 1) the inability to
stimulate T cells, 2) their resistance to degradation
in cells and tissues and 3) their absence of toxicity.

The many papers which we have heard presented in
this symposium have demonstrated that the phenomenology
classified under the general headings of specific tolerance or specific immunological unresponsiveness constitute in fact a variety of complex phenomena, many
with distinct mechanisms.

Recent progress in cellular immunology has permitted us to distinguish tolerance phenomena in defined
systems as operating either in T cells or B cells or in
both of these cell types. Different mechanisms have
been identified for the induction of tolerance in B
cells and in T cells. For instance, one of the major
advances at this meeting has been the recognition of
the importance of suppressor T cells in certain types
of tolerance phenomena. The experiments reported by
Gershon, Basten, Tada, Claman, Baker and by ourselves
have demonstrated the activity of a class of specific
T cells in suppressing immune responses specifically.

In certain of these studies it was further shown that the suppressor T cells exert their effects by acting on T cells concerned with cellular immunity or helper function, although the possibility that suppressor T cells may also act directly on B cells has not been ruled out, particularly in Baker's studies where B cell tolerance to SIII is obtained with low doses of the polysaccharide. The mechanism of action of suppressor T cells is one of the important mysteries to be resolved for the next Tolerance Conference. In fact, as far as tolerance mechanisms are concerned, practically nothing is known concerning the process or processes through which T cells are specifically inactivated. In contrast substantial progress has been achieved with respect to our understanding of B cell tolerance. This is not surprising since B cells have been much more amenable to analysis and the immunoglobulin nature of their receptors is not in doubt. It is reasonable to expect that further advances will be made in this area with the availability of purified B cell populations of known specificity and affinity. The studies of B cell tolerance to thymus-independent antigens of Feldmann and Diener have been very informative and have greatly clarified the importance of antigen dose and epitope density for the induction of this type of tolerance. Studies from many laboratories have also illustrated the critical role of helper T cells in inhibiting B cell tolerance. This result is achieved through the ability of activated helper T cells to increase considerably the range of antigen concentration which is immunogenic for B cells in the case of thymus-dependent responses. For this class of antigen, therefore, B cell tolerance should depend upon the previous induction of T cell tolerance or upon the absence of qualitatively or quantitatively adequate T cell helper function.

The studies of Katz, Howard, Paul, Unanue, Borel and Nossal have also indicated that there are probably two distinct mechanisms by which B cells may be rendered unresponsive in the absence of T cell function of either the helper or suppressor type. One of these mechanisms involves the binding by B cells of a critical amount of a non-metabolizable antigen such as DNP-D-GL or DNP-Levan. This form of tolerance may be viewed as a form of cell intoxication. At the present time, however, it is not clear whether this "intoxication", which is manifested by the cells being unable to reexpress receptors or to secrete antibody, is caused by the effect of the tolerogen on the cell membrane or on the protein synthetic machinery within the cell or both. Studies with purified specific cell populations should resolve these differences. The other tolerance mechanism for B cells involves the repeated interactions of the specific cell with an excess of metabolizable antigen over a period of time in the absence of T cell function. The ultimate result of such repeated inter-actions has not been ascertained precisely; however, there are indications that they may stimulate the cell towards terminal differentiation at the expense of clonal expansion as a mechanism of tolerance or possi-bly in some cases towards "abortive" differentiation.

I propose that we address ourselves to these var-ious issues in turn, but first to the question of whether the phenomena of self tolerance which operate to prevent immune responses to autologous components to which B and T lymphocytes are exposed in high or low concentrations proceed through the same mechanisms as the phenomena of acquired tolerance to foreign antigens which have been studied in the laboratory. Tolerance to those self components present in high concentration is generally considered to be the result of clonal dele-tions at the levels of both T and B lymphocytes. Tol-erance to self components present at low concentrations is usually believed to be primarily the result of T cell tolerance with the existence of B cells in peri-pheral lymphoid tissues capable of binding to the autologous components.

Another major issue to be discussed is whether the various tolerance phenomena where specific suppressor T cells have been shown to play a critical role have their counterpart in tolerance to self antigens, par-ticularly at the T cell level or whether the activity of suppressor T cells demonstrated in the laboratory should not be viewed rather as representing an aspect of the regulatory activity of T cells in immune res-ponses. The development and control of specific immune responses would according to this interpretation always depend upon the balance between the opposite effects of helper and suppressor T cells.

We should consider next what is known of the mechanism by which suppressor T cells exert their effects. Suppressor T cells stimulated by mitogens operate nonspecifically on all immune responses. However, the more interesting phenomena which have been discussed in this conference concern the effect of specific suppressor T cells which are stimulated by antigen and which also exhibit specificity for antigen in their suppressive activities. Such specificity can only result either from cell interactions mediated by antigen or from the activity of a "product" of the suppressor T cells possessing both specificity for the antigen and suppressive activity. The search for such products in several laboratories is already underway. We must also inquire whether suppressor T cells and helper T cells are indeed different cells with possibly different antigen receptors.

Last, but not least, we should discuss the possible therapeutic applications which can be derived from our basic knowledge of tolerance mechanisms. I sincerely believe that in immunology we are at the threshold of major applications of basic knowledge to relevant problems in clinical medicine. The detailed understanding of the cellular basis of immune responses and of the sophistication of their regulatory mechanisms which have been developed in the last few years will provide us with the tools to manipulate specific immune responses in various antibody classes for the benefit of the patients in many immunological diseases, allergic or auto-immune, and also in organ transplantation and tumor immunology.

Let us begin our discussion by considering the mechanisms of tolerance induction to autologous components.

E. MÖLLER: Do you suggest that there is no reason to believe that clonal deletion exists in no other situation than self tolerance?

BENACERRAF: I believe that clonal deletion can explain some phenomena of acquired tolerance to foreign antigens particularly as concerns B cell tolerance. What I was asking, rather, is the reverse question. That is, whether mechanisms such as suppressor T cells which have been demonstrated in tolerance to foreign antigens also operate in self tolerance at the T cell level with or without clonal deletion.

WAKSMAN: If you will accept studies of soluble protein antigens as a model for self-tolerance, our thymus experiments suggest that both deletion and suppression may
occur in the thymus. After neonatal induction of tolerance to BGG, transfer of whole thymus gave specific
tolerance lasting at least six weeks, the same duration
identified in Chiller and Weigle's experiments on T cell
tolerance. This length of time implies an actual deletion and the time required to regenerate competent T
cells reactive to BGG. On the other hand, when we transfer thymocytes shortly after an exposure to BGG, we
identify a clear-cut suppressor effect. This, however,
is short lived, no more than three or four days in Ha's
work and that of others.

I would suggest that these mechanisms involve different thymocyte populations. Clonal deletion may
affect the less mature cells, and suppression may affect
those cells which have already acquired peripheral T
cell properties. Suppression may provide the backup
mechanism protecting us against autoimmunization by
cells which have managed to escape the deletion mechanism.

ALLISON: I believe that the evidence I reviewed on Sunday
supports the view that suppressor T cells play a role
in the maintenance of self tolerance. For example,
deprivation of T cells in chickens, rats and mice leads
to or accentuates autoimmune thyroiditis. Similar evidence suggests that production of anti-nuclear factors
and autoantibodies against erythrocytes can be suppressed by T cells.

ADA: The work described by Allison shows clearly that functional B cells for thyroglobulin are present. The question then arises--are there functional T cells and if
so, do some of them have suppressor activity? I submit
that we do not have hard evidence at the present to
settle the question now. It should be one of the mes-
sages of this conference that work should now be done
to examine this point.

MITCHELL: Does Byron Waksman consider that short-lived
suppressor T cells act to clonally delete long-lived
helper T cells?

WAKSMAN: We have no evidence about this. Perhaps they do.

BRITTON: If suppressor T cells are responsible for maintenance of self tolerance, must we then assume that nude
mice are not athymic with regard to suppressor cells?
I think we yet have to restrict the possible function of
suppressor T cells to one of many regulating ones; not
operating in sustaining self tolerance.

PAUL: Clonal deletion seems an obvious mechanism for tolerance induction in cells which have a high affinity receptor. Perhaps in T cell tolerance to self antigens
which exist at high concentrations, active suppression
of cells with quite low affinity may be the major
mechanism.

HUMPHREY: The experiments carried out by Michael Feldman and
his colleagues (Cohen and Corniberg) showing that lymph
node cells cultured for 3 to 4 days will develop the
capacity for killing isologous target cells argues
strongly against clonal deletion of self-reactive T
cells in these nodes and more in favor of silent cells
or of suppressor cells.

LESKOWITZ: Doesn't the example of the obese chicken thyroiditis suggest that self tolerance does not exist because
of some genetic peculiarity and that other mechanisms
such as suppressor cells must now come into play?

WEIGLE: Our main line of defense against autoimmunity is
tolerance in the T cells. However, in order to have a
safeguard against autoimmunity, there has to be a backup system. One such system is to also have tolerance
in the B cells. When tolerance is present in both the
T and B cell, autoimmunity would be impossible unless
these cells were functionally abnormal. In the case
where tolerance to self components is present in only
the T cell, then there may be a necessity to have a
backup system involving suppressor T cells. Possibly we
may have suppressor cells to thyroglobulin, but I can
see no necessity to have suppressor cells to autologous
serum albumin.

G. MÖLLER: I want to emphasize Sven Britton's point made
earlier. The nude mouse shows that self tolerance does
not need suppressor T cells. A potentially self-reactive B cell is rather harmless because it will not be

turned on by mere contact with antigen. It seems sufficient to have tolerant T cells, tolerance in this case
being deletion.

BASTEN: Dr. Waksman implied that if antigen interacts with
an immature T cell (i.e. in the thymus), deletion may
occur. If, however, antigen interacts with a peripheral
T cell under appropriate conditions, suppressor cells
may develop. I would agree that this is a useful working distinction and would like to point out that suppressor cells have a number of properties which make
them potentially useful regulators of the immune response at the physiological level. For example, they
have a wide range of specificity and the capacity to
switch off cells already primed to antigen. In other
words, suppressor cells do indeed have the capability
of playing a role in in vivo self surveillance in the
Burnet sense rather than merely being an interesting
in vitro artifact.

SMITH: My point is that it is not possible at this time to
distinguish between self tolerance--putatively involving clonal deletion and the various identified regulatory mechanisms. This view is based upon the identification of components indicating the existence of recognition clones for nearly every "self" component examined thus far. Therefore, the question is how these
potentially responsive self clones, which presumably
are renewed throughout life, are tolerized, controlled
or suppressed rather than stimulated to proliferate and
differentiate or permitted to do so in a regulated fashion compatible with normal differentiation or repair
processes. Clone deletion, even if it occurs other
than in the case of the possibly poisonous antigens we
have heard about here, can only be a temporary process--
as the loss of soldiers in a battle in view of the
renewal mechanisms always providing reserves of new
recognition clones.

DRESSER: The point raised by Sven and Göran is very important if the observations made in the nude mouse can be
taken at face value. However, the idea that the nude
is totally deficient in T (helper or suppressor) cells
must depend on one's definition of T and B cell.
Perhaps lymphocytes should be looked on as a spectrum
with T and B being the two extremes; the dividing line
between the T and B half being largely arbitrary. The

cut-off in the nude may well leave T cells with helper or repressor activity albeit with an efficiency which in normal mice would be undetectable with the methodologies we have available.

ADA: I believe it is wrong to regard nude mice as mice without any functional T cells. It so happens that in our animal house recently our mice (but not rats) have become primed to the flagellar proteins we use. For example, they show an excellent DTH reaction (footpad swelling) to monomeric flagellin without repriming. This applied to our nude (nu/nu) mice. We have found that they give a clear-cut hapten-carrier response to DNP-flagellin but not to DNP-hemocyanin or DNP-HGG. This response is susceptible to anti-θ and complement (S. Kirov, unpublished). Kirov and Parish have now separated T and B cells from nu/nu mice; mixing one with the other reconstitutes the response.

The probable explanation of this phenomenon is that due to constant stimulation there has been built up in nude mice a population of T cells specific for flagellin. If this is so, there may be in nu/nu mice T cells with specificity for self antigens and they may have suppressor activity.

E. MÖLLER: I am afraid I might be stating the obvious. There is a certain affinity distribution curve of immunocompetent T and B cells. Every antigen injection, whether "immunogenic" or "tolerogenic" leads to tolerance in some cells, activation of others. Thus, in tolerance as we define it experimentally, clonal deletion as well as clonal expansion might occur. Therefore, the important issue is to define the biological relevance of those activated cells that we find in certain tolerant states. In the skin graft tolerance models, we have heard that "complexes" which are inhibitory exist. However, the biological relevance of these inhibitors is not yet established. They might be artifacts of our sensitive in vitro techniques. I do think that Baruj's elegant experiments with GAT might give a solution as to the relevance of suppressor cells.

BRITTON: Firstly, in response to Gordon Ada. If your nude mice are infected with an agent with potential B cell mitogenicity, you bypass T cell dependence and open up the possibility for the poor nude mouse to mount an

immune response to otherwise thymus-dependent antigens.
Secondly, as suppressor T cells undoubtedly show specificity, have they been specifically absorbed on anti-
gen-coated columns or perhaps even on antigen-immuno-
blobulin-coated columns as these cells appear to be in
a metabolically different state from helper T cells
thus possibly bearing surface immunoglobulins in such
a concentration that they allow binding onto an anti-
immunoglobulin-coated particle?

BASTEN: We have put murine spleen cells with suppressor activity through anti-immunoglobulin-coated columns.
The cells obtained which were at least 95% T cells
still possessed the capacity to abrogate an anti-hapten
response. In other words, specific receptors on suppressor T cells cannot be demonstrated by this technique.

E. MÖLLER: I think Tony Basten said that the suppressor
cells can be killed by radioactive antigen.

NOSSAL: We have not focused sufficiently on the central
dilemma of the academic immunologist, which is the
random, scattered way in which the generator of diversity functions. Nature faces us with a continuum, a
spectrum, yet our minds and more importantly, our experiments can function only in dualisms. Something is
antibody or not, a cell kills or doesn't and so forth.
As far as tolerance is concerned, there can be no
absolutes. We note that up to half a percent of B
cells bind a particular antigen. If there were true,
complete self tolerance for all self antigens, regardless of receptor affinity, there would be no immune
system. Everything would self destruct because of the
vast number of "self" antigenic determinants. As we
do have an immune system, this suggests that tolerance
is only relative. There may well be several levels,
e.g. clonal elimination of high affinity cells, suppressor mechanisms for those exigencies where lower
affinity cells slip through and become activated,
blockade, antibody feedback, antibody-antigen complex
tolerance and so forth, all acting as "fail-safes".
We must simply construct our artificial dualisms, iso-
late and refine each mechanism (e.g. suppressor T cells)
identify that they exist and then try to fit them into
the total picture. As regards T versus B cell tolerance, I do not deny that T cells may have lower thresh-

olds for tolerogenesis than B cells, but I deny the possibility of "absolutes" at the carrier-reactive cell level either. The same spectrum of possibilities faces us for T cell tolerogenesis.

ALLISON: The essential difference is that selective T cell tolerance is easily broken whereas B cell tolerance is not.

LESKOWITZ: Does the adult response to fetal antigens imply that clonal deletion does not exist as a mechanism for self tolerance since presumably clones to these antigens should be deleted in early life?

SMITH: In view of the built-in inevitability of tolerance induction in the continually generated clones capable of responses to "self", the only models in which to examine "self tolerance" may be those defined genetic deletions (i.e. C5 deletion) in which immunity can be shown. Here induction of tolerance to such proteins should be so circumscribed that the kinetics, induction, the cells involved and the mechanisms of maintenance should be easily defined and generalized to "self tolerance".

CLAMAN: The term "tolerant signal" must be looked at operationally. It is not measured by itself, but only be a failure to respond to an immunogenic signal.

BENACERRAF: I believe that we have discussed thoroughly all the important issues concerning the mechanism of tolerance to self components. The next questions which deserve your attention are the various mechanisms which have been identified as operative in B cell tolerance. Let us consider first the evidence for the presence or absence of antigen-binding B cells in tolerant animals. How reliable is the methodology and the results obtained?

ADA: Although it is not very difficult to detect antigen-binding B lymphocytes, many people have had trouble in detecting antigen-binding T lymphocytes. Even with B lymphocytes, quantitation is uncertain. We have recently found that there is a linear increase in the number of binding cells found as the labelled protein used is denatured. If the protein is not denatured, we (Lamelin, Vassalli and Ada, unpublished) have found

it is difficult to find antigen-binding T cells. Do T
cells only bind antigen if it has first been denatured?

BASTEN: I should like to support Dr. Ada's comments on the
problem of antigen-binding T cells. When we are studying antigen-induced suicide of T cells, we find appreciable numbers of cells binding highly substituted
antigens such as fowl gamma globulin. However, the
proportion of labelled cells declines linearly with
repeated washing. After 7 to 8 washes cell viability
is reduced preventing further analysis. This means
that one cannot say which antigen-binding cells are
significant in a functional sense.

UNANUE: The way to study the basic B cell defect in tolerance is to enrich for the specific cells. Studies with
whole populations will only give very limited results.

SISKIND: Recently, we have found, together with Dr. Young
TaiKim, that rabbits synthesize very large amounts
(perhaps several mg/ml) of very low affinity antibody
when immunized with optimal doses of DNP-BGG in complete Freund's adjuvant. This antibody is of such low
affinity that it cannot be absorbed on an immunoadsor-
bent column, but it clearly binds hapten in equilibrium
dialysis at higher affinity than does normal rabbit
globulin. Thus, this is an enormous range of antibody
heterogeneity of very low affinity antibodies. This
type of redundancy of the response is precisely what
one would expect from a random generation of diversity.
Thus, I would suggest that the large number of antigen-
binding cells which can be detected when studies are
carried out at high antigen concentration may truly be
demonstrating cells which can respond to antigen when
the animal is immunized under the right conditions.

On a more speculative note, I would suggest that
much of the low affinity antibody which is often made
by animals immunized experimentally may not be stimulated under conditions of normal biologic (natural)
stimulation of the immune response. It may be that in
nature only relatively higher affinity cells are stimulated. The type of "antibody-mediated tolerance" I
described yesterday may reflect such a situation. The
tolerance-inducing antigen injection stimulated a small
moderately high affinity response. This may really
correspond to the response to an antigen under natural

immunizing conditions. The small amount of high affinity antibody suppresses the formation of large amounts of low affinity antibody which is usually formed in the artificial situation of immunization with antigen in complete Freund's adjuvant.

E. MÖLLER: I have a comment on antigen-binding cells (ABC) and on the difficulty in finding them. You can easily find specific T and B-ABC in animals that have been immunized; both hapten-protein conjugates reacting with densely haptenated red cells. ABC are specific because they are sensitive to inhibition by free hapten. However, T cells irrespective of dose used for immunization or time after immunization is low, in contrast to B cells which show the expected increase in affinity. Avidity for multivalent ligands is high in both populations. However, when you inhibit with monovalent ligands, we found that the affinity of T-ABC for the homologous monovalent ligand is high, but for another carrier in a monovalent ligand is low. Thus, these data support the importance of the "local environment" for the activation of T cells by hapten-carrier conjugates, first suggested by Gell and Benacerraf. These affinity differences can explain difficulties in demonstrating hapten-binding T cells.

PAUL: One of the considerable problems which we must face in the evaluation of antigen-binding cells is that we determine the number and character of cells quite arbitrarily by the set of conditions we select for the antigen-binding test. What we must learn to do is to set the limits, so to speak, which allow us to examine the cells which are likely to be activated and to exclude, for the most part, those cells which are unlikely to be activated.

DRESSER: I suppose that when we put the remarks of Gus Nossal and Gregory Siskind together we can conclude that the mass of low avidity antibody is the penalty we must pay for needing a random generation of diversity.

BENACERRAF: Two distinct mechanisms of B cell tolerance have been identified by the studies presented at this conference. One of them involves what I have termed the "intoxication" of the B cell by the tolerogen (usually an unmetabolizable or poorly metabolizable molecule), which results in the inability of the cell to reexpress receptors and to secrete antibody. Let us now discuss this most intriguing phenomenon and its possible mechanisms.

HUMPHREY: The phenomenon described by Gus Nossal as effector blockade is certainly a reality. We do not know at present whether this blockade of already stimulated antibody-secreting cells is due to surface or to internalized antigen interfering with secretion or immunoglobulin synthesis. It is difficult to see how surface antigen can block continuous secretion. Whether this sort of blockade is equally relevant to the block which prevents the B cell being turned on in the first place remains to be shown. However, the difficulty then is to identify a cell which is not making the antibody which it might have made.

UNANUE: The basic defect in the B cell to D-GL binding is the apparent lack of synthesis of new receptors. Two possibilities have been raised to explain this: an abnormal signal that stems from the abnormal handling at the surface or a defect that results from the intracellular handling; I favor the first.

WAKSMAN: The question we are discussing was first posed by Möller and by Greaves with the statement that "the cell can count". A certain quantitative level of surface stimulation will stimulate and a higher level will turn the cell off. Diener and Feldmann's work suggests immobilization of the surface by a lattice. A parallel observation by the Edelman group is that concanavalin A in excess "freezes" the cell membrane, even inhibiting capping by unrelated agents. I doubt if we are in any position now to take the next step of asking how this surface effect alters cell function since basic cell biologists have not yet achieved any consensus on this class of problems. There is a large literature to show that increasing cyclic AMP levels within the cell (triggered by some types of surface stimulation) inhibit cell proliferation and inhibit some of its differentiated functions, e.g. cytotoxicity. Increased GMP gives opposite effects and the behavior of the cell is actually said to be determined by the balance between the two. It is possible that these provide the mechanisms leading to tolerogenesis and immunogenesis, respectively, as suggested recently by Mel Cohn. However, the assays of these molecules are highly unreliable and the data must be accepted with caution.

G. MÖLLER: Three points for Byron Waksman. 1) Immunologists are better equipped than cell biologists to study turning-on of cells because we know the receptor and the inducer. 2) The important events occur at the cell surface, and 3) There is no evidence for different signals being responsible for induction and tolerance. All the evidence suggest that the same signal is responsible and that cells are able to count. Large quantities of the signal turn off.

NOSSAL: I have three points in relation to John Humphrey's question. First, effector cell blockade is not just a trapping of secreted antibody as it floats past cell-associated antigen. This has been eliminated by two observations; first, the kinetic argument that blockade takes time and metabolism after antigen attachment and secondly, that mouse Ig is not present in abnormally high amounts at the cell surface. Secondly, we have no direct evidence for interiorization of attached antigen, but as so many complexes can blockade, this seems a very likely happening. Nevertheless, the pinocytosis as such may not be the thing that stops secretion. Thirdly, while secretion is clearly embarrassed, there is no evidence yet for inhibition of protein synthesis.

UNANUE: Dr. Coons showed that after injection of ferritin into rabbits immune to ferritin, plasma cells were found with ferritin inside vesicles, i.e. plasma cells can pinocytose.

CLAMAN: Since we do not know the detailed mechanism by which cells are turned on by immunogen, we are not in a strong position to figure out how a tolerogen prevents that turning on.

On a different but related point, there is no doubt that great progress has been made by looking at events at the cell surface. We should not forget that cell receptors may not be on the cell surface--for instance, the cortisol receptor is in the cytosol. And, it is not just receptor binding but the further signals sent to the nucleus for activation which counts.

624

FELDMANN: Our discussions on antigen binding in tolerance
have highlighted several important issues. First of
these is a philosophical one. Basically, the in vitro
studies of antigen binding like all in vitro studies
give us information about the cell biology of lymphocytes, telling us various possible mechanisms of suppression. They cannot tell us if these pathways are
actually expressed in vivo and so, in principle, it
seems essential to look at antigen binding in vivo
during tolerance induction (which differs markedly
from that in vitro as shown by Nossal, Mitchell, etc.).
That clearly is a difficult problem, but must be done
before we can understand the details of the mechanism
of tolerance induction. Secondly, there is the problem of heterogeneity in tolerance. By this I mean
both the heterogeneity of lymphocytes (classes and
their differentiation sequences) and of experimental
models used in these studies which makes conceptual
interpretations difficult. There is a need for com-
parative studies with different tolerogens before we
can generalize on antigen-handling mechanisms at the
cell surface in tolerance. It may differ with different antigens, e.g. POL versus DNP-D-GL or with cells
at different stages of differentiation and with antigens which can stimulate or those which cannot.

MITCHELL: Marc Feldmann has anticipated my point. When
talking of mechanisms such as intoxication, in vivo
events may dictate that an effector cell never sees
antigen simply because secreted antibody is preventing
access of antigen to the cell. Now by contrast, a B
cell with antigen reactivity will see much more antigen and will, therefore, be the target cell for tolerance. On the point of antigen-binding cells in tolerant mice, when we take cells out of tissues we immea-
surably wash them several times. If we were not to do
this but leave the cell in its high protein milieu,
would we have a more meaningful measure of antigen-
binding cells in tolerant and normal mice.

BENACERRAF: Let us now turn our attention to another mechanism of B cell tolerance which does not involve the
"intoxication" of the cell. This process appears to
result from the repeated interaction of specific B
cells with appropriate concentrations of metabolizable
antigens in the absence of adequate helper cell function from activated T cells. What are the possible

mechanisms of this phenomenon? Is there any evidence that it involves terminal differentiation or instead "aborted" differentiation, i.e. possibly blast transformation without the differentiation into antibody-secreting plasma cells?

G. MÖLLER: Baruj's question is very clear but also twisted. The answer to the question whether e.g. BGG in pure B cells could induce tolerance is no. BGG cannot by itself induce tolerance--in contrast, the strange molecules, SIII, Levan, as Baruj put it, can all do it. Clearly, this suggests that it is inherent properties of the molecules which determines the outcome. In my thinking molecules like BGG lack the property to deliver signals and this by the way, indicates that Ig receptors are not delivering any signal. In contrast, LPS, SIII, Levan, etc. are all competent to deliver a signal.

WEIGLE: I object to Göran Möller's suggestion that B cells cannot be made tolerant to HGG in absence of T cells. Jacques Chiller has been able to induce tolerance in B cells in lethally irradiated, thymectomized and bone marrow (treated with anti-theta and complement) reconstituted mice.

KATZ: I think a point that deserves emphatic consideration in our minds, and certainly a few minutes of discussion, is whether or not B cells exist which express specific receptors on their surface membranes capable of binding antigen but which for various reasons are unable to respond to the triggering signals delivered to it by antigen, T cells, etc. If you recall some of the experiments described yesterday in which exposure of B cells to DNP coupled to certain carriers (such as L-GL, OVA, etc.) under certain conditions resulted in functional unresponsiveness, we know that the experiments of Unanue and Ault indicate that the B cells involved are capable of binding DNP-proteins despite their functional refractoriness. More importantly, we know that certain maneuvers such as trypsin digestion release these cells from the refractory state. The question that intrigues me is, if these findings are not experimental artifacts, why are these cells refractory and what trypsin (and probably other comparable agents) does to reverse this state.

To raise a hypothetical point, it falls within my own personal bias to speculate that the missing link may be the absence of activation of other B cell surface sites than Ig--namely, the postulated "acceptor" molecule (J. Exp. Med. 137:1405, 1973)--at or near the time of antigen-receptor binding. Antigen binding with subsequent receptor movement, endocytosis, catabolism and resynthesis of surface Ig receptors can perhaps proceed in normal fashion without actual cell triggering, but in the absence of a temporally crucial signal at the acceptor site, this cell is now refractory--perhaps if a long time elapses in which this cell is in "limbo", permanent (irreversible) tolerance will ensue. However, for a finite period this cell is potentially "rescuable" and agents such as trypsin may act by altering the acceptor molecule in an appropriate manner so that the cell is then responsive. Furthermore, suppression by T cells or their products may also result in a receptor-bearing B cell that is not functionally responsive. Whatever mechanism(s) may be involved, the message seems clear to me that non-functional antigen-binding B cells do indeed exist in certain circumstances.

MAGE: The cells in rabbits recovering from total allotype suppression have membrane-associated Ig with the suppressed allotype. They are reminiscent of the B cells in some immuno-deficient patients who also have Ig-bearing cells which do not differentiate into productive cells. They may either be actively suppressed via suppressor cells or be intrinsicly blocked at a maturational step in B cell development. They might also be relatively normal "virgin B cells" which do not compete effectively with memory cells bearing Ig-receptors with lambda-type light chains.

ALLISON: There are some types of tolerance in which antigen-binding cells are present, as the Möllers and Gordon Ada pointed out. There are others in which the antigen-binding cells are reduced in number. This raises the possibility that some types of tolerance involve a block in maturation whereas others do involve clonal elimination. The Herzenberg machine makes it possible to obtain populations of B cells with surface receptors for a particular antigen. It would be interesting to see whether cells isolated in this way can be killed by exposure to certain antigens (e.g. levan) in

627

certain doses; whether they can be blocked in differentiation when transferred to irradiated syngeneic recipients or in what conditions they can recover their reactivity.

SISKIND: I am somewhat concerned about the significance of the observations that in some systems one can detect large numbers of antigen-binding cells in tolerant animals. Are these actually cells which in a normal animal would be stimulated to respond to antigen or are they actually all very low affinity cells? There are relatively large numbers of low affinity cells in a normal animal relative to very small numbers of high affinity cells. It is possible that the high affinity cells are actually deleted but one cannot detect their absence because of the large background of low affinity cells which are present. This type of technical problem might be particularly serious when the cell-binding studies are carried out with ligands of high epitope density where binding to low affinity cells would occur readily and with high avidity as a result of multi-point attachment.

E. MÖLLER: Precisely, Greg Siskind's point. I think that differences in findings of ABC in different tolerant situations are purely technical.

BASTEN: Following E. Möller's comments, I should like to ask whether any critical capping studies have been performed on tolerant cell populations where antigen-binding cells are detectable. In other words are the antigen-reactive cells detected or simply blocked? The answer to this question should enable us to decide what is the fate of a tolerant B cell.

E. MÖLLER: In response to Tony Basten, we have in fact incubated our RFC over night. Secondly, as I said the other day, all of our experiments indicated that ABC present in tolerant animals are low affinity cells; high affinity cells were not reactivated in vitro or by the polyclonal B cell activator, LPS.

NOSSAL: I should like to see more experiments of the type presented by Diener. He showed $80/10^5$ ^{3}H-POL-binding cells in normal spleen and proved the relevance of essentially all of these to anti-POL immune responses by showing that within 24 hours essentially all of these could be transformed into blasts following antigenic stimulation. This type of control of the relevance of particular antigen-binding cells is required in many of the tolerance models.

HUMPHREY: Even in mice tolerized by various tolerizing regimens (high or low) with heterologous albumins, there is no consistent evidence that cells capable of binding the tolerogen are absent--in fact, most experiments show them to be present. There is agreement that cells binding autologous albumin are absent.

Radioactive suicide experiments (Ada, our group, etc.) show that the antigen-binding cells include those which are capable of responding, but they do not show that all Ig-binding cells can respond.

DIENER: I want to address myself to the question as to whether or not a tolerant cell may exist with antigen receptors expressed. When we tried to find 3H-POL-labelled cells which, when having tolerogenic amounts of antigen on the surface, would, therefore, not cap, 12 hours later, they had disappeared. Yet the tolerant population could be made to respond again in the reversibility experiments using glucocorticosteroids, as I have described as a discussant.

SCOTT: All of us have been spending a great deal of time discussing antigen-binding cells in tolerant animals and what this implies. This, it seems to me, is off the point. We must not forget the elegant studies of Jacques Louis, Chiller and Weigle who showed that it is important to follow antigen-binding cells with time after tolerogen. There it is clear that ABC's are not detectable when, and only when, B cells are tolerant. Looking at antigen-binding cells during tolerogenesis as it proceeds in isolated cell populations is the only way to really answer this point.

ADA: The discussion during the last few minutes has really been directed towards the question--in B tolerant animals, are there functionally inactive specific B cells present? The antigen-binding technique is only one way of attempting to answer this question. If "normal" numbers of and the "normal" pattern of labelling is seen, this would suggest that functionally inactive B cells do exist and that their receptors are available for binding antigen.

BENACERRAF: To summarize this phase of the discussion, there appears to be general agreement, with naturally a few dissenting voices, that there are states of B cell tolerance characterized by the presence of antigen-binding cells. These cells may be indeed only cells with low affinity receptors or very possibly cells which have been rendered temporarily refractory to the differentiating stimuli of antigen and helper T cells. It is highly probable that the availability of purified specific B cells obtained with such devices as the Herzenberg separator will permit the resolution of many of the issues raised in this discussion, particularly when a combined approach is used involving both studies of cell binding, metabolism of antigen and re-expression of receptors and studies of immunocompetence carried out with the same cell population, as described by Unanue.

Let us turn our attention now to another very important set of phenomena, the activity of suppressor T cells. We should discuss whether suppressor cells are distinct from helper cells, whether they are specific in their action, whether they act on T cells, B cells or both and whether they act directly or through the production of specific suppressor molecules.

MAGE: In opening our consideration of specific suppressive effects, I would like to raise the issue mentioned by Phil Baker yesterday that B cell expression may be regulated by anti-idiotype. This may be the biologically significant form of suppression for which allotype-suppression is a model. Structural data indicate that some groups of antibodies with similar, though non-identical, specificities share structural features recognized by anti-idiotype antibodies. Auto-regulatory anti-idiotype could be an important mechanism for suppression. Autoanti-idiotype has been raised in individual rabbits and in mice of an inbred strain.

PAUL: I personally find the network concept for regulation most interesting but do have both theoretical and experimental difficulties. On the theoretical side, regulation by the production of antibody to the unique antigenic determinants implies that a new antibody

(or other type of receptor) with its own unique specificity will appear and this be subject to regulation
on the same basis. Thus, we have a situation of a
"mirrow into infinity" in this system. Of course, the
system may be highly damped. The experimental difficulty is the observation of Lieberman and Potter that
it is quite difficult to induce anti-idiotype antibodies to a BALB/c myeloma protein in a BALB/c mouse.
This would suggest it unlikely that a "fine-tuning"
mechanism could rely on the production of anti-idiotype antibodies to receptors.

MAGE: You are referring to the production of large amounts
of B cell product. The regulatory anti-idiotype could
even be on T cells or produced in very small amounts
by a regulatory B cell.

BAKER: The possible formation of anti-idiotype antibody
and antibody formed against it, etc. may not really be
a troublesome aspect of the Jerne model. It is a
common observation that specific antibody represents
only a small percentage (< 5% in most cases) of the
total amount of increased Ig produced; such a mechanism could well account for the development of much of
this seemingly "nonsense" Ig.

WAKSMAN: I think many apparently specific suppressor events
are really not specific except in their recognition
phase, e.g. experiments on tolerance. Yet, older
studies on competition established that a secondary
response to one antigen most frequently inhibits a primary response to another. Here recognition is specific yet the effect is not. Therefore, the "specificity" of tolerance experiments is open to doubt. A
quite different problem arises in cases where there is
(or appear to be) no antigen against which the suppressor T cell can react.

FELDMANN: There seems to be good evidence that specific
suppression is mediated by specific products released
by T cells, as described by Dr. Tada and myself, and
not by nonspecific products induced by specific antigen, as suggested by Dr. Waksman. I have tried to see
if nonspecific suppressor substances influence tolerance induction; so far without any success. So to
date, the evidence favors specific suppression by
specific cells and the molecules they release. The

locus of suppression by T cells varies in different
models, but suppression of other T cells is the most
sensitive in vitro as well as in vivo.

HUMPHREY: G.L. Asherson and M. Zembala's experiments (Proc.
Roy. Soc. B., in press and in preparation), similar to
those discussed by Henry Claman, clearly show that T
cells can elaborate a product which specifically inhibits a recognizable T cell function. Spleen and
lymph node cells of mice injected with picryl sulphonic
acid do become able to suppress contact sensitivity to
picryl chloride (active or passively transferred by
peritoneal cells from sensitized animals), as measured by the ear skin reaction or DNA synthesis in the
draining node. When lymph node cells from mice injected with picryl sulphonic acid, and skin painted one
week later with picryl chloride, are then cultured
in vitro for 24 to 48 hours, they release into the
supernatant material which is inhibitory--i.e. if
sensitized lymph node cells are treated with the
supernatant, they have much diminished capacity to
passively transfer sensitivity. The suppressor activity is also absorbed by peritoneal exudate cells
and these then acquire the ability to inhibit passive
transfer.

GERSHON: Of course, the isolation of effector suppressor
molecules which have antigen specificity should serve
to establish specificity at both the triggering and
effector level. I would just like to add that when
significant levels of specific T cell dependent suppression appears, the non-specific suppression disappears. Thus, four days after the last injection of a
sheep erythrocyte regimen which produces suppressor
factors that turn off the sheep response, the horse
cell response is better than it would be if only the
last injection of sheep cells had been given. Further,
GAT produces less antigenic competition in nonresponder mice, where specific suppression is seen than in
responder mice.

BASTEN: Dr. Benacerraf asked for comments on the site of
action and mediation of the suppressor effect. I
think it is clear from his data as well as those of
Tada's, Feldmann's and our own that a non tolerant T
cell is the target cell. The ability of suppressor T
cells to inhibit a) primed as well as normal T cells

and b) cross-reactive carrier-reactive cells implies that the suppressor phenomenon has real significance in regulation of immune reactivity particularly to self antigens. Concerning the mode of action of suppression, I would suggest that at the operational level, suppressor cells "protect" the B cell from immunogenic signals. Whether this is mediated by a soluble factor (Tada and Feldmann) or by "distraction" of helper cells remains to be established conclusively.

MITCHELL: Could I raise the "semi-philosophical" point that if the immune system is designed to remove foreign antigen, then if a mechanism is available which removes antigen, there is little reason to produce antibody. A hyperactive T cell or phagocyte axis may well compete with B cells for antigen. Perhaps we should look at the older methods of determining immunity (e.g. whole body clearance of labelled antigen) in order to assess whether a so-called suppressed animal is removing antigen in an accelerated fashion.

SISKIND: I would like to point out that the behavior of the specific suppressor described by Dr. Tada is very different from the suppression caused by the usual serum antibodies as in antibody-mediated suppression. In antibody-mediated suppression, it is the function of low affinity B lymphocytes that is inhibited. In contrast, the specific inhibitor described by Dr. Tada preferentially turns off high affinity B lymphocytes.

PAUL: There have now been several descriptions of suppressive factors with specific activities. Of these some notably Dr. Tada's have been resported to lack immunoglobulin determinants. I wish to inquire what is known of the precise specificity of these non-immunoglobulin factors and to raise the question of whether they may constitute candidates for the antigen-recognition units of T lymphocytes.

WAKSMAN: Can we ask Drs. Tada and Feldmann for a status report on the chemical nature of their specific immunosuppressive factors?

TADA: So far what we have found is the following: The suppressor component is a protein whose activity was destroyed by pronase and trypsin but not by DNase and RNase. The molecular weight is between 35,000 and

50,000. It has no immunoglobulin determinants, but nevertheless, has specificity and affinity for the antigen. It was contained in a fraction with a very small amount of polysaccharide. These are about all we know.

KATZ: Concerning the specificity of the non-immunoglobulin suppressor substance that you have identified in rat T cells, is it not true that you have only elicited this with the Ascaris carrier and that your specificity criteria are related to the capacity of an Ascaris-immunoabsorbent to completely remove this soluble product? The reason that I raise this is because I am intrigued by the possibility that components in the heterogeneous Ascaris protein extract might cross-react with membrane constituents of rat lymphocytes, such as histocompatibility antigens that may be involved in the regulation of lymphocyte responses. Have you any evidence that would speak to this--i.e. will other carrier proteins induce and elicit these suppressor substances or do you know whether or not any cross-reactivity between Ascaris and rat lymphocyte membranes exist?

TADA: Unfortunately, we could not induce good IgE antibody response with other DNP-derivatives, so we could not test the specificity by absorption with other antigens. For the second part of the question, we found that the suppressor factor was absorbed by heterologous anti-thymocyte serum, therefore, it is apparent that the molecule may contain T cell surface material in addition to the part which I personally think is an expression of Ir gene.

NOSSAL: Is the molecular weight of 35,000 to 50,000 for the native molecule or for reduced and alkylated material?

TADA: The molecular weight of the suppressor component was determined by gel-filtration with Sephadex G-100 under physiologic conditions. Reduction and alkylation were not performed.

HUMPHREY: The suppressor activities studied by Asherson and Zembala was susceptible to anti-θ and C but not to trypsin. It is absorbable onto macrophages. Since it is specific and required antigenic stimulation to cause release, it is likely to be a complex of the

antigen or hapten and some specific T cell product.
However, their preliminary observations suggest that
it is smaller than Ig.

FELDMANN: The evidence for two different types of suppressor molecules, one IgT and the other not seems to fit
in well with the results presented on many models of
T cell suppression in this symposium--some models
which fit in with the concept of excess help may be
caused by IgT complexes, whereas those which do not
seem to be due to excess help may be mediated by
Dr. Tada's factor. However, as yet we have no evidence
that IgT excess is a mechanism of T cell suppression
in vivo and because of the cytophilic nature of IgT,
IgT complexes in high concentrations would probably
be a mechanism of immunoregulation, rather than of
tolerance induction per se. Dr. Tada and I have planned to collaborate in order to compare the mode of
action of the two T cell suppressive factors, in vivo
and in vitro.

NOSSAL: Many of us would like to believe that the suppressor
molecule identified by Dr. Tada has something to do
with T cell surface molecules capable of recognizing
antigen. Others of us have speculated that the Ir
gene products may be T cell receptors for antigen. It
will have escaped no one that Dr. Tada's suppressor
and the molecules identified by Nathenson (and also by
Goding, myself and colleagues) on lymphocyte surfaces
which react with sera raised in mice differing in the
Ir region but possessing similar H-2K and H-2D genes,
have a similar molecular weight. Baruj, does it worry
you or anyone that these molecules which we hoped
might be the expression of Ir genes appear to be accessible in much larger amounts on B than on T cells?

BENACERRAF: I would have preferred that Dr. Tada's factors
be reversed. That is, that his factor with suppressor
activity be absorbable by anti-Ig and that his factor
with helper activity not be absorbable by anti-Ig as
only the latter one would be in my view a candidate
for the Ir gene product. With respect to Nossal's
concern that anti-I sera are predominantly specific
for B cells, I and my colleagues do not find this dis-
turbing. Indeed, the I region has been shown by Katz,
Hamaoka and ourselves to control physiological T-B
interactions (J. Exp. Med. 138:734, 1973). Indeed,

the hypothesis was offered by Katz and myself that the main specificities recognized by anti-I sera on B cells belong indeed to the acceptor molecules for the T cell or T cell products which regulate B cell responses to antigens. The relationship of the Ir gene to this product is a more complex problem which is not in the scope of this discussion.

PAUL: Our studies (Finkelman et al) of the guinea pig antigens against which alloantisera which specifically block Ir-gene-controlled functions indicate these antigens have a molecular weight of approximately 25,000 daltons and may be isolated from both B and T cell sources. Clearly, the goal must be to biochemically characterize this and related materials to determine whether a receptor function is possible for this molecule.

NOSSAL: Goding and I find that ^{125}I-labelled A.TH anti-A.TL sera bind much more strongly to B than to T cells. The differences in grain counts may be of the order of 10-20, but some cells are definitely and specifically positive. By the lactoperoxidase method, we find much less of this material on spleen cells than there is surface Ig. We have not yet investigated the relative amounts on T and B cells as judged by the lactoperoxidase technique. Of course, this may yield quite different relativities than the antibody-binding test.

ASOFSKY: Is there any evidence with respect to the site of synthesis of putative-Ir gene products? The anti-I antisera recognize something better on B than T cells by fluorescent or cytotoxic criteria. These antigens could be synthesized by other cells.

UNANUE: We have tested by immunofluorescence the anti-I antibodies produced by Shreffler. Our results indicate that such molecules are in B cells and in molecules that can be separated from those in the D and K end of H-2 or surface Ig.

LESKOWITZ: Marc Feldmann's evidence indicates that his suppressor substance is absorbed by macrophages and may act at that level. Does Dr. Tada have any evidence whether his suppressor substance adheres to macrophages with or without added Ascaris antigen? Conceivably, his suppressor molecule could represent an excess of IgT.

TADA: We have not tested it yet, but apparently this should be done.

HELLSTRÖM: I would like to bring up the thought that the blocking factors I discussed yesterday may represent at least some of the suppressor molecules elaborated by suppressor lymphocytes. Marc Feldmann told about the suppressor effects of supernatants (from suppressor lymphocytes) being removed by columns taking out either antigens or antibodies. The complexes he found thus appeared to be similar to the blocking antigen-antibody complexes seen in tumor-bearer serum. Another candidate for suppressor molecule could be antigen "processed" so that it is of the "right" type to prevent (or inhibit) lymphocyte reactivity rather than to stimulate it. I feel so because we could demonstrate a component in tumor-bearer serum which had the specificity of the given tumor and was capable of inhibiting lymphocyte-mediated cytotoxicity. Similarly, Dr. Smith found that a small molecule present in tumor antigen extracts could prevent the proliferative response of tumor-bearer lymphocytes exposed to the antigens of tumor cells.

BENACERRAF: There is ample evidence as our discussion has well documented that antigen-stimulated suppressor T cells are primarily specific in their suppressive activity. We should not forget, however, that "nonspecific" suppressor effects have been reported independently by Dutton and by Rich and Pierce caused by T cells activated by Concanavalin A. These nonspecific suppressive effects are operative both on the generation of plaque-forming cells and of specific killer T cells in culture. This activity can be demonstrated in supernatants from Con A-activated T cells.

I would like now to urge you to discuss our last and most important question, i.e. the possible clinical application of immunological technology on tolerance induction to allergic, autoimmune diseases and to organ transplantation. I trust that we shall thereby end this most rewarding and interesting meeting on a very hopeful note.

SMITH: Ample precedent exists for using classic tolerance-
         induction methods in humans in a therapeutic framework.
         In 1957 we reported that we could induce tolerance of
         foreign immunoglobulin antibody (horse GG anti-Tetanus)
         in newborn human infants. At intervals as long as one
         year later, those infants cleared this antigen in non-
         immune fashion and produced no antibody to horse GG.
         Chimpanzees were made tolerant of horse GG in the same
         fashion, and the tolerant state was more rigorously
         established. (Reviewed in R.H.S., Adv. Immunol. 1:1,
         1960). More recently, ALS has been used in transplan-
         splantation in the same context with induction later
         in life. Here tolerance seems to be complete as re-
         lates to the xenogenic source, and the antibody car-
         ried was retained; thus, the therapeutic effect
         sustained.

SISKIND: One can point out that Dr. Marc Weksler and his
          colleagues published that one could induce tolerance
          in humans with aggregate-free horse gamma globulin.
          This permitted the subsequent treatment of these renal
          graft recipients with horse anti-human lymphocyte anti-
          serum to be carried out without the stimulation of
          anti-horse globulin antibody. This permits more ef-
          fective use of ALS as an immunosuppressant without the
          risk of development of serum sickness.

TADA: I think it is appropriate to mention the suppression
        of IgE antibody formation. The activation of suppres-
        sor T cells may be hopeful in this respect, but at the
        same time induction of tolerance in IgG B cells seems
        to be also important. We recently found that DNP
        coupled to T cell independent carrier does not induce
        anti-DNP IgE antibody responses in mice. Furthermore,
        the pretreatment of animals with this antigen complete-
        ly prevented IgE antibody formation to the subsequent
        immunization with immunogenic DNP-Ascaris. This
        seems to me to show that IgE B cells are easily toler-
        ized by the hapten coupled to T cell independent anti-
        gen, which is analogous to that observed in B γ cells
        by Dr. Katz and by Dr. Mitchell.

KATZ: I would hate to inject any pessimism on the subject
        of clinically applicable possibilities based on the
        experimental models described here at this conference,
        but I think a note of caution is warranted lest we
        leave this beautiful place with ambitions of suppres-

sing everything in sight! We have observed very interesting differences in T cell regulation of IgE vs.
IgG B cells which we have interpreted to indicate a
greater sensitivity of IgE B cells to the regulatory
action of T cells. However, in keeping with the complexities of the immune system that we all thrive on,
it seems that IgE B cells although clearly more sensitive than IgG B cells to helper influences of T cells
are equally clearly less sensitive to suppressor T
cell functions. Hence, although some models may seem
to be potential candidates for therapeutic suppression
of allergic disorders in man, the means by which this
may be accomplished are not as readily clear. For
example, antigen-induced suppression of the type that
seems to work at the helper T cell level might be very
effective in suppressing IgG responses while failing
to diminish the level of IgE production. This could
upset a certain balance existing between these two
antibody classes (i.e. antibody feedback) with deleterious consequences to the patient.

It seems to me, therefore, that we may be more
prudent to keep our minds on the very unique molecules
such as D-GL, POL, etc. which for yet unknown reasons
do have the remarkable property of inducing rapid and
irreversible tolerance in B cells binding determinants
covalently coupled to the molecules. You will remember that I presented data two days ago showing that
IgE B cells as well as IgG B cells are effectively tolerized by DNP-D-GL. We are trying right not to determine whether protein D-GL conjugates will tolerize
specific B cells since this would be a necessary prerequisite to any therapeutic possibilities.

WAKSMAN: David, didn't Ishizaka show different helper cells
in IgG and IgE responses? I had the impression that
he recently showed that agents stimulating IgG were
suppressive to IgE.

KATZ: You are referring to the studies of Kishimoto and
Ishizaka (currently in press in the Journal of Immunology) in which they have tentatively identified distinct enhancing T cell products for IgE and IgG B
cells, respectively. The enhancing molecule for IgG
is m.w. 30,000 to 35,000 whereas that for IgE is
around 150,000, I believe. These are not antigen-
specific. However, you are wrong according to my

recollection in your impression that their enhancing molecule for IgG is suppressive for IgE--it is not.

LESKOWITZ: In devising a strategy for producing unresponsiveness in an allergic individual, it might be worth recounting an instance of the clinical difficulties involved. Some years back an attempt was made to induce such a state by cautious, continuous intravenous infusions of allergen into sensitive individuals. Despite the use of anti-histamines and steroids, it was very difficult to move up to levels of antigen capable of depressing sensitivity without precipitating uncomfortable anaphylaxis. The reservoir of IgE on mast cells in these individuals seems so large that the use of antigens which can trigger them is fraught with great difficulties. Perhaps molecules capable of shutting off IgE-producing cells without triggering IgE-bearing mast cells can be devised.

KATZ: This is precisely the goal I was alluding to when I referred to the use of molecules such as D-GL or POL as B cell tolerogenic moieties.

SISKIND: As a perhaps optimistic note, I recall a patient I was shown by Dr. Bernard Levine who had skin-sensitizing (IgE) antibody to minor determinants of penicillin. This patient was desensitized by increasing doses of penicillin over a roughly 10 hour period and then treated for many weeks with a high dose of penicillin for subacute bacterial endocarditis. This patient became skin test negative and remained so, as I recall now, for about six to eight months after termination of therapy. The patient then spontaneously redeveloped skin-sensitizing antibodies. I describe the case merely to point out that even with the simplest reagents, one can induce what may be called tolerance in humans who are already anaphylactically-sensitized. This should be a hopeful example in terms of future attempts at modifying immune responses.

CLAMAN: So far we have been talking about inducing unresponsiveness at the B cell level in immunized subjects making antibody. It appears that it can be done. In T cell hypersensitivity, however, prospects are still not so good. DeWeck showed years ago that a good tolerogen, $DNBSO_3$, is very poor at inducing tolerance in guinea pigs which have contact sensitivity. Even with

large doses at best we get a small and very transient
unresponsiveness.

KATZ: Henry has made an excellent point which reiterates
our discussion of yesterday where I mentioned our failure to tolerize determinant-specific T cell responses
with DNP or ABA coupled D-GL although these same conjugates are powerful tolerogens for B cells. As we
discussed at that time, these differences in results
probably reflect important differences in receptor-
binding events in the two lymphocyte classes and perhaps the manner in which signals are delivered to
these respective cells.

In closing this discussion I would like to offer
the following suggestive summation of where we might
well invest our energies towards clinically applicable
approaches based on what we have heard at this conference.

First, we can probably apply the capacity to render specific B cells unresponsive by the molecules
such as D-GL, POL, Levan, etc., in at least several
clinical problems. Thus, hypersensitivity to haptenic
allergens such as the benzylpenicilloyl (BPO) determinants of penicillin constitutes one such example.
Likewise, we have been recently successful in our laboratory in completely abolishing anti-nuclear antibody
production in immunized mice by administering nucleoside conjugates of D-GL (Eshhar, Katz and Benacerraf,
in preparation). A large collaborative effort with
Dr. Frank Dixon is underway to determine the effect
of such therapy in not only preventing, but more importantly, in alleviating progression of autoimmune
disease in NZB mice. This may open a dramatic therapeutic approach for the unfortunate patients with
systemic lupus erythematosus. Other possibilities
which we are currently studying include induction of
tolerance to ragweed antigen E coupled to D-GL, an
obvious potential benefit for hay fever victims. In
the same vein although less obvious is the possibility
of inducing tolerance to insulin coupled to D-GL which
would be of importance in therapy of patients with
diabetes who develop insulin-resistance due to high
levels of circulating antibodies. The latter two approaches require the demonstration that indeed small
proteins can be effective B cell tolerogens once

coupled in appropriate ratios to the D-GL backbone.

Secondly, and perhaps more difficult to approach at present, is the judicious therapeutic use of suppressor T cell mechanisms. It appears to me that this will be particularly essential in clinical situations where the desired therapeutic effect will require abrogation of T cell responses in the individual either due to a primary T cell-mediated disorder, i.e. some instances or stages of thyroiditis, allergic orchitis, sequelae of certain viral diseases (e.g. infectious mononucleosis) or when a deleterious humoral response is so heterogeneous or unknown in determinant specificity as to make use of specific conjugates to induce B cell tolerance untenable. Rheumatoid arthritis and certain allergic disorders might be immediate candidates in this category. It is also clear, to me at least, that the potential for successful organ transplantation will also be dependent upon our future success in utilizing suppressor T cells specifically induced by perhaps the appropriate solubilized histocompatibility antigens.

BENACERRAF: In bringing this conference to a close, it is most fitting that we introduce the man who introduced us to many of the theoretical concepts underlying the continuing pressing questions concerning immunological tolerance--Sir MacFarlane Burnet--after whose closing comments we will adjourn this most enjoyable and fruitful meeting.

CLOSING COMMENTS

SIR MACFARLANE BURNET

Department of Microbiology
University of Melbourne
Victoria, Autralia

All my points are at the level of the biological significance of the immune system as we see it in mammals today.

1) It is a highly complex homeostatic system which we can think of as a multi-dimensional net of interesting components--soluble or cellular--most of which are specifically patterned gene products. The system is both highly susceptible to disturbance by genetic or somatic changes and flexible in its responses. From its nature it may definitely resist any form of comprehensive analysis. One of my impressions from this meeting is that it is a universe within which an infinite number of two dimensional sections can be selected and studied effectively and reproducibly but yet throw very little light on most other aspects of the system.

2) It can be regarded primarily as a surveillance system to recognize abnormality in body components especially cell surface components. Some of these will be from parasitic or other intrusions from outside; others from deviation of normal patterns by somatic mutation and the like. Perhaps the immunological implications of pregnancy should be added.

3) In a similar sense, the immune system has a specially significant quality as a self-monitoring system, rather clearly devised by evolution to allow the possibility of any lymphocyte in the body making surface contact with cells of any subpopulations of lymphocytes that may be relevant. Many examples of this were implied in our three days of discussions.

4) The point of view I am adopting is essentially an expansion of Jerne's network theory and like him, I would guess that in due course there will be opportunities for sophisticated mathematical analysis of the system. It will presumably be in something equivalent to the algebraical formulation of information theory in a form that hopefully could eventually incorporate the results of

quantitative work in real experimental systems.

5) The immune system in view of its specific cell and product markers has unique advantages for the study of physiological development and control; effective formulation of immunological theory will provide an invaluable model for similar attack on the other homeostatic systems in the mammal, e.g. those concerned with circulatory control or morphological maintenance and repair.

In the broadest sense this is the direction in which I think immunology in the sense of a scholarly discipline must move. But, of course, that is only one side of immunology; there are two others equally important.

1) To restate the academic approach: Immunology is a branch of theoretical and experimental biology to be given its proper place in the evolutionary picture of life on earth.

2) We have the social obligation to apply all relevant advances as they arise to use in medicine or other humanly desirable ends, and

3) We must continue to seek understanding by the experimental study of model systems appropriate to our sense of where new knowledge can currently be gained. In short, to cultivate Medawars and of the soluble in our field.

I will confess that at times in this meeting I wondered whether we were not for the most part talking about laboratory artifacts rather than biological realities. It is not easy to work with tolerance situations which bear on matters of evolutionary survival. That, however, is an inadmissible attitude. Good experimental work can only be done on model systems deliberately abstracted from reality. And on the other side many of the situations where we may be called on to apply immunological discovery to medicine are matters of no significance to evolution, however important they may be at the human level. The immunological inadequacies of aging, the diseases with strong autoimmune components, the chronic infections and the genetic immuno-deficiencies. None of them really matter for human evolution. They are as far from the mainstream of life as any of our laboratory artifacts but we must seek one means of dealing with them.

All I would say is that however fascinating it is to follow our laboratory models where they lead us, we should not too infrequently look over one shoulder at the significance of what we are doing in its biological context and over the other for its possible human implication for good or evil.

As long as that habit persists the world will probably continue to think well of us.